NEW THERAPEUTIC STRATEGIES IN LOW-GRADE GLIOMAS

WHO GRADE 2 GLIOMAS

NEW THERAPEUTIC STRATEGIES IN LOW-GRADE GLIOMAS

WHO GRADE 2 GLIOMAS

LUC TAILLANDIER
LAURENT CAPELLE
AND
HUGUES DUFFAU

Nova Biomedical Books
New York

Library of Congress Cataloging-in-Publication Data
Taillandier, Luc.
  New therapeutic strategies in low-grade gliomas / Luc Taillandier, Laurent Capelle, and Hugues Duffau.
     p. ; cm.
  Includes bibliographical references and index.
  ISBN 1-60021-064-3
  1. Gliomas--Treatment. 2. Brain--Tumors. 3. Brain--Cancer--Treatment.
  [DNLM: 1. Glioma--diagnosis. 2. Glioma--therapy. 3. Patient-Centered Care--methods. QZ 380 T131n 2006] I. Capelle, Laurent. II. Duffau, Hugues. III. Title.
  RC280.B7T35   2006
  616.99'481--dc22   2006004655

Published by Nova Science Publishers, Inc. ✦ *New York*

CONTENTS

PREFACE

Low-grade glioma (LGG) (grade 2 or G2G) is a brain infiltrative neoplasia, often invading cortical and subcortical functional structures, while displaying as a rule a somewhat indolent course initially (no patent deficit). It affects essentially young, fully active patients, who usually present with seizures. However, these lesions progress relentlessly, and their final fate is anaplastic transformation, leading to neurological impairment and death, with an overall median survival of around 10 years since the onset of symptoms.

Due to their apparent biological variability, commonly admitted spontaneous prognostic factors are of limited use if not questionable; consequently, the management of LGGs remains difficult to define (individually), and subject to controversies in the literature. However, most studies have evaluated the eventual impact of treatment(s) independently of the individual natural history and of the global therapeutic strategy. Thus, the goal of the present review is to give new insights regarding the different therapeutic strategies that need to be considered for each patient, and the parameters that can help the decision making.

First, it is now possible to benefit from data allowing a better understanding of the natural history of a given LGG: (1) initial tumoral volume (2) tumoral growth rate evaluated on at least two MRIs (3) tumoral metabolic profile, using new radiological methods such as PET and SRM (4) tumoral molecular biology, completing the information provided by classical histopathology.

Second, it is mandatory to perform a complete neurological examination, extensive neuropsychological assessment and evaluation of the quality of life from the time of diagnosis throughout the follow-up. Moreover, the analysis of the brain functional (re)organization and connectivity is needed via the use of new neurofunctional imaging methods (PET, MEG, fMRI, DTI), in order to understand the individual mechanisms of functional compensation in reaction to the glioma growth – explaining the frequent lack of deficit despite a classical invasion of so called "eloquent" areas.

Third, the advantages and limits of each treatment have to be considered for each patient. In this way, the use of intraoperative electrical functional mapping as well as the integration, up to the operating room, of preoperative anatomo-functional data, has allowed the minimization of the risk of postoperative sequelae, while improving the quality of tumor removal, even in eloquent regions. However, the actual long-term impact of surgery on survival still remains to ascertain. Concerning radiotherapy, the adaptation of doses, fractionation and volume of irradiation has enabled to decrease its risks, especially regarding cognitive functions. Nevertheless, despite an impact on the progression free survival, the effect on the overall survival is not proven. Finally, the recent use of new chemotherapeutic drugs has allowed a better tolerance and a frequent improvement of the quality of life via an impact on seizures, with a stabilization or even partial regression of the LGG; however, the follow-up is still too short to conclude.

On the basis of these (non exhaustive) parameters, we propose in the last part of this article to consider not "a standard treatment", but rather alternative "multiple dynamic therapeutic strategies" adapted to each patient, to be evaluated according to the clinico-radiological evolution of the LGG.

Key words: Low-grade glioma, Tumor surgery, Brain mapping, Chemotherapy, Radiotherapy, Quality of life, Tumor biology

## Chapter I

INTRODUCTION

LGG – gliomas WHO grade II (353) – are slow-growing primary brain tumors representing approximately 15 to 35% of gliomas (average incidence around 2/100.000/year), which usually affect young adults between 30 and 40 years of age (732). They are generally revealed by seizures, in patients as a rule with no or slight neurological deficit in the first stage of the disease. However, recent extensive neuropsychological assessments have shown that most patients already have mild cognitive disorders at this time (671).

LGG can follow three ways of evolution: (1) local growth (2) invasion (3) anaplastic transformation. First, recent works demonstrated that before any anaplastic degeneration, LGG show a continuous, constant growth of their mean tumor diameter over time, with an average slope around 4 mm of mean diameter increase per year (435). Second, LGG have a tendancy to migrate along the main white matter pathways, both within the lesional hemisphere or even controlaterally essentially via the corpus callosum (174, 225). Third, LGG systematically changes its biological nature and evolves to a high grade glioma, with a median of anaplastic transformation around 7 to 8 years, invariably fatal (median survival around 10 years) (732, 747).

Such better knowledge of the natural history of LGG and their clinical consequences has lead, in the past decade, to propose a more active therapeutic strategy rather than a "wait and see" attitude. Indeed, the vision of a tumor with a "dynamic" behavior needs to be integrated in the therapeutic strategy, in order to adapt the treatment both to the actual biology of the glioma at the time of diagnosis ("tumor mapping"), and to the functional compensation of the brain already induced by the slow-growing glioma before any symptom ("cerebral mapping") – thus to their interactions.

The goal of this article is first to review the advances in the determination of the natural history for each LGG. Indeed, the definition of spontaneous risk factors remains very difficult for each patient using classical clinical and radiological parameters, as demonstrated by many retrospective studies and prospective trials in the literature [7-35 ou Wessels à Whitton]. Hence, the adjunct of complementary individual data allowing a "tumor mapping" is very useful, using recent developement in the field of metabolic neuroimaging, in addition to parallel progress in molecular biology (see chapter) and biomathematical modelisation (313, 435, 662).

Second, we will analyze the progress made in the precise evaluation of the consequences of tumour progression on brain functioning, thus on the quality of life. Indeed, in addition to the classical neurological examination, numerous recent studies have shown that it was mandatory to perform an extensive neuropsychological assessment in LGG. Furthermore, the study of the brain functional (re)organization and connectivity is needed via the use of new neurofunctional imaging methods (PET, MEG, fMRI, DTI), in order to understand the individual mechanisms of functional compensation in reaction to the glioma growth – explaining the frequent lack of deficit despite a frequent invasion of so called "eloquent" areas.

Third, on the basis of a better understanding of the individual dynamic interrelationships between tumor progression and brain compensation, we will discuss about new therapeutic strategies, i.e. combined and sequential treatments, adapted to each patient and to the clinico-radiological evolution, with the double goal to preserve (or even improve) the quality of life as well as to increase the median survival.

## Chapter II

ADVANCES IN THE STUDY OF THE NATURAL HISTORY OF LGG: TOWARDS AN INDIVIDUAL PROGNOSIS

A – INTRODUCTION - EPIDEMIOLOGY

Gliomas account for more than half of the primitive central nervous system tumors, and are the result of the abnormal proliferation of glial cells. They are classified according to the tumoral cell type, mainly astrocytes and/or oligodendrocytes, and to their relative aggressivity, reflected by two to four grades (1 to 4) in the WHO classification (353). Their incidence is usually reported around 5 to 7/100, 000/yr, with a greater frequency in males (especially for astrocytomas), caucasians, northern countries (Scandinavian, North American), rural zones (186, 196, 266, 322, 323, 657–CBTRUS-, 732), and increases with age (579, 691). There appears to be a true elevation of annual incidence of gliomas, and of the grade 2 forms (315), globally or among the oldest population (196). Its signification is still matter of discussion, but could not be the sole result of an easier detection.

The grade 1 astrocytomas are quite peculiar, comprising various oncotypes that share more or less a slow growth rate, a gross (spatial) delimitation, and on the whole a favorable prognosis. On the opposite, gliomas of other grades share an infiltrative (invasion, migration) potential which renders their radical and selective treatment uncertain, and a growing biological aggressivity from grades 2 to 4. It is noteworthy that, following the essentially pediatric prevalence of grades 1, grade 2 gliomas affect mainly young adults, and grade 3 then 4, representing more than 60% of all gliomas, affect middle-age and older patients. While the overall prognosis follows an inverse rule, with median survivals decreasing from around 10 years to less than 12 months from grades 2 to 4. Oligodendrogliomatous tumors are generally graded in two categories, low-grade (well differentiated) and high-grade (corresponding to a grade 3 glioma).

Grade 2 gliomas are glial neoplasias made of cells resembling their presumed original counterparts; astrocytomas derive from type 1A protoplasmic cortical astrocytes (GFAP+, A2B5-) or more frequently from perinatal progenitor cells O2-A giving rise to fibrillar astrocytes (GFAP+, A2B5+), like oligodendrogliomas (GFAP-) (84, 415). They present a slightly (or moderately) elevated cellularity and cellular atypia, and usually lack pleomorphism, (significant) cytoplasmic or nuclear atypia, vascular endothelial proliferation, mitosis (one/40 HPF accepted) or necrosis, that characterize high-grade gliomas (353). With few exceptions (130, 146, 319, 321), grade 2 gliomas are unique, sporadic, and do not metastazise, and familial forms outside neurocutaneous syndromes (86, 95), as well as causal environmental or external factors (301, 527, 584), are seldom recognized. They can sometimes grow in a manner resembling gliomatosis from an initially bulky tumor.

Astrocytomas can affect all age groups, with grossly 10% encountered before the age of 20, 60% between 20 and 45 years, and 30% after 45 years, the peak being at 30-40 years (713, 732). There is a male predominance of almost 1.2:1 (353). They are preferentially located in the supratentorial compartment, mostly in frontal and temporal sites, then in the brainstem and spinal cord, rarely in the cerebellum (353). If oligodendrogliomas can be encountered ubiquitarily among the neuraxis proportionally to the amount of white matter (183), they show a great predilection for frontal sites while intra-ventricular or posterior fossa locations are rare. Their distribution with age is more widespread, more often between 30 and 60 years, and the masculine predilection is more marqued at around 1.3:1 (353).

A meaningful peculiarity common to all these tumors is to favor locations in the immediate vincinity of, or originally within, eloquent cerebral areas («secondary» functional areas such as frontal SMA, insula), more frequently than de novo high-grade gliomas (162). By their infiltrative characteristic, they blurr anatomic boundaries, with a distorsion more than a destruction of invaded structures (137).

A categorical classification is by essence imperfect in terms of biological processes, and the situation with gliomas even more complicated. Indeed, there is an on-going controversy concerning the determination of the constituting cellular type, and even its neoplastic nature, and there are notable overlappings among the grades. Moreover, the natural tendancy of a glioma (grades 1 excepted) appears to be the acquisition/selection with time of a geno-phenotype of higher aggressivity (malignancy). That explains why the qualification of benign for grade 2 gliomas has been rightly abandonned. The progress made in the last decade(s) in various fields gives nowadays the opportunity to qualify differently these tumors than with the sole anatomopathologic examination, with the aim to reflect more closely the proper potential of a given glioma, and to evaluate more precisely its evolutive stage.

Until now, reflecting these difficulties, the biological diversity of gliomas, especially of grade 2, has long been recognized (28, 513, 555), and the poor knowledge of their natural history, the more so at an individual level, explains that the commonly accepted spontaneous prognostic factors are mostly imprecise or questionable, and that the impact of available treatments, if any, is still matter of debate (419, 497, 516).

B - METHODOLOGICAL BIASES

Our poor understanding of grade 2 gliomas, despite a prolific literature on the subject, results first of all from the different methodological approaches used in reported series, hampering the possibility of comparisons or pooling of available data (418).

Until the last (two) decades, the series of grade 2 gliomas comprised in fact «low-grade gliomas», ie. grouped grade 1 and 2 gliomas. This term should be abandoned once and for all, to ascertain that the focus is on grade 2 gliomas only. Moreover, among grade 2 gliomas, the gemistocytic oncotype, known to behave quite differently although this has been recently challenged, should be excluded from analysis or at least analyzed separately (383, 682, 748, 763). Similarly, the studies often encompassed cases of all age groups. Apart from the redundancy with the first point, since grades 1 affect primarily pediatric patients, this brought to study genuine grade 2 gliomas arising in children, but whose behavior, hence prognosis, is now well known to be fundamentally different than those arising in adults, as shown by clinical observation up to the study of genetic alterations (51, 101, 110, 194, 213, 511, 523, 524, 533, 612, 664). Also partly redundant with the first two points, is the mixture of the various possible locations inside the central nervous system in the populations studied; certain sites are essentially those of grade 1 gliomas and/or affects younger subjects (cerebellum, midline, in particular optic pathways and hypothalamus/diencephalon).

Controversy and natural evolution in histological concepts has lead to the use of various classifications in the series reported. Moreover, given the known important inhomogeneity of these tumors (119), and the frequent scarcity of tumoral specimen available, especially after sole biopsy, a misdiagnosis or underestimation of grade is always possible (43, 96, 361, 397, 448, 449, 454, 507, 512, 597, 637, 718). Another aspect of the problem would be the delay at which histological diagnosis is made. Some advocate, in the absence of necessity or will of oncologic treatment, to not perform systematically a diagnostic biopsy, and hence might exclude from analysis a given patient whose tumor will undergo malignant transformation and be histologically examined only at that time (713).

The relative rarity of grade 2 gliomas and their usually long history, result in series sometimes (too) small, or encompassing several decades, during which clinical, radiological, histological and therapeutic aspects have eventually greatly varied. Series are mostly retrospective in nature. Statistical methods used are also diverse and sometimes inappropriate, the value and sometimes definition of some parameters are frequently lacking or differ from one series to another, a multivariate analysis has frequently been done only in the last two decades. In the same manner, the evaluation of treatments has long suffered of imprecision, as for example the quality of resection only expressed as the surgeon's opinion, which is clearly unreliable for a tumor mostly difficult if not impossible to distinguish from normal parenchyma. Endpoints of the studies, as their definitions, can be a drawback to adequate comparisons (anaplasia, survival, recurrence, progression..) (570). Beginning a follow-up at diagnosis or treatment is first of all eventually quite different from a patient or a series to another, and secondly does not take into account in all cases the pre-diagnostic or pre–treatment period. Hence, post-diagnosis or post–treatment outcomes can simply reflect the fact that the patient was treated at a different delay or evolutive stage of his tumor, and not an eventual greater benefit of the therapeutic strategy (515). Last, the delay of effective observation is most of the time too short to draw reliable conclusions regarding a tumor whose natural history spans over several years to even decades (418, 515, 570).

For all those (non exhaustive) critics, «the bad results obtained from clinical research have contributed (..) to the notion that low-grade gliomas might represent a very heterogeneous population of patients, for which the prognostic factors could play a crucial role in the determinism of the evolution of the affection» (516). The vicious circle is about to close on itself, the prognostic factors appearing crucial but poorly known or not definitely adressed, and difficult to determine on populations that can not be adequatly subdivided (stratified) along reliable prognostic factors. Also because of the long observation period that would be needed, prospective, randomized studies are very difficult to realize, and a great number of cases would need to be included in the absence of homogeneous (a priori) risk-groups. Therefore, «the establishment of standards of care, or guidelines, is maybe not possible or not desirable» (25 refering to 464, 514, 610), and «another decade will probably be necessary to shift from a passive and defensive attitude (no significant gain so primum non nocere) to an active, aggressive, attitude» (80).

Nevertheless, thanks to a renewed interest in this pathology and technical progress, prospective, randomized trials have been, and are currently undertaken (EORTC/MRC, NCCTG/RTOG/ECOG), a common language begins to be adopted, significant progress has been made in the last decade and real advances should be definitely achieved in the coming years.

C - CLINICO-RADIOLOGICAL ASPECTS

Grade 2 gliomas are Constantly Evolving Tumors Menacing Life

Grade 2 gliomas, with the probable exception of «minute-gliomas» associated to – refractory- epilepsy and as a rule reported in series dealing with epilepsy rather than in an oncologic context (485), are constantly evolving lesions. More than half of the cases followed after withholding any oncologic treatment at diagnosis, will be ultimately treated at a median delay of around 2 years (541, 713), and the same proportion are expected to manifest significant clinical changes at a delay of 5 years after initial therapy (endpoint chosen for the EORTC trial 22845 –330-). The tendancy to progression does not show a plateau and continues at least during 10 years after treatment (752).

Another and not the least characteristic of grade 2 gliomas is their innate tendancy with time to undergo malignant transformation. It appears usually progressively (430) and is expected in about two-thirds of the progressions observed (469, 470), its risk growing with each recurrence (4, 469, 470). It is observed at a growing rate with time (no plateau either) (454, 710), affecting half of the cases at 5-6 years and more than 75% at 9 years (541), and on the whole its incidence increases with observation or survival time (253, 718), appearing «almost ineluctable» (5, 470). This process appears to be spontaneous, intrinsic, independant of any external stimulus (5). When transformed into their malignant (high-grade) counterparts (#20% of «secondary glioblastomas»), these gliomas carry the same prognosis that de novo forms (156–case control study -, in contrast to 753). With practical differences lying in a younger age (about 10 years less), that grade 3 forms predominate, and that a longer survival can sometimes be obtained, due to the fact in our experience that anaplasia can frequently be encountered at its beginning («intermediate forms»-123-), seen as microscopic foci among an otherwise seemingly histologically grade 2 tumor (448). If anaplastic transformation is by far the principal cause of fatal outcome (in this otherwise generally young then healthy population) (513), the sole volumetric evolution, especially in the case of deep-seated or axial tumors, can be responsible of the death of the patient (312, 448).

Life expectancy of (usually young) patients affected is greatly reduced, since overall survivals are in the order of 10 years from the clinical onset or 6-9 years after diagnosis or treatment for astrocytomas (316, 558, 706, 732), and up to 12 to even 16.7 years for oligodendrogliomas (497). In fact, reflecting their biological diversity (28, 513, 555), the reported survival rates at 5 and 10 years post-diagnosis or treatment vary greatly, first of all from one epoch to another (23, 316). Indeed, in older series, that is before the advent of CT or

MRI (and the easier access to these more performing radiological examinations), they were respectively of 17 to 53% and 6 to 11% (188, 193, 397, 514, 609, 637), while in more recent series they are around 40 to 80% and 20 to 50% for astrocytomas, and 60-85% and 30-60% for oligodendrogliomas (23, 260, 312, 351, 375, 405, 420, 448, 488, 512, 515, 591, 614, 718, 748). This difference in post-treatment survival rates is mainly the result of an earlier detection (407, 515), but apparently not only (316, 483). The malignant transformation rate is reported around 50% (20 to 80%) at 3 to 5 years post-diagnosis (63, 71, 339, 732), but its exact incidence is difficult to ascertain in the absence of repeated histological examinations.

Grade 2 Gliomas Show Grossly Two Clinical and Radiological Phases

The first phase is long when clinically perceptible, affecting a young subject; the lesion is initially asymptomatic or limited to epilepsy, which represents the most frequent symptom, inaugural in 2/3 to 90% of the cases, more frequent with oligodendrogliomas (33, 106, 750). This is in accordance with the low epileptic threshold of the regions most frequently affected by these tumors (limbic and temporal lobes, SMA, operculae and insulae). Radiological growth is slow, the lesion showing no particular vascularity. The progressive acquisition of genotypic and phenotypic characteristics ending up to malignancy leads to the second phase, with radiologically a faster growth, new or increasing contrast enhancement then edema, and biologically a different level of neoangiogenesis and proliferation (4, 93, 376, 427, 428, 540, 718).

The occurrence of focal neurological deficits or signs of raised intracranial pressure is usually associated with anaplastic evolution (320), as is the appearance of new types of seizures and/or the increase in intensity or frequence of epilepsy (204). Rarely, the inaugural symptomatology is due to a tumoral hemorrhage, as a rule with an oligodendroglioma (3, 55, 411).

The diagnosis and follow-up of grade 2 gliomas must rely now on MRI (621), with T1-weighted (and after contrast medium) and FLAIR images (78, 648). Grade 2 gliomas show as an area of hypointense signal on T1 and hyperintense on T2-weighted/FLAIR sequences, more or less homogeneous. Radiologically, they can appear well demarcated (bulky) or not delineated at all (infiltrative), and if they generate a mass effect, it is usually local (sulci, cortical surface) or relatively moderate with regard to the extension of the signal abnormality. Calcifications are frequent, especially with oligodendrogliomas, irregular, serpiginous more often than nodular (338, 727). Cystic tumors are rare (417), as the eventuality of a bony calvarial erosion (401).

Contrast enhancement should seldom be seen in grade 2 gliomas (8 to 15% of the cases – 81, 428, 513, 635, 718-), and diminishes in more recent series (25), is of faint or moderate intensity and thickness (4), patchy or in strands, and more often encountered with oligodendrogliomas which behold naturally a greater vascularization (183, 338, 420, 497, 727). When contrast enhancement is underscored by neoangiogenesis or disruption of the blood-brain barrier, it represents a strong indicator of a malignant phenotype, but a contrast enhancing tumor is not always malignant (apart cases of observed appearance and/or growth of the enhancement), and more importantly the reverse is also true, which stresses the importance of realising a sampling of a tumor focused on the enhancing or «hot» zones, whatever the radiological modalitiy (anatomic, vascular, metabolic). This two-way discrepancy is reported from 8 to 50% (4, 77, 96, 232, 361, 440, 449, 628, 718).

D – HISTOLOGY AND MOLECULAR ASPECTS

«To gauge therapy and advise patients with intracranial astrocytomas, an accurate measure of prognosis is needed. Histological grading has not been adequate to determine individual outcomes» (57). This is also true with the other oncotypes of gliomas for which none of the classification system is yet satisfying enough to reflect the natural history effectively observed, in particular at an individual level.

Histological Classification and Grading of Gliomas

Various histological classifications have been proposed, based on histogenesis, on cellular dedifferentiation or anaplasia, on the best fit to (histo)prognosis, on cytologic and spatial configuration criteria, or on the reproducibility of the classification. So anatomopathological classification can start with the histological (tissular) characterization and adjoin secondly an evolutive grade, or can be based on the assumption that the tumoral behaviour will reflect its histological aggressivity (540), grade 2 gliomas moving along an histological continuum that will lead them at the end to the glioblastoma multiforme (Kernohan, Sainte-Anne Mayo/revision).

Based on the WHO classification, oligodendrogliomas appear of better prognosis than astrocytomas, even though all authors did not observe significant differences (315, 374, 421). Mixed gliomas seem to carry an intermediate prognosis between oligodendrogliomas and astrocytomas, but this has been debated, based on the various definition of their oligoglial or astrocytic components and/or their grading (253, 384, 608, 610, 611, 635, 728). With time and new theories regarding glioma classification, and due to the partly subjective aspect of the WHO classification (134, 135, 136, 191), the reported respective proportions of the different oncotypes has varied, with a tendancy toward an overrepresentation in the more recent series of oligodendrogliomas, while astrocytomas largely predominated until the nineties. In the absence of specific marker of cellular lineage, the subject is still matter of debate.

Different studies, quantitative and/or qualitative, have been made of various cytological parameters, whose groupings allow a grading reflecting tumoral aggressivity, but the results are diverse among institutions, hence non reproducible. Some advocate a two-tiered system of grading only (360), with low- and high-grade tumors, for all oncotypes. One of the main problems lies in the relative part of subjectivity underlying an anatomopathological diagnosis, due to the lack of precision of the diagnostic criteria, the intra-tumoral heterogeneity, and the biological diversity of these tumors. As a consequence, intra- and inter-observer reproducibility is not as high as one would like, especially in terms of grading (327, central reviews of trials).

The presence of gemistocytes in high quantity in a grade 2 glioma indicates for most authors a more dismal prognosis, with a correlation with advancing age (96, 282, 381, 609, 738, 748), up to the gemistocytic astrocytoma which behaves frequently as a grade 3 glioma eventhough there are no cytological signs of anaplasia, or the proliferative index is low, but with a still ongoing controversy (282, 382, 383, 404, 548, 596, 682, 736, 738, 748, 763).

Complementary Methods of Grading

The proliferative potential of tumors was long thought to be more prognostic than the radiological evolution of the tumor or other commonly recognized prognostic factors (age, mitotic index...), evaluated by means of tritiated thymidine or bromodeoxyuridine incorporation or antibodies binding with cell-cycle antigens/enzymes (224, 281, 389). This has lead to sophisticated models. If a general relation exists between various proliferative indices and outcome, its actual value in terms of prognosis, eventually with the adjunct of flow cytometry data, varies among reported studies, ranging from no significance to superseding other variables (57, 114, 115, 117, 133, 218, 280, 303, 582, 583, 649, 650, 717). On the whole, the most widely used proliferation index utilizises an antibody directed against the Ki-67 antigen (nuclear DNA-polymerase α protein associated with actively dividing cells, present during phases G1 to M of the cell cycle). MIB-1 (monoclonal antibody directed against Ki-67 and usable on paraffin sections) index can be correlated with tumoral size but not location (399), with mitotic index (but more reliable and easy to use, especially on small samples) (601), with various cytological aspects (615), with histologic grade and age (255, 285). It is higher in oligodendrogliomas (255, 328). MIB-1 index (mean rather than maximal value) can complete, refine, the histological grading, at least in two classes (low vs. high-grade) (324, 349, 477, 685), but for some authors can even differentiate tumors of the same histological class (116, 195, 255, 279, 285, 345, 364, 380, 549, 580, 595, 682, 685), while other failed to recognize any significant interest in the MIB-1 index, at least at an individual level, frequently disappearing behind other prognostic factors (122, 267, 384, 463, 559, 595, 597).

The vascularity or angiogenetic status of a tumor should reflect its aggressivity (malignancy), since (neo)angiogenesis seems mandatory, if not causal, to the significant growth of a tumor (136, 197, 200, 201, 521). The density, size or aspect of tumoral microvessels, the intensity of, in particular, VEGF staining or of its epitopes and receptors, as well as radiologic studies studying vascularity or blood flow, have often uncovered correlations with prognosis (1, 89, 98, 183, 366, 367, 406, 505, 637), but this still needs confirmation (314).

Since tumoral growth results from the (im)balance between proliferation and cellular death, apoptotic ratios or the presence of molecules implicated in apoptotic pathways (inductors or protectors) have been studied, but does not seem to hold a significant prognostic value (89, 92, 365, 476, 554, 597, 598).

Histological grade of gliomas «grow» with time, spontaneously and/or after treatment, leading to the inexorable death of the patient. Hence tumor aggressivity and histobiological characteristics, of value but already insufficient individually from a static point of view, are even more highly variable when seen in a dynamic perspective, impossible to determine at different stages of the tumor history in the absence of repeated biopsy or resective surgery.

Molecular Biology

Gliomas are generally of the sporadic (vs. hereditary, by germinal mutation) type of neoplasia, as a result of an accumulation of DNA rearrangements (loss or gain of all or part of a chromosome, dysploïdy) and/or focal mutations (structural alteration of a specific locus), as hypothesized by the multi-hit concept (49, 450). The clonal theory (489) suggests a single cell of origin (335), while tumoral progression is the consequence of a genetic variability (instability) that autorizes the sequential selection of more aggressive cell lines (203, 207). Tumorigenesis is the consequence of a desequilibrium (at the DNA synthesis level) between inhibitory growth factors (tumor suppressor genes) and growth inducers (proto-oncogenes) (46). The oncogenes work in a dominant manner, while the former need the loss (functional or structural) of their two alleles. Ultimately, genetic deletions (allelic losses), inactivation (mutation) or gains of function (amplification, increased number of copies, activating mutation), ie. the genotype, will lead more or less to a quantitative and/or qualitative increase or decrease of its corresponding protein product, at the end defining the tumoral phenotype. It seems that «six essential alterations in cell physiology (..) collectively dictate malignant growth: self-sufficiency in growth signals, insensitivity to growth-inhibitory (antigrowth) signals, evasion of programmed cell death (apoptosis), limitless replicative potential, sustained angiogenesis, and tissue invasion (..)» (250).

There are numerous interconnections between the various processes and genetic and biologic parameters that account for the neoplastic transformation, progression (proliferation/apoptosis, angiogenesis, immunosuppression) and invasivity (invasion, migration) of gliomas. Neoplastic glial cells are able to secrete substances playing different roles. Certain components of the extra-cellular matrix can be induced by reparation mechanisms linked to neoangiogenesis and/or local production of substrates guiding locomotion. The extra-cellular matrix represents a reservoir of growth factors, proteases and their inhibitors that can also be expressed by the tumoral cells. Certain regulating agents are common to angiogenesis, migration and proliferation of endothelial as well as tumoral cells. The degradation of the extra-cellular matrix in turn liberates cytokines and growth factors. Last this whole microenvironment can induce activation or inactivation of genes promoting or suppressing tumors... (680). On the whole, glioma progression corresponds to the transformation of a slow growing, contact-inhibited, mildly tumorigenic and invasive tumor into a rapidly proliferating, anchorage-independant, highly tumorigenic and invasive tumor.

Oncogenesis of astrocytic and oligodendrocytic tumors obeys to different mechanisms, as well as the two types of grade IV astrocytomas (primary or de novo glioblastomas –for which the main genetic abnormalities concern the EGF receptor and its gene, in association with a loss of chromosome 10-, and secondary forms ie. malignant gliomas deriving sequentially from a grade II astrocytoma –eventhough the frequency of specific genetic modifications differ in the two types of glioblastoma, the same genetic pathways are altered, and the clinico-histologic pattern is similar-432-). To note that the already known genetic mechanisms/alterations involved in gliomagenesis that will be rapidly reviewed here do not account for all the gliomas encountered.

Astrocytoma Formation and Progression (111, 207, 353, 423, 480, 490, 538, 539, 705, 726).

The earliest reported chromosomal modifications consist in losses of genetic material on chromosomes 6, 7q, 13, 17p and 22, probably linked to the transformation of normal glia into a grade II astrocytoma. Allelic losses on 9p and 19q seem to parallel the transformation into an anaplastic astrocytoma (grade III astrocytoma), and chromosome 10 loss in fine into a glioblastoma (grade IV astrocytoma).

Astrocytoma formation appears to result from an original desequilibrium between an enhanced proliferation (PDGF-A & PDGFR-α -on 4q11-12- overexpressed in #60% of cases -262-) and a diminished apoptosis (LOH 17p13.1 –52, 182, 726- or TP53 mutation –402, 423, 623- in more than 65% of cases –352, 496-, the latter of increasing frequency with age, representing the only genomic alterations present with a similar frequency in all grades of astrocytomas –422-). Despite of a still slow growth capacity, there is a facilitation of the genomic instability that allows the transition to higher grades of malignancy.

Due to the various roles of (wild type) p53 (reviews in 209, 358), transcriptional regulator, its absence or mutation (poorly studied however in low-grade gliomas) leads to, among other effects, genomic instability reflected by amplifications and aneuploidy (623, 712), loss of DNA reparation capacity, diminished apoptosis probably more than an increased proliferation (alteration of the cell cycle control at the G1-S interface by the TP53-MDM2-p21(-p27-p14^{ARF}) pathway –297-), perturbation of chromosomal segregation (209, 490)... Mutations are essentially of the missense type affecting primarily residues crucial to DNA binding (423), the one at codon 175 being of worse prognosis (508); moreover, there might be a correlation of TP53 mutations with MGMT gene methylation (508). Progression appears similar whatever the p53 status (534), but the delay of anaplastic transformation seems shorter in case of p53 mutation (737), which could then be more associated with malignant progression of astrocytomas (296). TP53 mutation frequency is highest in gemistocytic astrocytomas, that usually progress more rapidly towards glioblastoma (Watanabe ANP1998).

On the other hand, PDGF-R (534) as well as EGF-R (on 7p12-13) overexpression are associated with a shorter survival of grade II astrocytomas, independantly of known prognostic factors (715, controversial for 556). Last, loss of 1p and 19q could concern about 15% of astrocytic tumors (74, 372, 544, 725).

The progression to anaplastic astrocytoma appears associated to the inactivation of tumor suppressor genes on chromosomes 11p, 19q, 9p and 13q (about 50%); the two latter contain the genes CDKN2/p16 (9p21) and Rb (13q14) (about 50% and 30% alteration respectively), resulting in the loss of one more critical pathway of cell cycle regulation at G1-S, hence an increased proliferation and mitotic activity (CDKN2/p16(-p15)-CDK4(/6)-cyclin D1-pRb1 and p27Kip1 pathway) (630). LOH 19q seems unique, restricted to gliomas and common to the three oncotypes, in a region containing genes implicated in DNA reparation (311).

Last, progression to glioblastoma seems associated to the inactivation of a putative tumor suppressor gene on chromosome 10 (331, 423) and the overexpression of EGFR (395), with sometimes PTEN mutations –at 10q23.3-, loss of DCC expression –at 18q21-... (295, 334, 539, 599).

To note that most non pilocytic astrocytomas in the pediatric age do not share the same genetic alterations as the adult forms (395, 416, 532, 724), except brainstem gliomas, that resemble secondary glioblastomas (424).

Oligodendroglioma Formation and Progression

These tumors present early and frequent losses (deletions) on 1p and 19q, in about 80% of the cases (respectively 40-100% and 50->80% -37, 74, 82, 372, 546, 725-). LOH 19q concerns mostly the totality of the long arm (546), a region where is suspected the presence of a gene implicated in astrocytoma progression, near DNA reparation genes (125), and LOH 1p can be complete or partial (189), of opposite prognostic signification (complete hemizygous loss strongly associated with 19q and oligoglial phenotype vs. partial deletions, essentially seen in astrocytomas, not associated with LOH 19q-298-). LOH 1p with or without LOH 19q is associated with a typical oligoglial phenotype (74, 536, 546, 590, 698, 725, 739), is more frequent in low-grade tumors and younger patients (472), is associated with a higher chemosensitivity to PCV protocol (82, 707), and/or Temozolomide, and even seemingly with a longer progression free survival after irradiation (73, 268, 636). The codeletion is associated with a longer overall survival (73, 82, 185, 189, 510), eventhough these prognostic effects seem less marked for low-grade than anaplastic oligodendrogliomas (189). These deletions are associated preferentially with frontal locations (390, 771, controversial for 189), and a lesser invasivity in vitro than their astrocytoma counterparts (501).

TP53 alterations or LOH 17p are rare in oligodendrogliomas (245), the accumulation of p53 protein being associated with a worsened prognosis (379). Overexpression of EGFR is on the contrary frequent in (low-grade mostly) oligodendrogliomas (545).

Oligodendroglioma progression seems associated with LOH 9p, 10q (telomeric end – 683-), gain on 12q, deletion of CDKN2A gene (p16) and mutation or deletion of CDKN2B (p15) on 9p21 (50, 236, 269, 636). PCR quantitative analysis of some proto-oncogenes confirms the early amplification (especially CDK4, MDM2, GAC1).

To note that, as with astrocytomas, pediatric oligodendrogliomas do not share the same genetic profiles as the adult forms (533).

Mixed Glioma Formation and Progression

Mixed gliomas seem to represent more clonal neoplasias of variable phenotypes rather than collision tumors (372), in which TP53 mutations and LOH 1p and 19q appear exclusive (546) or more precisely inversely correlated, associated with a preferential astrocytic or oligoglial phenotype respectively (434).

Combined immunohistochemical testing can help oncotype classification, as pure oligodendrogliomas show tumoral cells that are Olig2+/GFAP-, whereas two main populations Olig2+/GFAP- and Olig2-/GFAP+ are found in astrocytomas and mixed gliomas (461).

(Neo)Angiogenesis

Gliomas, especially the astrocytic forms, as invasive tumors moreover often limited to tumoral isolated cells in the normal parenchyma, incorporate initially the normal cerebral vasculature (135, 520, 679, 745). Eventhough progressive anaplastic transformation is associated with microvascular proliferation (136), since this neoangiogenesis is necessary for tumoral growth and facilitates invasion, and can even represent a self-limiting step in tumorigenesis (249), it does not appear in itself sufficient to define anaplasia (201), in part because anatomy can not reflect exactly the functional importance, leading to conflicting results in the correlations between vascularity and prognosis (65, 317, 406).

Angiogenesis implies angiogenetic factors directing endothelial cell migration (integrins) and proliferation, and vascular maturation, but first local disruption of the extra-cellular matrix by proteolysis (matrixmetalloproteinases, serin proteinases, cathepsins) (59, 124, 152, 198, 314, 317, 520, 521, 745).

Soluble growth factors and cytokines released by tumoral cells act in essentially a paracrine way on endothelial cells (199), and pericytes appear also very much implicated in angiogenesis (487, 746). Different growth factors are implicated in angiogenesis, as well in proliferation, tumor progression.. (EGF, PDGF, bFGF, TGF-β). VEGF is one of the main angiogenetic factors in gliomas, whose expression along with its receptors is correlated with histological grade, especially in hypoxic conditions (585, 622, 716); it could represent the final common pathway of neovascularization and progression towards grade IV astrocytoma (239, 692).

Last, angiogenesis could be initiated by the functional loss of (tumor) angiogenesis suppressor gene(s) (521, 711) and/or the upregulation of proangiogenic factors (64, 336). Or, on the contrary, VEGF expression, known to be hypoxia-induced, and onset of angiogenesis, could follow an initial regression of existing vessels due to angiopoietin-2 expression by tumor cells (432, 767, 768).

Invasion and Migration

Sub-population of glioma cells migrate away from the main tumor mass and invade the contiguous brain parenchyma (isolated cells of D-D or "guerilla-cells" of 517, 104, 627), along various possible routes (227, 229). This requires cell adhesion to extracellular matrix components (with loss of adhesion to the principal neoplastic mass), cell locomotion and the ability to create space into which to move (680). This process is facilitated by interaction with the extracellular matrix (233), in part provided by the neoplastic cells themselves (laminin, tenascin, hyarulonic acid providing substrates for invasion, cell adhesion to the latter being mediated by specific integrins and hyaluronan receptor CD44, SPARC, BEHAB), when stimulated by gangliosides, cytokines (TGF-β) and growth factors (EGF, PDGF, SF/HGF, insulin-like GF) (39, 102, 103, 237, 363, 393, 446, 517, 680). Modulation of these extracellular matrix components is facilitated by various proteases (matrix metalloproteinases, hyaluronidases, serine protease urokinase-type plasminogen activator, lysosomal cysteine peptidases or cathepsins) which degrade the surrounding stromal cells and extracellular proteins (35, 53, 107, 192, 409, 517, 537, 714, 693, 759). These proteases are regulated by biochemical pathways, especially protein kinase C (699). Individual cells are capable of deformation to fit in the extracellular brain spaces (640), and cell motility is an active process dependent on dynamic remodeling of the actin cytosqueleton (433). The process of motility/invasion is in fact a normal (regulated) capacity of astrocytes, in the mature (678) as well as developing brain (61, 537).

Factors controlling invasiveness also stimulate angiogenesis (36), tumoral cells taking advantage of neoplastic vascularisation for extension (684), but some anti-angiogenic drugs seem to increase invasion (392). Cellular migration and proliferation share common intracellular pathways (721), with major cross-links (PI-3 kinase and PTEN, focal adhesion kinase –FAK- and p53). Motility-related genes are often up-regulated in gliomas of advancing grade, and mobile cells show a decreased proliferation rate and a relative resistance to apoptosis (226, 229, 345). The balance of proteinases and their inhibitors varies from low- to high-grade gliomas (409, 537), while in vitro motility increases with histological grade (103). Deregulation of invasion gene expression can be an early event, under the dependance of p53 impairment with consequently activation of proto-oncogene Ets-1 dependent invasion-associated genes (225).

Hence, astrocytomas and/or oligodendroglial tumors grade 2 share a type II or III spatial configuration (138), and invasivity is not restricted to malignant forms of gliomas. This invasivity and migration is dependent on the tumoral location, frequently limited in the grey matter (peri-neuronal satellitosis), frequent at the level of superficial pia or subependymal zone (probably passively –680-), and along peri-vascular spaces and myelinated pathways of the white matter, facilitated by an eventual peri-tumoral edema (or cellular loss due for example to seizures) which increases the extra-cellular space (228). The glycolytic phenotype common to all malignancies seems to play a role in invasion since it allows an adaptation to the microenvironment (222).

Immunosuppression

Escape from immune survey is a particularity of glial tumors (571). Even though the central nervous system has long been considered as an immune sanctuary, the relative immunity of gliomas implies at least in part an interaction with immune cells (essential role of T lymphocytes). The antigenic presentation could be mediated by microglial cells, endothelial cells and pericytes, or even normal and neoplastic astrocytes (153). Immunosuppression is also linked to the capacity by neoplastic cells to secrete soluble immunologic mediators (as TGF-β2 initially called "glioblastoma cell-derived T-cell suppressor factor", Fas interacting avec Fas ligand on T cells leading them to apoptosis) (744), as well as to cytokines and/or growth factors, and even p53 (209).

First Results of Genomic, Transcriptional and Proteomic Studies

By cDNA (low density) arrays and DNA microarrays (high density arrays), several genetic alterations (up- and down-regulations), some already known and others novel (see 588), can be found in low- to high-grade gliomas, and between primary and recurrent tumors. On the whole, there are somewhat few differences between grades II and normal tissue as well as between grades II and III, the majority of differences in genetic expression being found in grade IV tumors (581).

Genetic alterations encountered in low-grade astrocytomas can be grouped in three main categories (288): cellular growth and differenciation/cell cycle control/apoptosis, cytokines/protein kinases/signal transduction/cell surface receptors and their corresponding proteins, and cellular adhesion/basal membrane and extra-cellular matrix proteins.

Some modifications are (quantitatively) associated with progression from low- to high-grade tumors, interesting for example p53 in astrocytomas (constant anomalies throughout, but increasing with, tumoral grades) (581, 709), CDKN2A and p14^{ARF} before CDK4 in primary glioblastomas (709), and vimentine and IGFBP2 for oligoglial tumors (581).

The most striking differences between low-grade astrocytomas (sharing similarities with secondary glioblastomas) and (primary) glioblastomas affect various categories of genes;

- genes suppressor of migration and implicated in cellular adhesion (and cytosqueleton) are more often expressed in low-grade tumors (235, 562)
- angiogenetic genes are up-regulated in primary glioblastomas (vs. grades II and secondary glioblastomas) (235, 709), while FGF2 is overexpressed in low-grade astrocytomas as in pediatric tumors (235)
- various genes implicated in inflammatory or immune response are differently expressed by grades II and secondary glioblastomas vs. primary glioblastomas (235)
- TGFβ2 and IGFBP3 also discriminate low- and high-grade gliomas (235), as well as genes implicated in proliferation, maintenance of minichromosomes, transcriptional family, inhibition of apoptosis, cellular motility (562, 709).

Low- and high-grade oligodendrogliomas also show striking differences, with even some «intermediate» forms eventually defined; dysregulations of genes implicated in cellular adhesion and signaling, immune response and cellular differentiation, down-regulated, and much less up-regulated in the anaplastic forms (740). Oligodendrogliomas with LOH 1p show similar expression profiles to the normal brain regarding the genes that they express differentially from their counterparts with intact 1p (468).

Another approach consists in defining small sets of highly discriminative genes (348 –for example subunit 2 of tansducine β2 in low-grade oligodendrogliomas-).

Generally, it appears that extensive genomic analysis allows to point out a relatively small subset of differentially expressed genes that can reliably discriminate different oncotypes and/or grades of gliomas (205, 210, 493, 605, 732), with a further refinement of classical histology in terms of classification or prognostic information. The same is applicable to the study of cell lines (291).

Since mRNA studies by microarrays does not accurately reflect the protein components (that result of transcriptional but also post-transcriptional controls, post-translational modifications and displacements), proteomic analysis are also of value. Again, protein clustering shows few differences between low-grade astrocytomas and normal tissue, can discriminate high-grade astrocytomas of different outcome, or point to modifications associated with progression or histological grade (proteins implicated in signal transduction, molecular chaperons, transcription and translation regulators, cell cycle mediators, linked to extra-cellular matrix and adhesion) (94, 305).

Last, pharmacogenomics of anti-epileptic drugs is also of importance, allowing a more comprehensive use if needed with greater safety.

Molecular imaging (with PET, MRI) will represent another valuable, in vivo tool (308).

Gliomas and Stem Cells (see 586)

The cell targeted for neoplastic transformation can be a differentiated, mature, cell (hence not representing a truly terminal event), but also an immature, yet undifferentiated one. Indeed, genetic factors involved in glioma genesis and progression are similar to the regulators of neural stem cells (553) and to developmental events (for example PDGF and PDGF-R, EGFR, pRb, p27 –742, see 432, 655-, Hedgehog pathway and transcription factors –126, see 586-, PTEN…), and their invasive propensity resembles glia and neuron migration during embryogenesis (254).

The frequent presence in gliomas of a biphasic tissue pattern (astrocytic and oligoglial differentiation or gliomatous and mesenchymatous differentiation –353-) argues in favor of (independant transformation of two differentiated cell types, or more likely) the neoplastic transformation of a (common) precursor cell presenting the ability of double differentiation (432). The more homogeneous genotype than phenotype in histologically heterogeneous tumors (730), the common LOH 1p/19q in both components of mixed gliomas (372), the genetic similarities of the glial and sarcomatous components of gliosarcoma (47, 467, 731), gives further arguments in favor of a common cellular origin, as well as results of cell culture studies (see 432).

In animals as well as humans, neural stem cells have been isolated from cerebral tumors of various phenotypes, identified by the expression of the cell surface marker CD 133 and nestin, that are without expression of neural differentiation markers, are necessary for proliferation and maintenance of tumors in culture, are capable of differentiation in vitro into cellular phenotypes identical to those of the tumor in situ (215, 631, 632, 633), as well as to non-glial, mesenchymatous, cell types (see 432). Stem cells and progenitor cells in the central nervous system (as in several other somatic or cerebellar sites) seem particularly more prone to tumoral/malignant transformation (as demonstrated in somatic neoplasms) than differentiated cells because they possess the ability to bypass apoptosis and senescence, and activated cellular mechanisms similar to those of initiating or progressing (maintained) tumors, especially through the abnormal functioning of developmental signaling pathways (586). It is then postulated that the state of glial cell differentiation can affect the biological effects of given genetic alterations, so primary malignant gliomas could represent the direct malignant transformation of primitive glial precursor cells (neural stem cell or glial progenitor), while secondary malignant gliomas may arise from somewhat more differentiated cells arising from the same precursors (432, 586).

Progenitor cells can be manipulated in rodents to differentiate into astrocytes and/or gliomas (19, 271), while mature astrocytes are more prone to gliomatous transformation unless dedifferentiated (586).

Models of Formation and Progression of Human Gliomas

Animal glioma models (genetically and/or phenotypically similar to human gliomas) combined with genomic and proteomic studies allow the study of the molecular mechanisms, and eventual treatment effects, of the formation, growth, invasivity, angiogenesis… of gliomas (34, 128, 242, 244, 285, 271, 272, 273, 275, 290, 294, 370, 408, 447, 700, 701, 743). The same is attempted with tumor models based on cell lines (127, 504, 620), eventually chimeric (473), eventhough there are also differences between cell lines and actual tumors in vivo (722), as well as in vitro tumor development (cell gene expression and thus phenotype as defined in vitro is affected not only by in vivo growth but also by orthotopic growth). In mice, genes more expressed in vitro reflect increased proliferation in a more favorable environment, while in vivo there is an upregulation of genes involved in extracellular matrix, cellular interaction and angiogenesis (120).

Nevertheless, in vivo models in close relations with clinical contingencies remain necessary as in other domains of cancer research (343). Spontaneous low-grade gliomas in animals and notably rodents resemble more or less human glioma growth patterns (238, 647). The historic model of sub-cutaneous heterotopic xenografts of human tumors with spontaneous immunosuppressed animals (like nude mice) showed its interest in the treatment research and allowed the selection of more than 50 drugs today used in general oncology for a great variety of cancers (446). It is indeed possible to use it by keeping, as in humans, all the usual response criteria (clinical signs variations, tumor measures and so the impact of the treatment on growth curves, treatment tolerance) while privileging survival as the main parameter. Applied to malignant heterotopic xenotransplanted glial tumors, the robustness of the model was confirmed with more than 60 % of graft success and a confirmed pathologic and genotypic stability of transplanted tumors (408). Models are now widely used, that can be globally considered as being able to reflect the efficiency of treatments in humans in spite of false positive results (revealing active drugs in the laboratory but not in clinical studies) due to various factors as the loss of the heterogeneity of the grafted samples, increased cell kinetics in the transplanted tumors, or the loss of the usual tumoral environment. The orthotopic transplant of these gliomas took gradually, as in other tumoral locations, a place of choice, in being more close to the reality than other models (270). The heterotopic transplant of human low-grade glioma in immunodeficient animals remains ineffective (666). Moreover, it appears obviously impossible to evaluate such parameters as survival because of the slow growth of this tumor type. On the contrary, recent data reflect the use of more and more complex animal models, with the aim of mimicking the greatest number of possible stages of the tumor progression, so to allow the evaluation of new drugs different from those acting in conventional chemotherapy, by their modulatory action of cellular signalisation at different stages of the developpment.

Experimental models of gliomagenesis have been performed (560, 639), mimicking, on normal human astrocytomas, the genetic alterations most often encountered in gliomas (alteration of p53 and Rb pathways, activation of telomerase maintenance and independance from growth factors), giving way to cells with a greatly expanded life-span, possessing a capacity of growth on soft agar and a tumorigenicity in mice resembling malignant gliomas (560). In cell cultures and in mice, overexpression of PDGF-B increased proliferation of astrocytes and neural progenitors, and neural progenitors transfered with PDGF can form oligodendrogliomas (127, 128), while GFAP+ astrocytes can form oligoglial or mixed gliomas, more often malignant when arising from Ink4a-ARF null progenitor cells (127). KRas and Akt can induce formation of astrocytomas and glioblastomas from neural progenitor cells (128), but not differentiated astrocytes unless there is a Ink4a-ARF deficiency (700). Many experiments give opportunities of new targeted therapies (eg. suppression of Rac1 activity leading to apoptosis of most glioma cells –603-, neural stem cells targeting gliomatous cells –2, 499-…).

Most of recent theoretical/mathematical modeling is based on the mutator phenotype, and as we have seen, on the multi-step acquisition and accumulation of gene alterations from normal cells to the most malignant phenotype. As well, a glycolytic phenotype is assumed generally for mammalian neoplasias, relying on the anaerobic metabolism of glucose to lactic acid, whose energetical inefficiency is compensated by an increase in glucose/blood flux (222). Other models rely on the frequent aneuploidy of cancers, with an increased cytogenetic instability in cases of hyperploidy, leading to the activation of growth promoting genes (604). There are numerous other proposed models of neoplasia, using population ecology approaches, game theory, the interaction of mutator phenotypes with environmental selection parameters (222), the spatial mobility of cells towards more growth-permissive places (agent-based model +/- game theory/geno-phenotype link –437, 438, 439-), the interaction of tumor-host interfacial morphology and physiology with tumor progression (reaction-diffusion model –220-).

There are also models proposed of blood-brain barrier (441), angiogenesis (770).

Drug- and Radiation-Resistance Genes

Correlations of genetic profiles and anticancer drug sensitivity can be tested on a panel of human cancer cell lines (129, 561, 568, 644, 733, 761, 769), on rodent models (248), which allows further novel anti-cancer compounds discovery and testing (306, 761), and help understanding mechanisms of drug action (292) and defining individual and new combinations therapies (22, 377). The same approach is currently underway for studying radiation sensitivity (687). Gene expression profiles determination will progressively lead to phenotypic outcome prediction (577). The transportome has been shown to play an important role in drug resistance (289), as well attachment or extracellular matrix genes explaining different drug sensitivity of solid tumors and their derived cell lines (646), or the SPARC protein or gene expression (665). Drug resistance seems closely linked to apoptotic pathways, while general drug sensitivity seems associated to genes linked to cell cycle control and proliferation (561), but also cell adhesion (642).

The drug efflux pump protein P-glycoprotein, multidrug resistance related proteins MRP1 to 5, lung-resistance protein (LRP), glutathiome S-transferase-pi (detoxification enzyme), DNA topoisomerase IIα, interferon receptor, interferon regulatory factors (IRF-1&2), dihydrofolate reductase, among others can protect the brain from xenobiotics, as well as cisplatine-resistance proteins (83, 465). Drug or xenobiotics metabolizing enzymes include various phase I (eg. cytochrome P450 or CYP) and II enzymes, whose gene expression is increased in response to inducers or xenobiotics triggering a global cellular stress (577). Endothelial cells of normal brain and tumors express differently the multidrug resistance genes and some matrixmetalloproteinases (543). Native drug resistance (acquired during tumorigenesis, then with different or common gene alterations for oncogenesis and drug response, or intrinsic property of the cell of origin ? –494-) appears more important than acquired resistance, no significant difference being evident from primary to recurrent tumors (primary glioblastomas show a higher ration MGMT/beta2-microglobulin than secondary forms or other tumors, while low-grade gliomas show a lower ratio –667-).

There could be a link between loss of p53 function and expression of multiple drug resistance in non-tumor CNS cells (442), p53 protein possibly contributing to the regulation of microtubule composition and function (its dysfunction generating complex microtubule-associated mechanisms of resistance to tubulin-binding agents like vinca alkaloids or taxanes –217-), but (experimental) modulation of chemosensitivity by p53 appears unlikely (690). This can be put in parallel to the role of defect or dysregulation of the apoptotic pathways (720).

There appear to exist broad cross-resistance secondary resistance mechanisms, involving altered expression in pro- and anti-apoptotic proteins, and primary resistance mechansims, specific to given anti-cancer agents. As for example depletion of alkylguanine alkyltransferase –AGT or MGMT- by O(6)-benzylguanine or MGMT hypermethylation increases the cytotoxicity of alkylating agents widely used against gliomas, of temozolomide (429) more than the BCNU efficacy (60), but mutant MGMT resistant to O(6)-BG have been identified (21), or the possible less growth inhibition of mutant p53 in the NCI anticancer drug screen, with the exception of anti-mitotic drugs (495).

Rat O-2A progenitors, astrocytomes and oligodendrocytes show various expressions of drug resistance genes, with higher expression of MGMT and MDR in astrocytes and of GSTµ and MT in oligodendrocytes (494), and wild-type p53 astrocytes show greater MGMT activity but a BCNU resistance (492). Human low-grade astrocytoma and oligodendrogliomas show the same proportion of methylation of MGMT gene (almost 50% -739-) or MGMT is more expressed in astrocytic tumors (494, 656) than in oligodendrogliomas and even more oligoastrocytomas or normal cerebral tissue (626), and there is a slightly but significantly lower MGMT expression in low-grade than high-grade gliomas (656). MGMT expression is inversely correlated with age and correlated with aneuploidy but not S-phase fraction (626), is associated with a shorter survival time (656), and BCNU (310) as well as temozolomide responsiveness of malignant astrocytomas (256).

E - TUMORAL SIZE AND ITS EVOLUTION

The careful monitoring, at the clinical and radiological levels, of the evolution of a patient harbouring a grade 2 glioma, is bound to reflect best the proper biological behavior of the latter interacting with the host, defined by his background and tolerance. Despite an apparent biological diversity, longitudinal clinico-radiological data enables to distinguish some common rules in this somewhat chaotic population of tumor/host pairs. The statements made here are derived mainly from our experience centered on supratentorial hemispheric gliomas affecting adults.

Tumor size has been evaluated in various one- to three-dimensional manners: greatest diameter, greatest surface, spherical or ellipsoid approximation, sommation of the actual surfaces on each sectional image, and now available, actual volume obtained by tumor segmentation on MRI that should be the only standard eventhough some have failed, in anaplastic gliomas, to find a prognostic relevance of post-operative volume when studying the mean geometrical while the planimetry method did (757). The FLAIR sequences appear the best to determine the margins of the glioma (78), especially in peripheral and periventiruclar regions (113 –absence of partial volume effect by the nulled CSF-). The three directions of growth should be taken in account since, due to the anatomico-biological characteristics of intra-cranial structures and the tendancy of most gliomas (depending on their site of origin) to grow towards the ventricular system and along white fibers, some tumors will demonstrate a preferential cranio-caudal growth that would be underestimated by one or two-dimensional estimations. Moreover, the determination of three diameters reduces the risk of error due to patient's positioning in the MRI unit, the angulation of the slice planes.. Every technique carries more a less a subjective dimension, and 2D or 3D evaluations overestimate the tumoral surfaces or volumes, the more so as the lesional volume is larger or more irregular (Mandonnet 2005, submitted). Nevertheless, a certain proportionality remains, in terms of volume or growth rates, which allows to draw some conclusions from our series, comprising mainly estimations using the ellipsoid approximation method (volume= half the product of the three biggest orthogonal diameters); indeed our preliminary results with segmentation volumetric measurement do not contradict the results obtained with the former method.

Grade 2 Gliomas are Constantly Evolving Tumors

The first notion is that all grade 2 gliomas grow with time. This means that any tumor image compatible with a grade 2 glioma that does not show any volumetric variation in one or two years, is probably a dysplasia or DNT. But since grade 2 gliomas grow at different rates, sometimes quite slow, one can be abused, comparing the last radiological exam with the second to last, without precise measurement, and believe that a given tumor is quiescent. There are hopefully attempts at developing pragmatic tools (quick and automated post-processing accessible to clinicians) to monitor eventual variations of volume (113).

The growth of human tumors depends on the cell cycle time, the proliferation index (cells in cycle/cells in G0 phase), and the cellular losses. During their period of possible observation, is follows usually a constant, exponential, type (in fact somewhat different due to cellular losses which result in the fact that the doubling-time is greater than the inter-mitotic or cell cycle time, and to the presence of aneuploid cells). Tumor doubling-times have been measured more often on CT-scans, ranging from 19.5=+/-1.9 to 48.1+/-20.9 or 69.7 days for grade 4 gliomas (57, 694 –regrowth-, 760), 66.5+/-29.4 to 140 days for grade 3 gliomas (57, 694 –regrowth-), and 937+/-66.5 days for regrowing grade 2 gliomas (694) while others have reported doubling-times for the latter, mixed with grade 1 gliomas (140 days –57-). By comparison, doubling-times of other oncotypes have been reported at around 30 days for embryonal tumors and lymphomas, 40 days for mesenchymatous sarcomas, 60 days for malpighian carcinomas, and 80 days for adenocarcinomas (695). Tumor doubling-times of gliomas do not differ greatly before and after treatment(s) (57). The tumor doubling-time has been shown to differ according to the ploidy of the tumor, much smaller in aneuploid(/multiclonal) than diploid than euploid tumors, whatever their histological grade (57). From a theoretical origin as a single neoplastic cell of 10 μm in diameter, it is commonly assumed that a tumor needs 30 doublings to attain 1 cc (2^{30} or around 10^9 cells) that is a minimal size to be detectable clinically (7, 112). At diagnosis, the tumor has progressed of a mean of little more than 5 doubling-times, and between diagnosis and death only slightly more than 3 doubling-times are necessary, whatever the histological grade of the glioma (57), since the average fatal volume of a (bulky) tumor seems to be around 100-150 cc.

The logistic growth model of Verhulst (1838), as the other models of Gompertz (1825, 24) or Bertalanffy (1941 –growth velocity is the difference between anabolism and catabolism-), are empirical models using mathematical equations (sigmoid) reflect probably more the fact that in the clinical phase of the tumors, the growth is somewhat slower when the tumoral volume is greater (9, 398), depending on the « carrying capacity of the environment, which is normally determined by the available resources» and/or waste product accumulation, with greater cellular losses, decreased proliferation fraction and longer mean G1 phase times, generating an exponentially decaying growth rate after an exponential growth of tumoral cells. The competition for nutrients in a avascular tumor could be a determining factor in generating papillary tumor morphology (190). Other modelisations are refined, for example with a focus on the emergence of clonal subpopulations in tumors (325, 326), a representation of stress distribution during an anisotropic growth with its consequences on vasculature (12), or are more molecular in nature (620).

But some have challenged the mathematical assumptions based on analysis of the growth of transplantable animal tumors and on averages of tumor growth in human populations (756). Tumoral growth could be more irregular, with dormant phases or plateaus separated by growth spurts (551). Other models are more functional, mechanistic, physiology- or biology-based, and offer other tumoral evolution laws (770) or focus specifically on one component of growth, for example proliferation, diffusion (697), invasion (437) eventually as a chemotaxis model (394, 587), angiogenesis (97), take in account ecology, or attempt to modelise at the molecular level the mutual exclusivity of proliferation and migration (16).

Derived from the observation of colonies issued from tumor cell lines, and indirectly confirmed on tumors developing in vivo, it has been shown that the spatio-temporal pattern of tumoral growth seems to obey to fractality, and that it follows a universal rule of linear growth (in terms of its radius), this dynamic behaviour in turn being compatible with the molecular beam epitaxy (MBE) universality class (69). In this setting, the main mechanism responsible for growth is cell diffusion at the interface with normal parenchyma, with a relatively great inhibition of cellular growth inside the tumor or colony (as attested by differential proliferative indices); while MBE dynamics implies surface diffusion of cells, ie. their movement along the tumor/colony border, and not their free movement away from it (69). Globally, the growth velocity is characteristic of the process, and not of the cell line, hence biological behaviour of similar tumors will vary depending on its external environment (the host), the major conditioner of tumor growth being space competition between tumor and host. So, the most commonly accepted mechanism conditioning tumor growth mainly to nutrient competition (between tumor cells and tumor and host cells), in accordance with a Gompertzian model, is insufficient to reproduce the main features of tumor growth (69). The linear regime of tumoral growth implies that there are less actively proliferating cells, and that these are homogeneously constrained to the border of the tumor and not randomely distributed throughout its whole volume. Moreover, newly generated cells move to sites with a higher number of neighbouring cells, while the inner cells are prevented from proliferating by the pressure exerted on them through the lack os space (69). Nevertheless, by analogy with pressure effects (solid state stress) in tumor spheroids, the pressure exerted by the host over the tumor could explain the deviation of the tumor growth rate from a pure linear regime.

Other models have been hypothesized, that explain an arrested tumoral growth at a volume around 100-150 cc, an irregular shape in the first stages of tumor development then a spheroidal shape, and a centripetal growth remission (479).

Since glial tumors are infiltrative, the cellular density of the more peripheral parts of the lesion will be insufficient to generate a signal abnormality on MRI, even with the most sensitive sequences. Hence, even if the total number of tumoral cells grows exponentially, the volumetric doubling time used to quantify the radiological growth of (high-grade) gliomas (57, 760) will not be appropriate. Instead, the growth curve of the tumoral volume is more likely cubic, or so to say the growth curve of the mean tumoral diameter will appear linear. That is in accordance with our observations, and with a biomathematical model (proposed initially by Murray in the 1990s –662- then others, 689, 754) of glioma growth as a conservation equation taking in account proliferation and diffusion of tumor cells, later refined (659, 660, 661, 662) to account for brain parenchyma heterogeneities and reflect asymmetric, nonspherical, tumor development and migration facilitated in white matter (227).

Representing then the growth rate of grade 2 gliomas as the slope of the curve reflecting the variations of the mean geometrical tumoral diameter with time, it could be shown, in a highly selected series, that the mean velocity of growth of grade 2 gliomas is around 4 mm/yr (435, 662). By contrast, for grade 4 gliomas, velocities of 30 mm/yr (662), or from 18 to 110 mm/yr (personal observation of four cases), have been observed before treatment.

In a larger series of unselected grade 2 gliomas in our experience, growth rates vary widely in contrast to a small confidence interval in the selected series. Nevertheless, the median growth rates were similar, of 3.8 mm/yr in the whole series against 4.1 mm/yr in the selected series.

The Growth Rate of Grade 2 Gliomas is Correlated with their Biological Behaviour

The slope of the mean diameter increase of a tumor can first help distinguish «true grade 2 gliomas» from particularly aggressive ones, which will soon demonstrate signs of malignancy (57, 542). Indeed, in our experience, some tumors that look like grade 2 gliomas on MRI (without any contrast enhancement suggestive of anaplasia), and even at the histological level, can in fact be ruled out in a few weeks or months as more aggressive, when their diameter growth rate exceeds 8 mm/yr, and more so at 10 mm/yr or more. This suggests that a period of radiological observation should be the rule before any therapeutic decision, since the absence of radiological signs of anaplasia does not rule out the possibility of a high-grade glioma. This remains valid even if a biopsy is realized, since the growth rate seems more reliable than histology, which can change dramatically in a few months (as the radiological features). Those particularly aggressive cases account for survival curves of grade 2 gliomas that show a decline in the first months or 1(-2) year(s), which seems paradoxical for a slow-growing, initially histologically benign, tumor. They account for almost 12% of our series, and in fact anaplastic gliomas with a radiological pattern suggestive of low-grade glioma have been reported in up to 50% of the cases (more frequently with advancing age).

This notion gives arguments to the practicians who do not advocate a systematic histological diagnosis in front of a suspected grade 2 glioma, even in the absence of oncologic treatment decision. Indeed, a (stereotactic) biopsy carries a functional risk (0-1% mortality, 2-5% morbidity –80b-, 3% morbidity in our series-), and the histological diagnosis can be mis- or underestimated (wrong diagnosis, or more frequently underestimation of the grade); this is also possible despite the thorough examination of a surgical (resection) specimen, as we have observed in some cases an anaplastic transformation a few months after extensive resection of a grade 2 glioma with no histologic «hint» of malignancy (proliferation index included).

In the same way, the growth rate (slope) appears constant throughout the evolution of a grade 2 glioma. But, when the tumor acquires a genophenotype of anaplastic (high-grade) glioma, its growth rate accelerates (Rees 2005 submitted). This change in the slope occurs, under the condition of a somewhat close follow-up (every 6 months for example), usually before other radiological signs of anaplasia (mainly contrast enhancement, which in turn can take up to 2 years to become patent and imply the most part of the tumor), and even preceed clinical signs (recurrent or increased epilepsy, overt deficit, signs of intracranial hypertension). Hence, aggressive therapeutic measures can be taken at the beginning of the anaplastic transformation, which offers in our series a better chance of result in terms of survival, and also helps maintain a patient in a better functional condition.

Also, quite logically, the growth rate of a grade 2 glioma reflects in part its biological behavior. There is indeed a correlation, on univariate analysis, between growth rates and outcome.

The Tumoral Volume is of Prognostic Importance

The determination of tumoral volume is important in more than one way. First of all, lesional volume, and its correlate of extension in terms of anatomical landmarks, is essential as it represents a major decisional factor for treatement decision-making, both in terms of feasibility (or ratio benefit/risk), and also in terms of chances of success.

But a tumoral volume, in conjunction of the tumoral growth rate, reflects also the evolutive stage of a given tumor at time of its observation. Indeed, when one evaluates one way or another the tumoral size, it represents an independant prognostic factor of outcome (43 –univariate-, 375, 516, our series). The cut-off value can vary from one series to another (20 ml –375-, 10 & 30 cc –43-, 5 to 6 cm of greatest diameter –516-). A greater volume, meaning a later stage of evolution of a (untreated) glioma, can thus undermean that the tumor is closer to its anaplastic transformation, the common terminal fate of grade 2 gliomas. Indeed, in our series, anaplastic transformation was never detected in (previously untreated) tumors whose mean diameter was less than 5 cm (62.5 cc –one exception at 4.7 cm-).

Hence, to accurately reflect the inherent biological potential of an individual tumor, or more precisely the result of the tumor/host interaction, one must take into account the volume as well as the growth rate of the lesion.

Tumoral Volumes and Growth Rates Are Also Valuable Post-Treatment Follow-Up Tools

Radiological follow-up of grade 2 gliomas after treatment(s) is as important as their pre-therapeutic evaluation (9), in terms of radiological aspect (enhancement, edema, mass effect, extension) as well as in terms of volume and growth rate.

It allows to evaluate objectively the quality of an eventual surgical resection, or more pratically the amount of residual MRI signal abnormality representing the residual tumoral tissue. This permits first to speak a common language, second to appreciate an eventual impact of resective surgery in the context of grade 2 gliomas. Indeed, when surgical cytoreduction is so quantified, and not described on the sole basis of the surgeon's impression, the everlasting debate on its prognostic value if any shows a trend towards a definite interest of surgery under the condition that the residual tumoral volume is less than 10 to 15 cc (43, our series), this cut-off appearing more interesting in practice eventhough the relation appears one the whole linear with the volume as a continuous variable. A simple law

(8) linked tumor doubling times and the amount of resection (50% resected offering a time survival gain of one doubling time, 75% two..), before a more thorough modelisation was made that proved valuable when applied to clinical data on high-grade gliomas (for review 662). Moreover, assuming that a given tumor follows a constant growth rate (mean diameter curve) pre-operatively, and that it resumes the same growth rate after surgery, which should represent a cytoreduction without any «side effect» that could alter tumor kinetics, one can calculate, and hence predict, the extra (progression-free) survival eventually provided by surgery. With the method of ellipsoid approximation, the post-operative diameter curves that we observe are of linear type, but with a slightly greater slope; this discrepancy could be due to the fact that this measurement technique overestimates more the volumes of (greater and) more irregular tumors (Mandonnet 2005, submitted).

Model predictions as well as spatial classification of gliomas (137) show that diffusion represents a paramount, if not predominant, component of gliomas. Hence, ideally the coefficient diffusion should be determined before any surgical decision, since essentially lesions with a low diffusion coefficient will benefit from a large resection. In this respect, oligoglial tumors with LOH 1p/19q could be more suitable to surgical treatment since they grow more as circumscribed lesions (501).

Quantitative static and dynamic evaluation of tumoral volume allows to monitor the effect of chemotherapy if any, along with mathematical modeling (661, 689). In our experience, the first effect of a «successfull chemotherapy» is to arrest the tumoral growth (horizontalization of the diameter curve). Then, there is is a more or less slow and rarely important decrease of the tumoral extension, in a centripetal manner, which can even continue well after the termination of chemotherapy (446, 645, personal observations). This evaluation of the efficacy of chemotherapeutic drugs on low-grade gliomas seems at the moment the only effective monitoring method (645), since even spectro-MR is not fully tested in this context (reduction of choline seemingly parallel to the volumetric effect –471-).

When it is admitted that the growth of grade 2 gliomas obey a linear regime, that is based on fractality and MBE laws, the proliferative cells as discussed upper are mainly associated with the surface of tumors. Since they represent the cells sensitive to antiproliferating agents, one can deduce two main consequences. The first is that the killed cellular population will be at the periphery of the radiological image, as we have observed (as in other models proposed –479-). Second, the effectiveness of chemotherapy will decrease with tumor size (as described with glioblastomas –340-), on the opposite of the current log-kill concept assuming a constant effect at random (on cells in proliferation). Moreover, it is well known that hypoxia plays a role in radio- as well as chemoresistance, which can be explained by cells following MBE dynamics and hence migrating to positions where oxygen is less available (higher celleular concentration, lower pH due to lactate production). Other models aim to reflect (and understand) that heterogeneity in drug delivery due to variability in vascular density can lead to an apparent tumor reduction in certain areas while there remains a persistent growth in other areas, eventually beyond the resolution of imaging (661), or attempt to represent drug resistance (502), or attempt to predict in the preclinical phase of development of oncology drugs, empirical (mathematical equations), functional (mechanistic, physiology-based hypotheses) or mixed (629).

The effect of radiotherapy is also monitored in the same way. Even if the importance of tumoral reduction is of no prognostic importance on outcome (29), one can rule out early, as under chemotherapy, an absence of effect of the therapeutic modality, allowing to change the strategy more precociously. As is the rule in the field of oncology, we have observed that the quicker and the more important is the tumoral volumetric reduction after chemotherapy essentially, but frequently after radiotherapy also, the greater the probability that the tumor was more aggressive, as reflected as a rule by a greater pre-treatment growth rate.

In this field too, modelisation is of importance (350).

But there still remains a biological diversity or hazardous aspect in the natural history of grade 2 gliomas

Despite the common rules described above as lessons learned from the (trivial) radiological follow-up of grade 2 gliomas, we are still unable to predict the outcome, moreover at the individual level, of patients harbouring a suspected or proven grade 2 glioma.

In terms of functional prognosis, even if the tumoral site and extension, hence volume, are of paramount importance, there is a well known anatomo-functional variability (tolerance, plasticity) that hampers the possibilities of a precise individual functional prognosis. More importantly, anaplastic transformation is an event that appears yet unpredictable, at least in the terms described in this chapter. The modification or value of the slope of the tumoral diameter curve is a constant predictor of imminent anaplasia, but we have observed cases of malignant transformation, in the absence of, as well as after treatment, without significant changes of the tumoral growth rate. Anaplastic transformation seems indeed to be a spontaneous, intrinsic process, independant of any external stimulus (5).

Tumor growth modeling is also limited by individual factors that appear prognostic in clinical series, such as age, performance status (662).

In all event, progress has to be made in this aspect of tumoral dynamic evaluation, and maybe the actual volumetric measurement now accessible to everyone will help to refine and extend these observations.

Nevertheless, the notions of volume and growth rates should already be included in the evaluation and studies of grade 2 gliomas, providing additional information that can help defining risk groups a priori after a short period of observation of the natural history of these tumors. This should allow the realization of valuable clinical trials, soon probably spanning shorter times of follow-up to obtain results of comparable quality. Every effort in refining volumetric analysis of tumors should then be encouraged (660).

F - METABOLIC NEUROIMAGING

In addition, the use of various brain radioactive tracers has shed invaluable light on the pathophysiology of gliomas: nature and degree of heterogeneity of the tumor, patterns of growth and extension, risk and delay of anaplastic transformation.

First, Single Photon Emission Computed Tomography (SPECT) studies showed a relationship between tracers uptake and tumor grade, using both Thallium-201 (302, 498) or ^{99m}Tc-MIBI (32, 38, 259, 386, 592, 641, 643, 741, 766). Thus, determination of regions with the highest metabolic activity within the tumor was used to guide surgical biopsy in a stereotactic frame (259). Some authors also suggested that ^{99m}Tc-MIBI SPECT might help in predicting the response to chemotherapy in patients with gliomas (766), and in establishing the prognosis of survival after radiation therapy (32). However, despite the development of new tracers such as ^{99m}Tc- Tetrofosmin (641) or ^{123}I-Alpha-Methyl Tyrosine (IMT), potentially useful for identifying postoperative tumor residue (741) and recurrence (386),

SPECT still lacks reliability, and cannot be used as the sole noninvasive diagnostic or prognostic tool in gliomas (38).

Second, less widely available and more expensive, Positron Emission Tomography seems to represent a more reliable and accurate method of metabolic imaging in brain tumors (592). Beyond recent studies with positron emitters presenting definite research interest in molecular imaging (265), e.g. [I-124]Iododeoxyuridine (58) or [F-18]Fluorothymidine proposed to measure tumor proliferation rate (616), or FIAU as an indicator of gene expression in glioma useful for gene therapy (307), most clinical works have focused their efforts on metabolic substrates such as ^{11}C-choline (252, 619), and above all ^{18}Fluoro-2-deoxy-2-glucose (FDG) and ^{11}C-methyl-methionine (MET). Indeed, FDG PET can predict tumor grade (347, 457), while low-grade oligodendrogliomas and pilocytic astrocytomas can be quite FDG avid – so FDG uptake in such lesions does not necessarily imply a poorly differentiated histology (333). Also, the metabolic activity of gliomas as shown by the PET-FDG method seems to have a good prognostic significance (143, 277), independent from histology (142, 144). Furthermore, because brain tumors are histologically heterogeneous, PET-FDG was used to guide stereotactic biopsies (410, 445). Indeed, while LGG are noted to have low levels of FDG uptake, areas of malignant degeneration show increased metabolic activity (204), associated with an unfavorable prognosis (143). Finally, FDG-PET has been used to document the extent of tumor resection (234), and differentiate brain tumors from necrosis after radiation and/or chemotherapy (72). In a pilot study, it has even been reported that FDG-PET could differentiate responders from non responders after one cycle of temozolomide in recurrent high-grade gliomas (76). However, since FDG-PET has limited value in defining the extent of tumor involvement and recurrence of LGG, MET-PET may be preferable for this group of lesions (108). Indeed, MET-PET appears to be related to tumor aggressivity (148), with a high uptake statistically associated with a poor survival time (141, 149, 261, 557) and allows to delineate the invasion of tumors (especially LGG) much better than FDG-PET – thus representing a better choice for PET guidance in neurosurgical procedures (518) an for assessing response to therapy (723). Furthermore, the value of the combination of FDG-PET and MET-PET has been suggested (283), in particular in LGG with a low methionine uptake (144), for instance in astrocytomas – which have lower levels of MET uptake in comparison to oligodendrogliomas (147). Finally, recent development of ^{18}F-labeled amino acid tracers such as ^{18}F-alpha-methyl-tyrosine, with promising preliminary results in the evaluation of gliomas (300), opens the field for wider use of PET scanning in the management of brain tumors (455, 458).

Third, Proton MR spectroscopy (MRS) represents a new, noninvasive tool recently used in clinical practice to investigate the spatial distribution of metabolic changes in brain tumors (140). Indeed, several authors have reported increased levels of choline-containing compounds (Cho, a marker of increased membrane turnover or higher cellular density –458-) and a reduction in the signal intensities of N-Acetyl Aspartate (NAA, a neuronal marker mainly contained within neurons –703-) and Creatine (a marker of energy metabolism –342-) in gliomas (264, 478). The ranges of Cho increase and NAA decrease seem compatible with the range of tumor infiltration (121, 284). The calculation of metabolic maps by integrating the peak area of a metabolite of interest or some ratios such as the Cho-NAA index for each voxel is currently a common method to visualize these changes (154, 452, 673). Metabolite profiles have been used to differentiate various types of tumor from one another (284), in particular LGG (519) and gliomatosis (214). Metabolite maps have also helped to determine brain tumor grade (263) and to predict the length of survival (387), notably using : the phosphocholine / glycerophosphocholine ratio which increases with the grade of glioma (578); Cho levels which correlate with proliferative potential as determined by immunohistochemical analysis of tumors biopsies using the KI-67 labelling index for gliomas (617); Cho/Cr ratio which increases with grade (284) while myo-Inositol (91) and Glycine (100) decrease with grade; and the lipids which correlate with necrosis (385) then are increased in high-grade tumors (18). Also, MRS can monitor response to therapy, since the typical change that occurs when a tumor responds to treatment is a reduction of Cho with possibly an increase in lactate and/or lipids (241), indicating the transformation of viable tumor cells towards necrosis. Following radiotherapy, glioma progression could be predicted on the basis of MRS abnormalities (in particular an increase of Cho/Cr ratio) that were outside the MRI-defined treatment region, and can occur prior to subsequent increase in contrast enhancement (241). However, the sensitivity of MRS to detect tumor progression drops when there is a mixture of necrosis and recurrent tumor (566). The improved spatial resolution and more detailed spectral information using higher field MR systems could optimize the discrimination between radiation damage and glioma recurrence (531). Progression to higher grade could be equally documented using MRS (675). Finally, a combined used of PET and SRM in the evaluation of tumor metabolism was recently proposed (704).

To be noted that the biological behavior of brain tumors can also be indirectly studied using complementary sequences of MRI (525), i.e. diffusion weighted imaging (DWI) (542) and perfusion weighted imaging (344). In particular, apparent diffusion coefficient values for LGG are higher than those for high-grade gliomas, because more highly cellular gliomas would have a smaller interstitial space and hence more restricted diffusion (362, 654, 762). Perfusion weighted imaging provides information about tumor tissue perfusion by measuring cerebral blood volume (CBV), and might be used in the preoperative classification and grading of gliomas (653). Indeed, CBV has been shown to correlate with microvessel cell density (403, 565), and varies with tumor grade in that maximum CBV values of LGG seem significantly lower than those of high-grade gliomas (357, 426, 529). Moreover, perfusion MR imaging could be helpful in predicting LGG response to radiotherapy (211). Nevertheless, this technique still lacks sensitivity (391). Thus, it was suggested that a combination of the perfusion image results with those of DWI and SRM could improve the reliability of these methods, notably for tumor grading (762).

G - CONCLUSIONS

Grade 2 gliomas are to be considered as continuously evolving tumors, as a continuum along a spectrum beginning long before their discovery, as initially a very slow-growing, indolent, neoplasia, but ending as a highly malignant, and lethal tumor, with overall a short period of clinico-radiological observation. Most of our diagnostic armamentarium is static in essence, and it is indeed mandatory to reflect the status of the tumor and the host at a given time. But the dynamic dimension of tumoral progression has to be evaluated as well, since it probably represents a paramount factor to take into account in the definition of the most appropriate therapeutic strategy.

Along with the other parameters available (clinical, radiological, histological, biological), the evaluation of tumoral volume and growth rate, which does not demand the obtention of repeated tumoral samples (eventhough a biopsy at least at some stages of tumoral evolution – recurrences requiring a treatment for example- would prove very interesting), allows already in daily practice to rule out the most aggressive tumors that in fact behave as anaplastic gliomas. It also provides additional information essential for therapeutic decision making (urgency of treatment, evaluation of the individual efficacy and overall prognostic influence of a therapeutic modality, indication of retreatment, prediction of anaplastic transformation), as well as the building and conduct of clinical trials.

In the meantime, progress in genomics to proteomics, albeit accessible only if a surgical act is performed, should provide additional tools to classify, grade and envision the prognosis of an individual tumor. Non invasively, metabolic examinations will also probably complete the possibilities of evaluation of a given tumor. We will at last be able to differentiate the proper aggressiveness of a tumor a priori, and this will provide the basis for studies aiming to define the most appropriate therapeutic strategy to propose to a given patient.

Animal models allow to study in vivo tumoral behaviour, spontaneous as well under different environmental and therapeutic conditions, but models of low-grade gliomas are nevertheless difficult to establish (666).

## Chapter III

Advances in the Study of the Individual Dynamic Organization of the Brain

A – The Functional Brain: A Plastic Potential

Despite the description by some pioneers of several observations of post-lesional recovery, the dogma of a static functional organization of the brain was settled for more than a century. This vision was essentially based on anatomo-functional correlations performed in lesional studies, which led to the view of a brain organized in so-called « eloquent » regions, for which any lesion induced a neurological deficit (such as the central, Broca's and Wernicke's areas, early identified), and in « non-functional » structures – with no clinical consequence despite their damage. However, through regular reports of improvement of the functional status following damages of cortical and/or subcortical structures considered as « critical », this conception of a « fixed » central nervous system was called in question in the past decades. Consequently, many investigations were performed, initially in vitro and in animals, then more recently in humans since the development of functional mapping methods, in order to study the mechanisms underlying these compensatory phenomena: the concept of cerebral plasticity was born.

Therefore, cerebral plasticity could be defined as the continuous processings allowing short, middle and long-term remodelling of the neurono-synaptic organization, in order to optimize the functioning of the networks of the brain – during phylogenesis, ontogeny, physiological learning and following lesions involving the peripheral as well as the central nervous system (157). On the basis of the recent literature, several hypothesis about the pathophysiological mechanisms underlying plasticity can be considered. At a microscopic scale, these mechanisms seem to be essentially represented by: synaptic efficacy modulations (79), unmasking of latent connections (309), phenotypic modifications (304) and neurogenesis (243). At a macroscopic scale, diaschisis (481), functional redundancies (177), cross-modal plasticity with sensory substitution (31) and morphological changes (155) are implicated. Moreover, the behavioral consequences of such cerebral phenomena have been analyzed in human in the last decade, both in physiology – ontogeny (318) and learning (332) – and in pathology (99, 359). In particular, the ability to recover after a lesion of the nervous system, and the patterns of map reorganization within eloquent area and/or within distributed network, allowing such a compensation (especially regarding sensorimotor and language functions), have been extensively studied – notably in stroke (247, 412, 491, 563, 569, 677).

Such knowledge allows a better study of the dynamic reorganization of the eloquent maps induced by LGG, and to select the optimal therapeutic management adapted to each patient.

B – Linkage between LGG Progression and Functional Brain Reshaping

Most patients with LGG present with seizures and have no neurological deficit (145). This is puzzling considering the frequent invasion of eloquent structures (162). This means that these slow-growing lesions have likely induced progressive functional brain reshaping (159). Preoperative neurofunctional imaging supports this claim (187). Interestingly, the patterns of reorganization may differ between patients, a notion very important to know by the neurosurgeon with the goal to optimize both indication of surgery and surgical planning (87, 219). Indeed, despite the limitation of the preoperative neurofunctional imaging previously detailed, these methods have shown that three kinds of preoperative functional redistribution are possible, in patients without any deficit.

In the first one, due to the infiltrative feature of gliomas, function still persists within the tumor, thus with a very limited chance to perform a good resection without inducing postoperative sequelae (17, 594). In the second one, eloquent areas are redistributed around the tumor (258, 755), thus with a reasonable chance to perform a near-total resection despite a likely immediate transient deficit – but with secondary recovery within a few weeks to months. In the third one, there is already a preoperative compensation by remote areas within the lesional hemisphere (602, 676, 702) and/or by the controlateral homologuous (20, 85, 187, 276, 573, 668): consequently, the chances to perform a real total resection of this kind of gliomas are very high, with only a slight and very transient deficit.

Therefore, in cases of brain lesions involving eloquent areas (i.e. the structures supporting the sensorimotor, language or other cognitive functions), plasticity mechanisms seem to be based on an hierarchically organized model, i.e.: first with intrinsic reorganization within injured language areas (indice of favorable outcome) (258); second, when this reshaping is not sufficient, other regions implicated in the functional network are recruited, in the ipsilateral hemisphere (close and even remote to the damaged area) then in the controlateral hemisphere if necessary.

C – The Limit of Brain Plasticity

Nevertheless, despite this potential of compensation, LGG growth and migration, even before anaplastic transformation, may induce functional deficits. While sensorimotor and/or language disorders are very unusual (around 10% of cases) (145), cognitive deficits are more frequent than previously thought. Indeed, recent works using extensive neuropsychological assessment in patients harbouring a low-grade tumor, have shown impairments of cognitive functioning in most cases (around 90%) at the time of diagnosis (388, 671, 696). More precisely, an impact of the glioma on verbal fluency performance (240), picture and word recognition memory (240b), attention (240c) and executive functions (240d) has been demonstrated. It is worth noting that, in addition to the tumor itself, epilepsy may interfer with higher function and quality of life (354b). Furthermore, it seems that cognitive dysfunction might constitute a prognostic factor (68b). As a consequence, such a deficit of higher functions needs to be accurately evaluated for each patient before making a therapeutic decision, since the treatment may have a positive or negative impact on cognitive, emotional and even social (dys)function (10, 11, 14, 15, 68, 68c, 257, 354, 355, 388, 526, 528, 547, 593, 658, 663, 669, 670, 671, 672, 686), depending on the individual interrelationships tumor / function (159). Longitudinal neuropsychological assessment can also be useful in the early detection of brain tumor recurrence following a first treatment (13) – thus should be incorporated in the systematic follow-up, in order to adapt a specific dynamic (multistage) therapeutic strategy to each patient, with an optimization of the oncological impact, but also with a preservation of the quality of life.

## Chapter IV

ADVANCES IN THERAPEUTIC MANAGEMENT

A – THE CLASSICAL VIEW

1. The Wait and See Attitude

When the management of a disease implies a choice between different therapeutic strategies with a seemingly similar effect in terms of survival, and in the absence of an actual curative treatment, the quality of life can help decision making, the iatrogenic risks of treatment representing the basis of the controversia (25, 81, 497, 541, 635). Under the condition that the diagnosis can be confidently made on clinical and radiological data, and that outcome is independant of the timing of treatment(s) (541).

In the grade 2 glioma setting, evidence-based decisions are difficult to make in the absence of definite proofs of the efficacy of the available treatments and/or of their timing, with the exception of radiotherapy whose role and modalities have been explored by prospective randomizeds trials. Hence some authors advocate therapeutic abstention in cases of a typical radiological aspect, a medically controlled epilepsia, without significant neurological deficit in a younger patient (80b, 81, 430, 541, 609, 635, 713), the treatment being delayed until it is deemed «clearly indicated» (430).

Nevertheless, some prone the systematic practice of a biopsy for histological confirmation of the diagnosis (23, 93, 405, 513), since there is always, albeit rarely a risk of misdiagnosis (5 to 10% -232, 323, 361, 541-), and more frequently a risk of underdiagnosis, a great proportion of non enhancing lesions mimicking a grade 2 glioma can be in fact anaplastic (eventhough the reverse can also be true, as we have seen), the risk rising with advancing age (26). Biopsy guided by anatomical, vascular or metabolic examinations as practiced nowadays seems nevertheless reliable, the target consisting of an enhancing, hypervascular or hypermetabolic region of the tumor (with PET -204-, spectro-MR -518-, vascular MR maps –357-), but also sampling the entire extension of the lesion and even its periphery because the undelimited, infiltrative nature of these tumors and their heterogeneity (137, 356, 732). The tumoral aggressiveness can further be studied, even on small biopsy specimen, by different convergent means (histology, proliferation indices, apoptosis, karyometry, immunohistochemistry, molecular biology..). An alternative to a systematic biopsy would be a close clinical and radiological follow-up (81), to rule out tumoral evolutions somewhat incompatible with the diagnosis/prognosis of a grade 2 glioma. The more so since there is no difference observed, in terms of survival or quality of life, whether the diagnostic has been ascertained or not (535, 547).

When dealing with a recurrent tumor, the tendancy to obtain a new histological diagnosis should be encouraged, notwithstanding the ethical issues, knowing the possibility of modifications with time of the cellular components (astrocytic and/or oligoglial) of a tumor, of its aggressivity (malignancy), eventually mixed with iatrogenous changes. This attitude represents the best way to tailor the therapeutic aggressivity according to the evolutive stage that the tumor has attained, and to monitor reliably the effect of treatments (ie. stratifying according to the tumoral aggressivity).

There is indeed no available evidence that a «wait and see» (541, 713) or «primum non nocere» (80) attitude is better or worse than a more active, (oncologically) therapeutic strategy, in the absence of prospective and even retrospective comparative studies, and of the knowledge a priori of relatively precise risk-groups or reliable prognostic classes. The variable therapeutic indications among series, among teams/institutions, practicians, patients, and epochs, hamper the possibility of comparisons. Most if not all authors of course agree to be more proactive in front of an older patient (>40 or 50 years), the presence of significant neurological deficits or refractory epilepsy, an extensive tumor with mass effect or evolutive contrast enhancement, but these subgroups account for a small proportion of the cases diagnosed by modern and easily available radiological examinations (and in most cases correspond to an advanced stage, "pre-anaplastic"). On the other hand, a subgroup of patients whose tumor is (para-)limbic/temporal, presenting clinically at a young age, with a long-standing isolated epilepsy (with a normal neurologic examination), has been identified with a good prognosis (27, 397, 513, 514); to note that these radio-clinical aspects resemble those of DNETs.

2. Surgery

Most authors agree on the (functional more than oncological) indication, initially, of resective surgery, if by its volume and extension the tumor at diagnosis exerts a significant mass effect (corresponding as a rule to a tumoral diameter of 4-5 cm) (427), as well as when a midline site or extension compromises CSF (out)flow, or when the radio-clinical aspect is suggestive of a (pre-)anaplastic state, or when one thinks that the follow-up of the patient will prove difficult and/or depending on the wish of the patient (80b).

Some authors prone undelayed resective surgery when a large (subtotal or complete) resection appears feasible, claiming that it has a prognostic value and that it is safe (at least under certain conditions/technical adjuncts). By contrast for others, when surgery carries a greater risk (eloquent areas) and especially in the eventuality of an oligoglial tumor, its indication should be carefully weighted, since there are alternative therapeutic modalities. On the opposite, some do not advocate surgery initially in the absence of pejorative factors as we have seen previously.

The rationale for a surgical cytoreduction is to reduce the number of proliferating cells («greater log-kill»), so to diminish the risk of successive genetic alterations leading to anaplastic transformation, thereby delaying progression and malignancy (448); moreover, this can facilitate the effect of other treatments. Because of the everincreasing infiltrative behaviour of these tumors, surgery should logically be proposed as soon as possible (smaller volume, lesser migration). But the infiltrative, undelimited, mode of growth of gliomas precludes their cure by surgery (see above), and some have stressed the tenuous concept of an even (sub)total resection of the radiologically apparent part of these tumors, which could be attained by radiotherapy for example (427). Unfortunately, for practical and even ethical reasons, a prospective randomized study of the impact of surgery seems impossible to accomplish, in part also because there would be to many selection bias that could not be overcome (339).

The everlasting debate on the prognostic influence, if any, of resective surgery of grade 2 gliomas is fueled for most part by the absence of objective estimation of the post-operative residual tumor (which is preferable to the report of the proportion of tumor removed, particularly when the pre-operative volume is not stated). Among the numerous reports relating the effect of surgery as based on the surgeon's impression, one can find from no interest at all of a surgical resection (80b, 614), to a prognostic influence, on univariate and sometimes even multivariate studies, only in terms of tumoral progression, and/or in terms of survival (303, 337, 397, 405, 464, 475, 482, 488, 506, 513, 591, 607, 637, 732), rarely prospectively (184, 330).

More recently, there has been reports evaluating objectively (and statistically) the amount of resection (on CT then MRI), among which the majority seem to show a benefit of extensive surgery (review in 339), only studied or more often apparent in univariate analysis (43, 45, 482, 506) than in multivariate analysis (23, 312, 418, 591). The principal differences shown relate to resection vs. no resection, or (sub)total resection vs. biopsy and/or clearly partial surgery, and to a benefit especially apparent in the first years (no or important reduction of progressions and recurrences after complete resection in the 4-5 years after surgery –43, 482, 506-), the survival curves converging at about 10 years (312). To note is the fact that (sub)total resections are in general achieved predominantly with smaller tumors (591), more easily accessible and less invasive tumors (488), preceeding determination of the spatial configuration of the tumor is warranted (591), lesions not crossing the midline (516). In our experience, complete radiological removal, eventhough more frequent with smaller tumors, has similar influence whatever the size or location of a tumor. A difference is indeed difficult to demonstrate, especially when one recalls that a small surgical specimen (biopsy, partial removal) can be underscored in terms of aggressivity (516), eventhough the value of cytoreductive surgery can appear more important with more aggressive lesions (123). Last, the quality of resection might influence only the delay of a surgery for recurrence (in the absence of other intervening treatment) but not the incidence of anaplastic transformation (600, in contradiction with an initial report of the same team –43- and our experience), which recalls the seemingly effect of radiotherapy in our experience. Hence, for the moment no conclusive evidence is clearly demonstrated about the prognostic impact of resective surgery in grade 2 gliomas (749), but the improvement in the surgical techniques (and quality) has allowed a reduced functional risk for the patients (316).

The extent of surgery favorably influences the immediate functional outcome (506, even more linked to age), not solely when it allows the alleviation of signs of raised intracranial pressure or focal deficits (rarely) due to a compressive mechanism. Epilepsy benefits from surgery in the majority of cases, without even the use of specialized approaches/techniques of corticectomy (with improvement of the quality of life), even in eloquent areas (150), and more so with (sub)total resections (206). But there are unchanged epilepsies, and the initial efficacy seems to decrease often over the years of follow-up, especially in temporal locations, whatever the pre-operative duration of seizures (750). It is difficult in this setting to appreciate the role of the slowly-growing tumor, sometimes infra-radiological only, in the mid/long-term effect of resective surgery on epilepsy.

The functional risk of surgery is notable/evident, in this context of tumors that show a high propensity to arise or extend in eloquent areas, with persistance of functional cerebral parenchyma within the tumor (especially in primary eloquent areas) and/or at the tumor/brain interface (159, 161, 165, 167, 168, 169, 174, 594, 634. The recent advent of pre- and intra-operative anatomo-functional techniques have allowed a reduction of the surgical risk while permitting a more extensive tumoral removal (see after).

3. Radiotherapy

Historically, radiotherapy was necessary as the first standard postoperative additional treatment.

Modalities

Initially, main recommendations concerning radiotherapy were based on heterogeneous retrospective studies (443) and led to propose systematically an additional radiotherapy for biopsied patients or those having benefited from a partial surgery all the more if they were more than 40 years old (404, 609).

The most often proposed dose was from 50 to 55 Gy with fractions of 1, 8 to 2 Gy at the rate of 5 fractions per week. Target volume was first the brain *in toto* and then the X ray scan hypodensity or the T2 MRI signal raised by a 2 (to 3) cm safety margin (609, 735).

This "standard" prevailed until the recent realization of prospective multicentric studies, as two trials allowed to clarify the optimal dose of radiotherapy.

The North Central Cancer Treatment Group / Radiation Therapy Oncology Group / Eastern Cooperative Oncology Group trial compared 50, 4 Gy in 28 fractions versus 64, 8 Gy in 36 fractions for 203 eligible patients included between 1986 and 1994. No survival difference was noted, and a recent actualisation has even demonstrated a better survival, but not statiscally significant, in the low dose group after a median follow-up of 6.43 years for the 120 surviving patients; toxicity seems besides greater in terms of radionecrosis in the high dose group (613).

European Organisation for Research and Treatment of Cancer (EORTC) 22844 trial compared 45 Gy in 5 weeks versus 59, 4 Gy in 6, 6 weeks for 379 (343 eligible) patients included between 1986 and 1997 (330). No significant difference between the two groups was observed. The median follow up is now greater than 6 years (706). The five year survival rates were around 60 % for the two groups, median survival a little more than 7 years. The quality of life seems besides better in the low dose group (346, 516).

These last two trials plead clearly in favor of a low dose radiotherapy (45-50 Gy) in terms of efficiency and of toxicity, notably neurocognitive.

Optimal Timing

The timing question was recently analyzed by a European multicentric study. European Organisation for Research and Treatment of Cancer 22845 trial compared a conventional 6 weeks/54 Gy radiotherapy immediate versus delayed in 311 (290 eligible) patients included between 1986 and 1997 (329). It was clearly shown that immediate radiotherapy allowed an increase of the five year progression free survival (five year estimates for time to progression of 44 % for the treated group and 37 % for the control group) while it had no impact on the global survival (five year overall survival estimates of 63 % for the treated arm and 66 % for the control arm). Data concerning the quality of life and toxicity are nevertheless not available.

So, the choice of treatment strategy is still not so evident (368) and relies mainly on the therapist convictions. The theoretical risk of long-term radio-induced side effects in terms of radionecrosis or cognition, all the more when large volumes are irradiated, would rather plead in favour of withholding radiotherapy initially.

Short, Middle and Long Term Effects of Radiotherapy

We saw that radiotherapy had no significant impact on survival, but increases the progression-free survival.

Radiotherapy can also improve epilepsy or pre-existent neurological deficits (in 70-80% of cases), although the data of the literature remain on this point very marginal (29, 40, 427, 428, 522, 606).

These positive effects must be opposed to the negative effects represented by alopecia (sometimes definitive), late endocrinopathies, radionecroses (risk of 2.5 to 5% -607-) and especially neuro-cognitive decline (correlated with the degree of leuco-encephalopathy even sometimes difficult to differentiate from a tumoral spread) being able to alter considerably the quality of life. Eventhough studies on this subject are contradictory (70, 567, 672, 719, 764), these cognitive side effects seem bound to the total dose, the dose by session, target volume, age of the patient, vascular risk factors like arterial hypertension or diabete melitus and existence of concomitant treatments like chemotherapy. Most of these factors can be partially controled or limited with the modern focal techniques of radiotherapy.

To be noted that chemotherapy was used for a long time only in case of anaplastic transformation, and when the glioma continued to grow or recurred after radiotherapy.

B – NEW THERAPEUTIC STRATEGIES

1. Methodological Developments

Surgery

In addition to a systematic preoperative planning by non invasive neurofunctional imaging (now also possible during surgery via the recent development of intraoperative anatomical and functional MRI), an essential advance in the surgery of LGG was the use of intraoperative direct cortical stimulation (DCS), under general or local anesthesia – due to the frequent location of these tumors in eloquent areas and their infiltrative feature (44, 56, 131, 132, 166, 167, 175, 179, 180, 208, 278, 378, 396, 436, 456, 484, 507, 509, 550, 552, 589, 624, 625, 652, 674, 729, 734, 751). DCS allows the mapping of motor function (possibly under general anesthesia, by inducing unvoluntary motor response if stimulation at the level of an eloquent site), somatosensory function (by eliciting dysesthesia described by the patient himself intraoperatively), and also the mapping of cognitive functions such as language (spontaneaous speech, oject naming, comprehension, etc…), calculation, memory, reading or writing, performed in these cases on awake patients – by generating transient disturbances if the electrical stimulation is applied at the level of a functional "epicenter". It is important that a speech therapist be present in the operative room, in order to interpret accurately the kind of disorders induced by DCS, for instance speech arrest, anarthria, speech apraxia, phonological disturbances, semantic paraphasia, perseveration, anomia, dysculia, and so on. Thus, DCS is able to identify in real-time the cortical sites *essential for the function (i.e. to be imperatively preserved)*, following the dura-matter opening but before the beginning of the resection, in order to both select the best surgical approach and to define the cortical limits of the glioma removal (175).

Intra-operative mapping has also allowed a better understanding of brain functioning, notably with regard to the cortical organization of the areas involving language, memory, and calculating, as well as the role of the supplementary motor area, the insula and the premotor cortex (163, 164, 164b, 170, 173, 176, 202, 223, 425, 459, 572, 573, 575).

This stimulation also allows study of anatomo-functional connectivity, through the detection of bundles for sub-cortical, motor, somatosensory, language pathways and those for other cognitive functions (41, 42, 45, 168, 171, 172, 178, 181, 231, 246, 341, 634, 765).

Finally, repetition of electrical stimulation gradually during resection allowed the existence of reorganization phenomena of the functional cortical maps to be documented over the short and long term, making it possible to consider a second surgical intervention with the addition of resecting lesions located in the eloquent zones that could not be removed during the first intervention (158, 159, 160, 161, 165, 169, 177, 371). Indeed, the mechanisms of such a plasticity induced by surgical resection within eloquent areas were studied, by performing postoperative neuroimaging once the patient has recovered his preoperative functional status (371). In particular, several patients were examined following the resection of gliomas involving the supplementary motor area (SMA), which has elicited a transient postsurgical SMA syndrome (see below). Functional MRI showed in these cases, in comparison to the preoperative imaging, the occurrence of activations of the SMA and premotor cortex contralateral to the lesion: the contrahemispheric homologuous then likely participated to the post-surgical functional compensation and recovery (371). Integrating this plastic potential into the interventional strategy has thus opened the door to surgery for removing lesions traditionally considered to be "unresectable", in particular within the primary motor areas, primary somatosensorial areas, the Broca's area, the dominant insula, the striatum or the corpus callosum (for a review, see 159).

In summary, the integration of a systematic functional mapping, of the on-line study of the effective connectivity and of the individual plastic potential during each surgical procedure has enabled (1) to extend the indications of the surgery for LGG within the so-called eloquent areas, (2) to maximize the quality of the resection and (3) to minimize the risk to induce postoperative permanent neurological sequelae – i.e. to optimize the benefit to ratio risk of the surgery.

Radiotherapy

In practice, the current attitude, although still controversial, is rather to withhold radiotherapy, at any stage after eventual surgery, for a documented clinical progression and/or "significative" radiological progression.

An ongoing tendancy is rather to use, before radiotherapy, chemotherapy, eventhough the question of the role/efficacy of the latter treatment option remains open as witnessed by the soon to be opened EORTC phase III trial aiming to compare, in a randomised way, radiotherapy versus chemotherapy at time of progression, with a stratification on the 1p status (708).

Target volume remains the hypersignal T2 or flair more or less increased by a safety margin of 2 cms. Fractionation remains at the moment classical (<=2 Gy by session, 5 sessions per week). Finally a dose between 45 and 50 Gy must be discussed.

Open Questions

A lot of questions persist concerning radiotherapy.

What could be the criteria of beginning such a treatment : age, epilepsy, general status, neurological status, specific neurocognitive status, tumor volume, curve of growth, new functionnal imaging data, histologic or biologic data ?

When a treatment other than surgery is indicated, must radiotherapy be systematically moved in second line after chemotherapy ?

When the treatment is ended, what could be the criteria of response: clinical criteria, radiological criteria such as volume or impact on the growth curve? Which is the optimal moment to estimate the response ?

In case of response, would be it possible to reconsider an initial contraindication of surgery ?

With new focal techniques, what is the risk to expose a patient to delayed toxicities ?

What about radiosurgery for small postoperative residual tumors ?

What about new fractionation modalities ?

What about radiotherapy and brain plasticity ?

Chemotherapy

Modalities

The place of chemotherapy has yet to be defined.

Many theoretical arguments must be considered against its potential efficiency like subnormal blood-brain or blood-tumor barrier or low proliferation indices.

On the contrary, it is classic to consider chemotherapy as generally more effective when delivered before radiotherapy. In this situation, it could allow, if effective, to delay radiotherapy and its potential side effects (necrosis, cognitive decline). It could also, in case of an objective radiological response, to reduce the fields of radiotherapy.

Finally we know, eventhough it is possible to obtain radiological responses, that the quantification of the latter seems particularly difficult and that the classical Mac Donald criteria used for malignant gliomas are not applicable.

The first and only randomised phase III trial concerning chemotherapy for low-grade gliomas was conducted by the Southwestern Oncology Group. Were compared radiotherapy alone versus radiotherapy plus lomustine chemotherapy after subtotal/partial surgery or biopsy. No benefit was showed and the trial was prematurely terminated (184, 749).

Macdonald has, the first, evoked the possibility of an objective response in low-grade tumors within a serie of aggressive oligodendrogliomas (431). Six years later, Mason was able to note 9/9 responders (8 patients at presentation and 1 patient for a recurrence after radiotherapy) under Procarbazine + CCNU + Vincristine (PCV) (444) while Soffiety (638) reported 13/13 patients stabilised or responders, also under PCV.

More recently, Buckner reported a series of 29 patients treated by PCV and noted 28 % of objective response (73), but in this series chemotherapy was followed immediately by radiotherapy.

Brada treated 10 patients with temozolomide for newly diagnosed oligodendrogliomas and observed 2 partial responses and 3 minor responses (62).

The multicentric serie reported by Quinn based on temozolomide chemotherapy comprised 46 patients with tumoral progression, with a majority of astrocytomas (14 radiotherapy and chemotherapy pretreated patients). 61 % of objective responses were noted. The PFS for the all group was 22 months. 76 % were in PFS at 12 months from the beginning of treatment (530).

Hoang-Xuan and al reported their experience concerning the treatment of 60 patients by conventional temozolomide schedule (200 mg/m^2/day for 5 days every 28 days). The median number of chemotherapy cycles delivered was 11. More than half of the patients were improved clinically. A radiological objective response was noted in 1/3 of the cases. Only 8 % of the patients were considered in progression during the treatment period. The only factor correlated with the response was the loss of the chromosome 1p (268).

Finally, Stege et al reported their experience with PCV chemotherapy for low grade gliomas. They treated 16 newly diagnosed patients and 5 patients at recurrence, and observed respectively 13 and 3 responses with a median time to disease progression up to 24 months. The 1p19q status did not predict, in this small series, the response (645).

Optimal Timing

Nevertheless, since the princeps publications (431, 444), the interest carried in such a treatment is increasing (88).

The majority of teams suggest to propose chemotherapy as first and early treatment (62, 73), or at the time of progression (after surgery and before radiotherapy) eventhough the clinical or radiological criteria of progression remain to be defined with more precision than at present (268, 500, 530, 645).

Short, Middle and Long Term Effects of Chemotherapy

We know that "historic" association of Procarbazine + CCNU + Vincristine (PCV) or more recent monotherapy with temozolomide can allow clear symptomatic improvements concerning epilepsy or pre-existent neurological deficits or headache in more than 50 % of patients. In a general way, chemotherapy seems to bring an improvement of the quality of life in spite of insufficient studies concerning this subject (62, 73, 268, 400, 645). These treatments, contrary to radiotherapy, do not possess informed cognitive toxicity.

Nevertheless, the tolerance is not perfect. The "PCV" association possesses a cumulative hematologic toxicity rendering difficult the administration of more than 4 or 6 courses without serious adverse events. Not to be neglected are the peripheral neurological risk of the vincristine or the risk of lung fibrosis with CCNU. The patients complain frequently of an intense asthenia and/or a loss of weight. Gonadic toxicity seems also frequent.

The prescription of temozolomide would eventually be more adapted to this type of tumor with an absence of cumulative hematologic toxicity in spite of very prolonged treatments. It will be necessary to consider the risk of lymphocytopeny especially with continuous treatment plans and to consider a preventive treatment of opportunistic infections and notably pneumocystosis (212). The risk of cutaneous eruption and even of liver toxicity is not to be underscored, and no data is available concerning potential gonadic toxicity. The future EORTC trial will help answering these questions. Moreover, various modalities of prescription could be discussed (66).

In Practice

In practice, the tendancy is, at present, to favor this type of treatment first line for non operable tumors, in case of actual clinical and/or radiological evolution, all the more if there is a 1p deletion, since then expecting a clinical and an even radiological efficiency, while delaying radiotherapy because of its potential neuro-cognitive side effects.

It is nevertheless imperative to confirm these hypotheses, to set up clinical trials and to associate to it number of ancillary works connected to biologic, pathologic, radiological, functional and neurocognitives and also economic questions.

Open Questions

Finally, like for radiotherapy, numerous and essential questions surround the problem of chemotherapy.

Must the treatment be proposed very prematurely ?

Otherwise, what can be objective criteria of beginning such a therapy : age, epilepsy, general condition status (WHO Performance Status or Karnofsky scale), neurological status, specific neurocognitif status, tumor volume, curve of growth, functionnal imaging data, histologic or biologic data ?

When the treatment is begun, what can be the criteria of response: clinical criteria (efficacy and tolerance), radiological criteria such as volume or impact on the growth curve, functionnal imaging criteria ?

What is the optimal duration of chemotherapy before this evaluation ?

In case of clinical and radiological stabilization or response, how long must the treatment be pursued ?

Would be it possible in this case to reconsider an initial contraindication of surgery ?

In case of response to chemotherapy, is it licit to propose systematically a radiotherapy at the end of the chemotherapy or is it preferable to postpone until a new progression ? What would be the criteria to take that kind of decision ?

If one decides to treat "for a long time", what is the risk to expose the patient to delayed onco-hematologic or gonadic toxicities ?

Can this treatment have an impact on survival by modifying radically the natural history of these tumors ? Will the results be the same as radiotherapy with an impact on the progression free survival without modification of the overall survival ?

What about chemotherapy and plasticity ?

2. Sequential Combined Strategies: Adapted to the Natural History of the Tumor and the Brain Reaction

What Do We Know and What Do We Want to Achieve ?

Since the last two decades we are collectively learning to apprehend better the natural history of WHO grade 2 gliomas, which, since it is a continuously evolving tumor interacting with the brain, an adaptative organ but to a certain extent only to its environment, leads to a initially overt (epilepsy) or insidious (functional impairment) deterioration of the quality of life. We know that, inexorably, a grade 2 glioma will, covertly during a long period, acquire genotypic alterations that will ultimately transform its phenotype into that of an overt high-grade glioma, for which we have still no effective enough treatment. In the same way, we are refining our knowledge of the limits and advantages of each of the three treatment modalities available, and are learning how to evaluate them in terms of quality, and duration of, life, more than simply in terms of, for example, a radiological response judged according to habits developped for higher grade tumors. We are learning how to dismember this rather chaotic and biologically diverse group of lesions, and envision that we should soon be able, on clinico-radiological and/or biological grounds, to define homogeneous and finite risk-groups. From then on only will we be able to really appreciate an (almost) individual spontaneous prognosis a priori at the clinical onset or discovery of a lesion compatible with a grade 2 glioma. And tailor according to cumulated data during a short period of observation, a therapeutic strategy aiming, with a minimized risk, to significantly prolong at least (if not definitely cure) a (young) patient's life span; while preserving or even ameliorating his quality of life, and interfering as little as possible with his productive socio-professional as well as personal life.

Significant progress has yet to be made, which demands to pool data because of the relative rarity of the disease and its long duration of evolution, and because of its biological variety, expressed from the clinical to the genomic or proteomic levels. When prognostic factors will be reliable at (almost) the individual level and our methods of evaluation of efficacy adequate, prospective studies and trials will allow to test the efficacy of elementary treatments as well as different therapeutic strategies.

What do we know we can achieve, by what means ?

At the moment, the medical community can probably agree on several facts. That a WHO grade 2 glioma is definitely not a benign tumor, since it interferes with a young subject's quality of life from the start (of its clinical overt phase), and will be responsible of a fatal outcome in gene"ral in the 5 to 15 years after its discovery. That, if administered, radiotherapy should be done with the best technique available (conformal, fractions of no more than 2 Gy, total dose of no more than 45 to 50 Gy) to avoid significant, (essentially) cognitive risks, and that its timing does not significantly alter its overall influence on outcome. That resective surgery could probably effect the functional and probably vital outcome of a patient under certain conditions; it should also be performed with the best anatomo-functional techniques available, allowing the preservation, and even often the amelioration of, function, and aiming to leave only a small, or no residual signal abnormality on the systematic post-operative control MRI (at two-three months in particular). Last, that chemotherapy seems to represent a valuable tool, already occupying a previous therapeutic «no-man's land» between eventual surgery and radiotherapy, when the latter was withheld until «clearly indicated».

But since all these facts need to be further explored, ascertained and/or refined, we need to collaborate for additional and rapid progress. World-wide collaboration underscores that we talk the same language (or that everyone is understandable, readable, «translatable» by everybody else) when reporting on a patient's clinical condition, on the (radiological) behavior of his tumor, on the monitoring of his evolution, in the pre- as well as post-treatment periods. With that level of comparability, we can exchange, oppose different attitudes, and lessen the need for formal trials, as long as the prognostic (stratification) criteria are reproducible/exportable from one series to another, giving an actual value to smaller coherent cohorts. At the end, we will be thru only when the timing and various combinations of treatments will be explored.

What Can We Propose to a Patient Harbouring a WHO Grade 2 Glioma ?

A «primum non nocere» attitude is of course laudable and represents one of our main concerns as physicians. Nevertheless, that is not ineluctably synonymous with a «wait and see» attitude, the latter denying any effect to treatment(s).

There are two intermingled levels of medical reflexion in front of a patient, focusing on his functional and life-expectancy status. There again, no inherent contradiction precludes the simultaneous quest of the two goals, since an active as well as an expectative attitude both carry the same kind of risks, albeit dissimilar factually, menacing an individual harbouring a grade 2 glioma.

With what we know nowadays, we can argue in favour of a proactive strategy, since even if some therapeutic measures do not at the end really prolong a patient's life, they can first of all protect, and even improve his functional status, and second prolong his «disease-free» lifetime (recurrence-free period). Meanwhile, we will be able to collect enough homogeneous, convergent data from multiple sources, to prove as we have the intuition, that active strategies also prolong somewhat, if they are still unable to cure, the life expectancy of a patient, significantly shortened at the announcement of this sort of diagnosis.

In the absence of a definitive method to avoid and predict anaplastic transformation, the therapeutic strategy(ies) can only aim to try to «confine the tumor to a grade 2 stage», by limiting the number and/or activity of tumor cells, leading to the progression of the tumor and moreover its progressive (multi-step, clonal ?) acquisition of a malignant geno-phenotype. In this setting, radiotherapy has a definite effect on grade 2 progression (with its functional favorable consequences, and a good ratio benefit/risk with up-to-date irradiation techniques), surgical sub- and total radiological resection has the same efficacy, and probably is also capable of delaying anaplasia; if pushed to its functional limits, that is the wall of the surgical cavity abuting essential (non compensable) eloquent areas and pathways, we know that we create or worsen focal deficits, which will take several days to months, under adapted physiotherapy at best, for the patient to recover. Chemotherapy, for which less is known, could have a similar capacity of delaying progression, of grade 2 as well as anaplasia as it seems, with an «acceptable» level of risk (ie. low toxicity rate, while considering also its side-effects). When combined in a one-stage or multi-stage temporal associative strategy, we have learned from our personal experience that radiotherapy, but not chemotherapy, carries the risk, if done after «maximal surgery», to hamper functional recovery, and even to reduce the chance of complete recovery, giving the impression that it reduces somewhat brain plasticity capacity. This has not been our experience with chemotherapy, at least with a single regimen. Chemotherapy (and probably soon other treatment modalities –immunologic, genetic..-) can be delivered locally during surgery, with the aim of a higher local (concentration, distribution, therefore) efficacy while diminishing or avoiding the risk of somatic deleterious effects. Last, radio- and chemotherapy can, as is done with high-grade gliomas, be delivered simultaneously, in an attempt to obtain synergestic, potentialisating or facilitatory effects.

Then, When Should We Propose What to Which Patient ?

The discussion with a patient presupposes that we have exposed what we know or envision of his common history with his tumor, and foreseen the different offerable possibilities, with their pros and cons, and the risks attached to the instauration as well as the withholding of a treatment.

For our part, the first step is to be as sure as possible, with the greatest inocuity but also reliability, that we are dealing with a grade 2 glioma, and to evaluate its evolutive stage (in the continuum from a slow, indolent tumor, to its malignant counterpart). At the moment, before genotypic or proteomic reliable data, the close MRI follow-up of the lesion during three months or more if necessary, allows to improve the diagnostic accuracy by eliminating the probability of other possible diagnoses, and to appreciate the individual tumoral growth rate. Imminent or already anaplastic lesions mimicking a low-grade glioma can thereby, with very few exceptions, be ruled out, that mandate aggressive, multimodality treatment from the beginning. In the meantime, a thorough anatomo-functional evaluation can be performed (neuropsychological/language examinations, fMRI, perfusion MR, spectroscopic-MR/PET scan, DWI, DTI, MEG).

A second step to be discussed early, because the ratio surgical usefulness/statistical unsignificance is tenuous considering even the slow growth/extension of the vast majority of these tumors, is to evaluate the possibilities of surgical resection, by cumulating a priori static anatomo-functional and dynamic data, combined to a patient's background, and his opinion. If a (sub)total resection seems feasible, we would propose it as first choice treatment. If not, but if the a priori impossibility lies only in an extension «slightly to far» in eloquent areas (confer to the probability map), we might propose a neoadjuvant chemotherapy that could, in case of even a small centripetal effectiveness in the reduction of the FLAIR area, render an extensive resection possible.

If a initially surgical strategy seems impossible, there is in general no urgency in initiating other types of treatment, namely radio- or chemotherapy, unless the glioma is discovered at a late satge, either clinically or radiologically (refractory epilepsy, cognitive or focal neurological deficit, large volume, mass effect, bilateral extension). One can usually take some time more to refine the dynamic (with time) estimation of the result of the everchanging tumor/host interaction before decision making. Grossly, since radiotherapy can be delivered only once, and since it works so well on the grade 2 progression that the recurrence is immediately or very quickly of the anaplastic type, allowing most of the time no intervening treatment before this event, we prefer to delay it as much as possible. Then chemotherapy would be the prefered «second choice», whatever the genetic status with our current knowledge since LOH 1p seems only indicative of a greater chance of efficacy and does not indicate a tautologic mode of sensitivity, and since the role of MGMT and other drug resistance factors status has not been clarified in low-grade gliomas. In all cases, a close clinico-radiologic monitoring of the effective efficacy of a chemotherapy regimen is mandatory, in order to switch treatment modality early (other chemotherapy protocol or other therapeutic modality), but taking into account the generally slow efficiency in this context, and in order to decide the duration of chemotherapy according to the apparent chemosensitivity of the tumor.

In our opinion, an important aspect of the treatment of grade 2 gliomas is the notion of repetitive treatments, in a rather «preventive» manner albeit without precipitation, ie. not waiting for the presence of neurologic impairment, in order to try to delay the evolutive stage of the tumor that generates significant brain function alterations, which usually puts it closer to malignant transformation. The same order by which the various treatment modalities were initially discussed is applied to progression, namely considering surgery, then chemotherapy or radiotherapy. Even more than at first treatment, the results of anatomopathological and (molecular) biological thorough examination of an eventual tumoral specimen, crossed with the clinico-radiological tumor kinetics and tolerance of the patient, are the main ingredients of decision making. At progression more than initially given the amount of our ignorance at the moment, could be discussed simultaneous treatment associations, like for example the focalised irradiation of a small post-operative tumoral residue (in particular by radiosurgery, brachytherapy), or the local delivery of a chemotherapeutic (carmustine implant, other by convection…) or radiosensitizing drug (or in the near future an immuno- or genotherapeutic agent).

All along follow-up, functional and quality of life monitoring is mandatory as well as the collection of «classical» clinical and radiological parameters. It allows to refine the evaluation leading to decision making, to explore brain plasticity as a resultant of tumoral growth and treatment imputation(s), and ultimately judge the appropriateness of the therapeutic strategy applied.

Last but not least, as much as possible the treatment should be tailored to the individual at risk, or even more to the couple host/tumor and its state at a given time (but considered in perspective, ie. with the past evolution and what can be foreseen). But in parallel every effort should be made to pool data, and include the patients taken in charge into homogenous cohorts or eventual ongoing trials.

REFERENCES

[1] Abdulrauf, S.I., et al., Vascular endothelial growth factor expression and vascular density as prognostic markers of survival in patients with low-grade astrocytoma. *J Neurosurg*, 1998. 88(3): p. 513-20.

[2] Aboody, K.S., et al., Neural stem cells display extensive tropism for pathology in adult brain: evidence from intracranial gliomas. *Proc Natl Acad Sci U S A*, 2000. 97(23): p. 12846-51.

[3] Abrahams, N.A. and R.A. Prayson, The role of histopathologic examination of intracranial blood clots removed for hemorrhage of unknown etiology: a clinical pathologic analysis of 31 cases. *Ann Diagn Pathol*, 2000. 4(6): p. 361-6.

[4] Afra, D. and E. Osztie, Histologically confirmed changes on CT of reoperated low-grade astrocytomas. *Neuroradiology*, 1997. 39(11): p. 804-10.

[5] Afra, D., et al., Preoperative history and postoperative survival of supratentorial low-grade astrocytomas. *Neuroradiology*, 1999. 13(3): p. 299-305.

[6] Alavi, J.B., et al., Positron emission tomography in patients with glioma. A predictor of prognosis. *Cancer*, 1988. 62(6): p. 1074-8.

[7] Alvord, E.C., Jr., Why do gliomas not metastasize. *Arch Neurol*, 1976. 33(2): p. 73-5.

[8] Alvord, E.C., Jr., Simple model of recurrent gliomas. *J Neurosurg*, 1991. 75(2): p. 337-8.

[9] Alvord, E.C., Jr., Patterns of growth of gliomas. *AJNR Am J Neuroradiol*, 1995. 16(5): p. 1013-7.

[10] Andrewes, D.G., et al., Emotional and social dysfunction in patients following surgical treatment for brain tumor. *J Clin Neurosci*, 2003. 10: p. 428-33.

[11] Andrewes, D.G., et al., The ESDQ: a new method of assessing emotional and social dysfunction in patients following brain surgery. *J Clin Exp Neuropsychol*, 2003. 25: p. 173-89.

[12] Araujo, R.P. and D.L. McElwain, New insights into vascular collapse and growth dynamics in solid tumors. *J Theor Biol*, 2004. 228(3): p. 335-46.

[13] Armstrong, C.L., et al., The predictive value of longitudinal neuropsychologic assessment in the early detection of brain tumor recurrence. *Cancer*, 2003. 97(3): p. 649-56.

[14] Armstrong, C.L., et al., Late cognitive and radiographic changes related to radiotherapy: initial prospective findings. *Neurology*, 2002. 59: p. 40-8.

[15] Ashby, L.S. and W.R. Shapiro, Low-grade glioma: supratentorial astrocytoma, oligodendroglioma, and oligoastrocytoma in adults. *Curr Neurol Neurosci Rep*, 2004. 4(3): p. 211-7.

[16] Athale, C., Y. Mansury, and T.S. Deisboeck, Simulating the impact of a molecular 'decision-process' on cellular phenotype and multicellular patterns in brain tumors. *J Theor Biol*, 2005. 233(4): p. 469-81.

[17] Atlas, S.W., et al., Functional magnetic resonance imaging of regional brain activity in patients with intracerebral gliomas: findings and implications for clinical management. *Neurosurgery*, 1996. 38(2): p. 329-38.

[18] Auer, D.P., et al., Improved analysis of 1H-MR spectra in the presence of mobile lipids. *Magn Reson Med*, 2001. 46(3): p. 615-8.

[19] Bachoo, R.M., et al., Epidermal growth factor receptor and Ink4a/Arf: convergent mechanisms governing terminal differentiation and transformation along the neural stem cell to astrocyte axis. *Cancer Cell*, 2002. 1(3): p. 269-77.

[20] Baciu, M., et al., Presurgical fMRI evaluation of cerebral reorganization and motor deficit in patients with tumors and vascular malformations. *Eur J Radiol*, 2003. 46(2): p. 139-46.

[21] Bacolod, M.D., et al., Mechanisms of resistance to 1, 3-bis(2-chloroethyl)-1-nitrosourea in human medulloblastoma and rhabdomyosarcoma. *Mol Cancer Ther*, 2002. 1(9): p. 727-36.

[22] Baharith, L.A., A. Al-Khouli, and G.M. Raab, Cytotoxic assays for screening anticancer agents. *Stat Med*, 2005.

[23] Bahary, J.P., et al., Low-grade pure and mixed cerebral astrocytomas treated in the CT scan era. *J Neurooncol*, 1996. 27(2): p. 173-7.

[24] Bajzer, Z., Gompertzian growth as a self-similar and allometric process. *Growth Dev Aging*, 1999. 63(1-2): p. 3-11.

[25] Bampoe, J. and M. Bernstein, The role of surgery in low grade gliomas. *J Neurooncol*, 1999. 42(3): p. 259-69.

[26] Barker, F.G.2nd, et al., Age and the risk of anaplasia in magnetic resonance-non enhancing supratentorial cerebral tumors. *Cancer*, 1997. 80(5): p. 936-41.

[27] Bartolomei, J.C., et al., Low-grade gliomas of chronic epilepsy: a distinct clinical and pathological entity. *J Neurooncol*, 1997. 34(1): p. 79-84

[28] Bauman, G., et al., Pretreatment factors predict overall survival for patients with low-grade glioma: a recursive partitioning analysis. *Int J Radiat Oncol Biol Phys*, 1999. 45(4): p. 923-9.

[29] Bauman, G., et al., Low grade glioma: a measuring radiographic response to radiotherapy. *Can J Neurol Sci*, 1999. 26(1): p. 18-22.

[30] Bauman, G.S., et al., Allelic loss of chromosome 1p and radiotherapy plus chemotherapy in patients with oligodendrogliomas. *Int J Radiat Oncol Biol Phys*, 2000. 48(3): p. 825-30.

[31] Bavelier, D. and H.J. Neville, Cross-modal plasticity: where and how? *Nat Rev Neurosci*, 2002. 3(6): p. 443-52.

[32] Beauchesne, P., et al., 99mTc-sestamibi brain SPECT after chemoradiotherapy is prognostic of survival in patients with high-grade glioma. *J Nucl Med*, 2004. 45(3): p. 409-13.

[33] Beaumont, A. and I.R. Whittle, The pathogenesis of tumour associated epilepsy. *Acta Neurochir (Wien)*, 2000. 142(1): p. 1-15.

[34] Begemann, M., G.N. Fuller, and E.C. Holland, Genetic modeling of glioma formation in mice. *Brain Pathol*, 2002. 12(1): p. 117-32.

[35] Bellail, A.C., et al., Microregional extracellular matrix heterogeneity in brain modulates glioma cell invasion. *Int J Biochem Cell Biol*, 2004. 36(6): p. 1046-69.

[36] Bello, L., et al., Angiogenesis and invasion in gliomas. *Cancer Treat Res*, 2004. 117: p. 263-84.

[37] Bello, M.J., et al., Allelic loss at 1p and 19q frequently occurs in association and may represent early oncogenic events in oligodendroglial tumors. *Int J Cancer*, 1995. 64(3): p. 207-10.

[38] Benard, F., J. Romsa, and R. Hustinx, Imaging gliomas with positron emission tomography and single-photon emission computed tomography. *Semin Nucl Med*, 2003. 33(2): p. 148-62.

[39] Berens, M.E. and A. Giese. "those left behind." Biology and oncology of invasive glioma cells. *Neoplasia*, 1999. 1(3): p. 208-19.

[40] Berg, G., E. Blomquist, and E. Cavallin-Stahl, A systematic overview of radiation therapy effects in brain tumours. *Acta Oncol*, 2003. 42(5-6): p. 582-8.

[41] Berger, M.S., Lesions in functional ("eloquent") cortex and subcortical white matter. *Clin Neurosurg*, 1994. 41: p. 444-63.

[42] Berger, M.S., Functional mapping-guided resection of low-grade gliomas. *Clin Neurosurg*, 1995. 42: p. 437-52.

[43] Berger, M.S., et al., The effect of extent of resection on recurrence in patients with low grade cerebral hemisphere gliomas. *Cancer*, 1994. 74(6): p. 1784-91.

[44] Berger, M.S., G.A. Ojemann, and E. Lettich, Neurophysiological monitoring during astrocytoma surgery. *Neurosurg Clin N Am*, 1990. 1(1): p. 65-80.

[45] Berger, M.S. and R.C. Rostomily, Low grade gliomas: functional mapping resection strategies, extent of resection, and outcome. *J Neurooncol*, 1997. 34(1): p. 85-101.

[46] Besson, A. and V.W. Yong, Mitogenic signaling and the relationship to cell cycle regulation in astrocytomas. *J Neurooncol*, 2001. 51(3): p. 245-64.

[47] Biernat, W., et al., Identical mutations of the p53 tumor suppressor gene in the gliomatous and the sarcomatous components of gliosarcomas suggest a common origin from glial cells. *J Neuropathol Exp Neurol*, 1995. 54(5): p. 651-6.

[48] Bigner, S.H., et al., Gene amplification in malignant human gliomas: clinical and histopathologic aspects. *J Neuropathol Exp Neurol*, 1988. 47(3): p. 191-205.

[49] Bigner, S.H., et al., Specific chromosomal abnormalities in malignant human gliomas. *Cancer Res*, 1988. 48(2): p. 405-11.

[50] Bigner, S.H., et al., Molecular genetic aspects of oligodendrogliomas including analysis by comparative genomic hybridization. *Am J Pathol*, 1999. 155(2): p. 375-86.

[51] Bigner, S.H., et al., Chromosomal characteristics of childhood brain tumors. *Cancer Genet Cytogenet*, 1997. 97(2): p. 125-34.

[52] Bigner, S.H. and B. Vogelstein, Cytogenetics and molecular genetics of malignant gliomas and medulloblastoma. *Brain Pathol*, 1990. 1(1): p. 12-8.

[53] Binder, D.K. and M.S. Berger, Proteases and the biology of glioma invasion. *J Neurooncol*, 2002. 56(2): p. 149-58.

[54] Bishop, M. and S.M. de la Monte, Dual lineage of astrocytomas. *Am J Pathol*, 1989. 135(3): p. 517-27.

[55] Bitoh, S., et al., Cerebral neoplasms initially presenting with massive intracerebral hemorrhage. *Surg Neurol*, 1984. 22(1): p. 57-62.

[56] Black, P.M. and S.F. Ronner, Cortical mapping for defining the limits of tumor resection. *Neurosurgery*, 1987. 20(6): p. 914-9.

[57] Blankenberg, F.G., et al., The influence of volumetric tumor doubling time, DNA ploidy, and histologic grade on the survival of patients with intracranial astrocytomas. *AJNR Am J Neuroradiol*, 1995. 16(5): p. 1001-12.

[58] Blasberg, R.G., et al., Imaging brain tumor proliferative activity with [124I]iododeoxyuridine. *Cancer Res*, 2000. 60(3): p. 624-35.

[59] Blood, C.H. and B.R. Zetter, Tumor interactions with the vasculature: angiogenesis and tumor metastasis. *Biochim Biophys Acta*, 1990. 1032(1): p. 89-118.

[60] Bobola, M.S., et al., O6-methylguanine-DNA methyltransferase, O6-benzylguanine, and resistance to clinical alkylators in pediatric primary brain tumor cell lines. *Clin Cancer Res*, 2005. 11(7): p. 2747-55.

[61] Boudreau, N. and M.J. Bissell, Extracellular matrix signaling: integration of form and function in normal and malignant cells. *Curr Opin Cell Biol*, 1998. 10(5): p. 640-6.

[62] Brada, M., et al., Phase II study of primary temozolomide chemotherapy in patients with WHO grade II gliomas. *Ann Oncol*, 2003. 14(12): p. 1715-21.

[63] Brandes, A.A., F. Vastola, and U. Basso, Controversies in the therapy of low-grade glioma: when and how to treat. *Expert Rev Anticancer Ther*, 2002. 2(5): p. 529-36.

[64] Brat, D.J., et al., Genetic and biologic progression in astrocytomas and their relation to angiogenic dysregulation. *Adv Anat Pathol*, 2002. 9(1): p. 24-36.

[65] Brem, S., The role of vascular proliferation in the growth of brain tumors. *Clin Neurosurg*, 1976. 23: p. 440-53.

[66] Brock, C.S., et al., Phase I trial of temozolomide using an extended continuous oral schedule. *Cancer Res*, 1998. 58(19): p. 4363-7.

[67] Brock, C.S., et al., Early evaluation of tumour metabolic response using [18F]fluorodeoxyglucose and positron emission tomography: a pilot study following the phase II chemotherapy schedule for temozolomide in recurrent high-grade gliomas. *Br J Cancer*, 2000. 82(3): p. 608-15.

[68] Brown, P.D., et al., The neurocognitive effects of radiation in adult low-grade glioma patients. *Neuro-oncol*, 2003. 5(3): p. 161-7. [68b] Brown, P.D., et al., Importance of baseline mini-mental state examination as a prognostic factor for patients with low-grade glioma. *Int J Radiat Oncol Biol Phys*, 2004. 59: p. 117-25. [68c] Brown, P.D., et al., Effects of radiotherapy on cognitive function in patients with low-grade glioma measured by the Folstein Mini-Mental State Examination. *J Clin Oncol*, 2003. 21: p. 2519-24.

[69] Bru, A., et al., The universal dynamics of tumor growth. *Biophys J*, 2003. 85(5): p. 2948-61.

[70] Bruehlmeier, M., et al., Effect of radiotherapy on brain glucose metabolism in patients operated on for low grade astrocytoma. *J Neurol Neurosurg Psychiatry*, 1999. 66(5): p. 648-53.

[71] Buatti, J.M., et al., Low-grade gliomas: answering one question in a myriad of new questions. *J Clin Oncol*, 2002. 20(9): p. 2223-4.

[72] Buchpiguel, C.A., et al., PET versus SPECT in distinguishing radiation necrosis from tumor recurrence in the brain. *J Nucl Med*, 1995. 36(1): p. 159-64.

[73] Buckner, J.C., et al., Phase II trial of procarbazine, lomustine, and vincristine as initial therapy for patients with low-grade oligodendroglioma or oligoastrocytoma: efficacy and associations with chromosomal abnormalities. *J Clin Oncol*, 2003. 21(2): p. 251-5.

[74] Burger, P.C., et al., Losses of chromosomal arms 1p and 19q in the diagnosis of oligodendroglioma. A study of paraffin-embedded sections. *Mod Pathol*, 2001. 14(9): p. 842-53.

[75] Burger, P.C., et al., Glioblastoma multiforme and anaplastic astrocytoma. Pathologic criteria and prognostic implications. *Cancer*, 1985. 56(5): p. 1106-11.

[76] Burger, P.C. and R.T. Vollmer, Histologic factors of prognostic significance in the glioblastoma multiforme. *Cancer*, 1980. 46(5): p. 1179-86.

[77] Butler, A.R., et al., Computed tomography in astrocytomas. A statistical analysis of the parameters of malignancy and the positive contrast-enhanced CT scan. *Radiology*, 1978. 129(2): p. 433-9.

[78] Bynevelt, M., et al., FLAIR imaging in the follow-up of low-grade gliomas: time to dispense with the dual-echo? *Neuroradiology*, 2001. 43(2): p. 129-33.

[79] Byrne, J.H., Synapses. Plastic plasticity. *Nature*, 1997. 389(6653): p. 791-2.

[80] Cairncross, J.G., Understanding low-grade glioma: a decade of progress. Neurology, 2000. 54(7): p. 1402-3. 80b. Cairncross, J.G., Low-grade glioma: the case for delayed surgery. *Clin Neurosurg*, 1995. 42: p. 391-8

[81] Cairncross, J.G. and N.J. Laperriere, Low-grade glioma. To treat or not to treat? *Arch Neurol*, 1989. 46(11): p. 1238-9.

[82] Cairncross, J.G., et al., Specific genetic predictors of chemotherapeutic response and survival in patients with anaplastic oligodendrogliomas. *J Natl Cancer Inst*, 1998. 90(19): p. 1473-9.

[83] Calatozzolo, C., et al., Expression of drug resistance proteins Pgp, MRP1, MRP3, MRP5 and GST-pi in human glioma. *J Neurooncol*, 2005. 74(2): p. 113-21.

[84] Cameron, R.S. and P. Rakic, Glial cell lineage in the cerebral cortex: a review and synthesis. *Glia*, 1991. 4(2): p. 124-37.

[85] Caramia, M.D., et al., Ipsilateral motor activation in patients with cerebral gliomas. *Neurology*, 1998. 51(1): p. 196-202.

[86] Caroli, E., et al., Familial gliomas. Analysis of six families with cerebral gliomas and without other inheritable syndromes. *Neurosurg Rev*, 2003. 26(4): p. 280-2.

[87] Carpentier, A.C., et al., Patterns of functional magnetic resonance imaging activation in association with structural lesions in the rolandic region: a classification system. *J Neurosurg*, 2001. 94(6): p. 946-54.

[88] Carpentier, A.F., *Neuro-oncology: the growing role of chemotherapy in glioma. Lancet Neurol*, 2005. 4(1): p. 4-5.

[89] Carroll, R.S., et al., KDR activation in astrocytic neoplasms. *Cancer*, 1999. 86(7): p. 1335-41.

[90] Carroll, R.S., et al., Apoptosis in astrocytic neoplasms. *Acta Neurochir (Wien)*, 1997. 139(9): p. 845-50.

[91]   Castillo, M., J.K. Smith, and L. Kwock, Correlation of myo-inositol levels and grading of cerebral astrocytomas. *AJNR Am J Neuroradiol*, 2000. 21(9): p. 1645-9.

[92]   Cavalla, P. and D. Schiffer, Cell cycle and proliferation markers in neuroepithelial tumors. *AntiCancer Res*, 1997. 17(6B): p. 4135-43.

[93]   Celli, P., et al., Cerebral oligodendroglioma: prognostic factors and life history. *Neurosurgery*, 1994. 35(6): p. 1018-34; discussion 1034-5.

[94]   Chakravarti, A., et al., Prognostic and pathologic significance of quantitative protein expression profiling in human gliomas. *Clin Cancer Res*, 2001. 7(8): p. 2387-95.

[95]   Challa, V.R., H.O. Goodman, and C.H. Davis, Jr., Familial brain tumors: studies of two families and review of recent literature. *Neurosurgery*, 1983. 12(1): p. 18-23.

[96]   Chamberlain, M.C., J.A. Murovic, and V.A. Levin, Absence of contrast enhancement on CT brain scans of patients with supratentorial malignant gliomas. *Neurology*, 1988. 38(9): p. 1371-4.

[97]   Chaplain, M. and A. Anderson, Mathematical modelling of tumour-induced angiogenesis: network growth and structure. *Cancer Treat Res*, 2004. 117: p. 51-75.

[98]   Chaudhry, I.H., et al., Vascular endothelial growth factor expression correlates with tumour grade and vascularity in gliomas. *Histopathology*, 2001. 39(4): p. 409-15.

[99]   Chen, R., L.G. Cohen, and M. Hallett, Nervous system reorganization following injury. *Neuroscience*, 2002. 111(4): p. 761-73.

[100] Cheng, L.L., et al., Correlation of high-resolution magic angle spinning proton magnetic resonance spectroscopy with histopathology of intact human brain tumor specimens. *Cancer Res*, 1998. 58(9): p. 1825-32.

[101] Cheng, Y., et al., Genetic alterations in pediatric high-grade astrocytomas. *Hum Pathol*, 1999. 30(11): p. 1284-90.

[102] Chicoine, M.R., C.L. Madsen, and D.L. Silbergeld, Modification of human glioma locomotion in vitro by cytokines EGF, bFGF, PDGFbb, NGF, and TNF alpha. *Neurosurgery*, 1995. 36(6): p. 1165-70; discussion 1170-1.

[103] Chicoine, M.R. and D.L. Silbergeld, The in vitro motility of human gliomas increases with increasing grade of malignancy. *Cancer*, 1995. 75(12): p. 2904-9.

[104] Chicoine, M.R. and D.L. Silbergeld, Assessment of brain tumor cell motility in vivo and in vitro. *J Neurosurg*, 1995. 82(4): p. 615-22.

[105] Chicoine, M.R. and D.L. Silbergeld, Mitogens as motogens. *J Neurooncol*, 1997. 35(3): p. 249-57.

[106] Chin, H.W., et al., Oligodendrogliomas. I. A clinical study of cerebral oligodendrogliomas. *Cancer*, 1980. 45(6): p. 1458-66.

[107] Chintala, S.K., J.C. Tonn, and J.S. Rao, Matrix metalloproteinases and their biological function in human gliomas. *Int J Dev Neurosci*, 1999. 17(5-6): p. 495-502.

[108] Chung, J.K., et al., Usefulness of 11C-methionine PET in the evaluation of brain lesions that are hypo- or isometabolic on 18F-FDG PET. *Eur J Nucl Med Mol Imaging*, 2002. 29(2): p. 176-82.

[109] Cillekens, J.M., et al., A histopathological contribution to supratentorial glioma grading, definition of mixed gliomas and recognition of low grade glioma with Rosenthal fibers. *J Neurooncol*, 2000. 46(1): p. 23-43.

[110] Ciurea, A.V., et al., Neurosurgical management of cerebral astrocytomas in children. *Ann N Y Acad Sci*, 1997. 824: p. 237-40.

[111] Collins, V.P., Genetic alterations in gliomas. *J Neurooncol*, 1995. 24(1): p. 37-8.

[112] Collins, V.P., R.K. Loeffler, and H. Tivey, Observations on growth rates of human tumors. *Am J Roentgenol Radium Ther Nucl Med*, 1956. 76(5): p. 988-1000.

[113] Connor, S.E., et al., Magnetic resonance image registration and subtraction in the assessment of minor changes in low grade glioma volume. *Eur Radiol*, 2004. 14(11): p. 2061-6.

[114] Coons, S.W., J.R. Davis, and D.L. Way, Correlation of DNA content and histology in prognosis of astrocytomas. *Am J Clin Pathol*, 1988. 90(3): p. 289-93.

[115] Coons, S.W., P.C. Johnson, and D.K. Pearl, Prognostic significance of flow cytometry deoxyribonucleic acid analysis of human astrocytomas. *Neurosurgery*, 1994. 35(1): p. 119-25; discussion 125-6.

[116] Coons, S.W., P.C. Johnson, and D.K. Pearl, The prognostic significance of Ki-67 labeling indices for oligodendrogliomas. *Neurosurgery*, 1997. 41(4): p. 878-84; discussion 884-5.

[117] Coons, S.W., et al., Prognostic significance of flow cytometry deoxyribonucleic acid analysis of human oligodendrogliomas. *Neurosurgery*, 1994. 34(4): p. 680-7; discussion 687.

[118] Coons, S.W., et al., Improving diagnostic accuracy and interobserver concordance in the classification and grading of primary gliomas. *Cancer*, 1997. 79(7): p. 1381-93.

[119] Coons, S.W., P.C. Johnson, and J.R. Shapiro, Cytogenetic and flow cytometry DNA analysis of regional heterogeneity in a low grade human glioma. *Cancer Res*, 1995. 55(7): p. 1569-77.

[120] Creighton, C., et al., Profiling of pathway-specific changes in gene expression following growth of human Cancer Cell lines transplanted into mice. *Genome Biol*, 2003. 4(7): p. R46.

[121] Croteau, D., et al., Correlation between magnetic resonance spectroscopy imaging and image-guided biopsies: semiquantitative and qualitative histopathological analyses of patients with untreated glioma. *Neurosurgery*, 2001. 49(4): p. 823-9.

[122] Cunningham, J.M., et al., Analysis of proliferation markers and p53 expression in gliomas of astrocytic origin: relationships and prognostic value. *J Neurosurg*, 1997. 86(1): p. 121-30.

[123] Curran, W.J., Jr., et al., Does extent of surgery influence outcome for astrocytoma with atypical or anaplastic foci (AAF)? A report from three Radiation Therapy Oncology Group (RTOG) trials. *J Neurooncol*, 1992. 12(3): p. 219-27.

[124] D'Amore, P.A. and R.W. Thompson, Mechanisms of angiogenesis. *Annu Rev Physiol*, 1987. 49: p. 453-64.

[125] Dabholkar, M.D., et al., Malignant and nonmalignant brain tissues differ in their messenger RNA expression patterns for ERCC1 and ERCC2. *Cancer Res*, 1995. 55(6): p. 1261-6.

[126] Dahmane, N., et al., The Sonic Hedgehog-Gli pathway regulates dorsal brain growth and tumorigenesis. *Development*, 2001. 128(24): p. 5201-12.

[127] Dai, C., et al., PDGF autocrine stimulation dedifferentiates cultured astrocytes and induces oligodendrogliomas and oligoastrocytomas from neural progenitors and astrocytes in vivo. *Genes Dev*, 2001. 15(15): p. 1913-25.

[128] Dai, C., et al., The characteristics of astrocytomas and oligodendrogliomas are caused by two distinct and interchangeable signaling formats. *Neoplasia*, 2005. 7(4): p. 397-406.

[129] Dan, S., et al., An integrated database of chemosensitivity to 55 anticancer drugs and gene expression profiles of 39 human cancer cell lines. *Cancer Res*, 2002. 62(4): p. 1139-47.

[130] Daneyemez, M., et al., Multiple oligodendroglioma: case report. *Minim Invasive Neurosurg*, 2000. 43(1): p. 51-2.

[131] Danks, R.A., et al., Craniotomy under local anesthesia and monitored conscious sedation for the resection of tumors involving eloquent cortex. *J Neurooncol*, 2000. 49(2): p. 131-9.

[132] Danks, R.A., et al., Patient tolerance of craniotomy performed with the patient under local anesthesia and monitored conscious sedation. *Neurosurgery*, 1998. 42(1): p. 28-34; discussion 34-6.

[133] Danova, M., et al., Prognostic significance of nuclear DNA content in human neuroepithelial tumors. *Int J Cancer*, 1991. 48(5): p. 663-7.

[134] Daumas-Duport, C., Histoprognosis of gliomas. *Adv Tech Stand Neurosurg*, 1994. 21: p. 43-76.

[135] Daumas-Duport, C., et al., [Gliomas: WHO and Sainte-Anne Hospital classifications]. *Ann Pathol*, 2000. 20(5): p. 413-28.

[136] Daumas-Duport, C., et al., Grading of astrocytomas. A simple and reproducible method. *Cancer*, 1988. 62(10): p. 2152-65.

[137] Daumas-Duport, C., B.W. Scheithauer, and P.J. Kelly, A histologic and cytologic method for the spatial definition of gliomas. *Mayo Clin Proc*, 1987. 62(6): p. 435-49.

[138] Daumas-Duport, C. and G. Szikla, [Definition of limits and 3D configuration of cerebral gliomas. Histological data, therapeutic incidences (author's transl)]. *Neurochirurgie*, 1981. 27(5): p. 273-84.

[139] Daumas-Duport, C., et al., Oligodendrogliomas. Part II: A new grading system based on morphological and imaging criteria. *J Neurooncol*, 1997. 34(1): p. 61-78.

[140] De Edelenyi, F.S., et al., A new approach for analyzing proton magnetic resonance spectroscopic images of brain tumors: nosologic images. *Nat Med*, 2000. 6(11): p. 1287-9.

[141] De Witte, O., et al., Positron emission tomography with injection of methionine as a prognostic factor in glioma. *J Neurosurg*, 2001. 95(5): p. 746-50.

[142] De Witte, O., et al., FDG-PET as a prognostic factor in high-grade astrocytoma. *J Neurooncol*, 2000. 49(2): p. 157-63.

[143] De Witte, O., et al., Prognostic value positron emission tomography with [18F]fluoro-2-deoxy-D-glucose in the low-grade glioma. *Neurosurgery*, 1996. 39(3): p. 470-6; discussion 476-7.

[144] De Witte, O., et al., [Contribution of PET to the management of patients with low-grade glioma]. *Neurochirurgie*, 2004. 50(4): p. 468-73.

[145] DeAngelis, L.M., Brain tumors. *N Engl J Med*, 2001. 344(2): p. 114-23.

[146] Delattre, J.Y., R.W. Walker, and M.K. Rosenblum, Leptomeningeal gliomatosis with spinal cord or cauda equina compression: a complication of supratentorial gliomas in adults. *Acta Neurol Scand*, 1989. 79(2): p. 133-9.

[147] Derlon, J.M., et al., [11C]L-methionine uptake in gliomas. *Neurosurgery*, 1989. 25(5): p. 720-8.

[148] Derlon, J.M., et al., Non-invasive grading of oligodendrogliomas: correlation between in vivo metabolic pattern and histopathology. *Eur J Nucl Med*, 2000. 27(7): p. 778-87.

[149] Derlon, J.M., et al., The in vivo metabolic pattern of low-grade brain gliomas: a positron emission tomographic study using 18F-fluorodeoxyglucose and 11C-L-methylmethionine. *Neurosurgery*, 1997. 40(2): p. 276-87; discussion 287-8.

[150] Devaux, B., et al., Chronic intractable epilepsy associated with a tumor located in the central region: functional mapping data and postoperative outcome. *Stereotact Funct Neurosurg*, 1997. 69(1-4 Pt2): p. 229-38

[151] Dexter, D.L., et al., Chemotherapy of mammary carcinomas arising in ras transgenic mice. *Invest New Drugs*, 1993. 11(2-3): p. 161-8.

[152] Diaz-Flores, L., R. Gutierrez, and H. Varela, Angiogenesis: an update. *Histol Histopathol*, 1994. 9(4): p. 807-43.

[153] Dietrich, P.Y., et al., Immunobiology of gliomas: new perspectives for therapy. *Ann N Y Acad Sci*, 1997. 824: p. 124-40.

[154] Dowling, C., et al., Preoperative proton MR spectroscopic imaging of brain tumors: correlation with histopathologic analysis of resection specimens. *AJNR Am J Neuroradiol*, 2001. 22(4): p. 604-12.

[155] Draganski, B., et al., Neuroplasticity: changes in grey matter induced by training. *Nature*, 2004. 427(6972): p. 311-2.

[156] Dropcho, E.J. and S.J. Soong, The prognostic impact of prior low grade histology in patients with anaplastic gliomas: a case-control study. Neurology, 1996. 47(3): p. 684-90.

[157] Duffau, H., Short-term cortical sensorimotor plasticity in humans: a study using intraoperative electrical stimulation. 2000: Paris.

[158] Duffau, H., Acute functional reorganisation of the human motor cortex during resection of central lesions: a study using intraoperative brain mapping. *J Neurol Neurosurg Psychiatry*, 2001. 70(4): p. 506-13.

[159] Duffau, H., Lessons from brain mapping in surgery for low-grade glioma: insights into associations between tumour and brain plasticity. *Lancet Neurol*, 2005. 4(8): p. 476-86.

[160] Duffau, H., et al., Functional compensation of the left dominant insula for language. *Neuroreport*, 2001. 12(10): p. 2159-63.

[161] Duffau, H. and L. Capelle, [Functional recuperation after resection of gliomas infiltrating primary somatosensory fields. Study of perioperative electric stimulation]. *Neurochirurgie*, 2001. 47(6): p. 534-41.

[162] Duffau, H. and L. Capelle, Preferential brain locations of low-grade gliomas. *Cancer*, 2004. 100(12): p. 2622-6.

[163] Duffau, H. and L. Capelle, Incontinence after brain glioma surgery: new insights into the cortical control of micturition and continence. Case report. *J Neurosurg*, 2005. 102(1): p. 148-51.

[164] Duffau, H., et al., The role of dominant premotor cortex in language: a study using intraoperative functional mapping in awake patients. *Neuroimage*, 2003. 20(4): p. 1903-14. 164b. Duffau, H., et al., The insular lobe: physiopathological and surgical considerations. *Neurosurgery*, 2000. 47: p. 801-10.

[165] Duffau, H., et al., Functional recovery after surgical resection of low grade gliomas in eloquent brain: hypothesis of brain compensation. *J Neurol Neurosurg Psychiatry*, 2003. 74(7): p. 901-7.

[166] Duffau, H., et al., Usefulness of intraoperative electrical subcortical mapping during surgery for low-grade gliomas located within eloquent brain regions: functional results in a consecutive series of 103 patients. *J Neurosurg*, 2003. 98(4): p. 764-78.

[167] Duffau, H., et al., Intra-operative direct electrical stimulations of the central nervous system: the Salpetriere experience with 60 patients. *Acta Neurochir (Wien)*, 1999. 141(11): p. 1157-67.

[168] Duffau, H., et al., Intraoperative mapping of the subcortical language pathways using direct stimulations. An anatomo-functional study. *Brain*, 2002. 125(Pt 1): p. 199-214.

[169] Duffau, H., D. Denvil, and L. Capelle, Long term reshaping of language, sensory, and motor maps after glioma resection: a new parameter to integrate in the surgical strategy. *J Neurol Neurosurg Psychiatry*, 2002. 72(4): p. 511-6.

[170] Duffau, H., et al., Intraoperative mapping of the cortical areas involved in multiplication and subtraction: an electrostimulation study in a patient with a left parietal glioma. *J Neurol Neurosurg Psychiatry*, 2002. 73(6): p. 733-8.

[171] Duffau, H., et al., The articulatory loop: study of the subcortical connectivity by electrostimulation. *Neuroreport*, 2003. 14(15): p. 2005-8.

[172] Duffau, H., et al., New insights into the anatomo-functional connectivity of the semantic system: a study using cortico-subcortical electrostimulations. *Brain*, 2005. 128(Pt 4): p. 797-810.

[173] Duffau, H., et al., Transient Foix-Chavany-Marie syndrome after surgical resection of a right insulo-opercular low-grade glioma: case report. *Neurosurgery*, 2003. 53(2): p. 426-31; discussion 431.

[174] Duffau, H., et al., Surgical removal of corpus callosum infiltrated by low-grade glioma: functional outcome and oncological considerations. *J Neurosurg*, 2004. 100(3): p. 431-7.

[175] Duffau, H., et al., Contribution of intraoperative electrical stimulations in surgery of low grade gliomas: a comparative study between two series without (1985-96) and with (1996-2003) functional mapping in the same institution. *J Neurol Neurosurg Psychiatry*, 2005. 76(6): p. 845-51.

[176] Duffau, H., et al., Delayed onset of the supplementary motor area syndrome after surgical resection of the mesial frontal lobe: a time course study using intraoperative mapping in an awake patient. *Stereotact Funct Neurosurg*, 2001. 76(2): p. 74-82.

[177] Duffau, H., J.P. Sichez, and S. Lehericy, Intraoperative unmasking of brain redundant motor sites during resection of a precentral angioma: evidence using direct cortical stimulation. *Ann Neurol*, 2000. 47(1): p. 132-5.

[178] Duffau, H., et al., Intra-operative mapping of the subcortical visual pathways using direct electrical stimulations. *Acta Neurochir (Wien)*, 2004. 146(3): p. 265-9; discussion 269-70.

[179] Ebel, H., et al., Surgery of intrinsic cerebral neoplasms in eloquent areas under local anesthesia. *Minim Invasive Neurosurg*, 2000. 43(4): p. 192-6.

[180] Ebeling, U., et al., Safe surgery of lesions near the motor cortex using intra-operative mapping techniques: a report on 50 patients. *Acta Neurochir (Wien)*, 1992. 119(1-4): p. 23-8.

[181] Eisner, W., et al., Use of neuronavigation and electrophysiology in surgery of subcortically located lesions in the sensorimotor strip. *J Neurol Neurosurg Psychiatry*, 2002. 72(3): p. 378-81.

[182] el-Azouzi, M., et al., Loss of distinct regions on the short arm of chromosome 17 associated with tumorigenesis of human astrocytomas. *Proc Natl Acad Sci U S A*, 1989. 86(18): p. 7186-90.

[183] Engelhard, H.H., A. Stelea, and E.J. Cochran, Oligodendroglioma: pathology and molecular biology. *Surg Neurol*, 2002. 58(2): p. 111-7; discussion 117.

[184] Eyre, H.J., et al., A randomized trial of radiotherapy versus radiotherapy plus CCNU for incompletely resected low-grade gliomas: a Southwest Oncology Group study. *J Neurosurg*, 1993. 78(6): p. 909-14.

[185] Fallon, K.B., et al., Prognostic value of 1p, 19q, 9p, 10q, and EGFR-FISH analyses in recurrent oligodendrogliomas. *J Neuropathol Exp Neurol*, 2004. 63(4): p. 314-22.

[186] Fan, K.J., J. Kovi, and K.M. Earle, The ethnic distribution of primary central nervous system tumors: AFIP, 1958 to 1970. *J Neuropathol Exp Neurol*, 1977. 36(1): p. 41-9.

[187] Fandino, J., et al., Intraoperative validation of functional magnetic resonance imaging and cortical reorganization patterns in patients with brain tumors involving the primary motor cortex. *J Neurosurg*, 1999. 91(2): p. 238-50.

[188] Fazekas, J.T., Treatment of grades I and II brain astrocytomas. The role of radiotherapy. *Int J Radiat Oncol Biol Phys*, 1977. 2(7-8): p. 661-6.

[189] Felsberg, J., et al., Oligodendroglial tumors: refinement of candidate regions on chromosome arm 1p and correlation of 1p/19q status with survival. *Brain Pathol*, 2004. 14(2): p. 121-30.

[190] Ferreira, S.C., Jr., M.L. Martins, and M.J. Vilela, Reaction-diffusion model for the growth of avascular tumor. *Phys Rev E Stat Nonlin Soft Matter Phys*, 2002. 65(2 Pt 1): p. 021907.

[191] Figarella-Branger, D. and C. Bouvier, [Histological classification of human gliomas: state of art and controversies]. *Bull Cancer*, 2005. 92(4): p. 301-9.

[192] Fillmore, H.L., T.E. VanMeter, and W.C. Broaddus, Membrane-type matrix metalloproteinases (MT-MMPs): expression and function during glioma invasion. *J Neurooncol*, 2001. 53(2): p. 187-202.

[193] Firsching, R., et al., Long-term prognosis of low grade astrocytoma. *Zentralbl Neurochir*, 1994. 55(1): p. 10-5.

[194] Fisher, B.J., et al., Results of a policy of surveillance alone after surgical management of pediatric low grade gliomas. *Int J Radiat Oncol Biol Phys*, 2001. 51(3): p. 704-10.

[195] Fisher, B.J., et al., Ki-67: a prognostic factor for low-grade glioma? *Int J Radiat Oncol Biol Phys*, 2002. 52(4): p. 996-1001.

[196] Fleury, A., et al., Descriptive epidemiology of cerebral gliomas in France. *Cancer*, 1997. 79(6): p. 1195-202.

[197] Folkerth, R.D., Descriptive analysis and quantification of angiogenesis in human brain tumors. *J Neurooncol*, 2000. 50(1-2): p. 165-72.

[198] Folkman, J., How is blood vessel growth regulated in normal and neoplastic tissue? G.H.A. Clowes memorial Award lecture. *Cancer Res*, 1986. 46(2): p. 467-73.

[199] Folkman, J. and M. Klagsbrun, Angiogenic factors. *Science*, 1987. 235(4787): p. 442-7.

[200] Folkman, J., et al., Isolation of a tumor factor responsible for angiogenesis. *J Exp Med*, 1971. 133(2): p. 275-88.

[201] Folkman, J. and Y. Shing, Angiogenesis. *J Biol Chem*, 1992. 267(16): p. 10931-4.

[202] Fontaine, D., L. Capelle, and H. Duffau, Somatotopy of the supplementary motor area: evidence from correlation of the extent of surgical resection with the clinical patterns of deficit. *Neurosurgery*, 2002. 50(2): p. 297-303; discussion 303-5.

[203] Foulds, L., The experimental study of tumor progression: a review. *Cancer Res*, 1954. 14(5): p. 327-39.

[204] Francavilla, T.L., et al., Positron emission tomography in the detection of malignant degeneration of low-grade gliomas. *Neurosurgery*, 1989. 24(1): p. 1-5.

[205] Freije, W.A., et al., Gene expression profiling of gliomas strongly predicts survival. *Cancer Res*, 2004. 64(18): p. 6503-10.

[206] Fried, I., Management of low-grade gliomas. Results of resections without electrocorticography. *Clin Neurosurg*, 1995. 42:

[207] Fueyo, J., et al., The functional role of tumor suppressor genes in gliomas: clues for future therapeutic strategies. *Neurology*, 1998. 51(5): p. 1250-5.

[208] Fukaya, C., et al., Intraoperative wake-up procedure with propofol and laryngeal mask for optimal excision of brain tumour in eloquent areas. *J Clin Neurosci*, 2001. 8(3): p. 253-5.

[209] Fulci, G., N. Ishii, and E.G. Van Meir, p53 and brain tumors: from gene mutations to gene therapy. *Brain Pathol*, 1998. 8(4): p. 599-613.

[210] Fuller, G.N., et al., Molecular voting for glioma classification reflecting heterogeneity in the continuum of cancer progression. *Oncol Rep*, 2005. 14(3): p. 651-6.

[211] Fuss, M., et al., Tumor angiogenesis of low-grade astrocytomas measured by dynamic susceptibility contrast-enhanced MRI (DSC-MRI) is predictive of local tumor control after radiation therapy. *Int J Radiat Oncol Biol Phys*, 2001. 51(2): p. 478-82.

[212] Gajewski, T.F., Temozolomide for melanoma: new toxicities and new opportunities. *J Clin Oncol*, 2004. 22(4): p. 580-1.

[213] Gajjar, A., et al., Low-grade astrocytoma: a decade of experience at St. Jude Children's Research Hospital. *J Clin Oncol*, 1997. 15(8): p. 2792-9.

[214] Galanaud, D., et al., Use of proton magnetic resonance spectroscopy of the brain to differentiate gliomatosis cerebri from low-grade glioma. *J Neurosurg*, 2003. 98(2): p. 269-76.

[215] Galli, R., et al., Isolation and characterization of tumorigenic, stem-like neural precursors from human glioblastoma. *Cancer Res*, 2004. 64(19): p. 7011-21.

[216] Galmarini, C.M. and F.C. Galmarini, Multidrug resistance in cancer therapy: role of the microenvironment. *Curr Opin Investig Drugs*, 2003. 4(12): p. 1416-21.

[217] Galmarini, C.M., et al., Drug resistance associated with loss of p53 involves extensive alterations in microtubule composition and dynamics. *Br J Cancer*, 2003. 88(11): p. 1793-9.

[218] Ganju, V., et al., Prognostic factors in gliomas. A multivariate analysis of clinical, pathologic, flow cytometric, cytogenetic, and molecular markers. *Cancer*, 1994. 74(3): p. 920-7.

[219] Ganslandt, O., et al., Magnetic source imaging supports clinical decision making in glioma patients. *Clin Neurol Neurosurg*, 2004. 107(1): p. 20-6.

[220] Gatenby, R.A. and E.T. Gawlinski, A reaction-diffusion model of cancer invasion. *Cancer Res*, 1996. 56(24): p. 5745-53.

[221] Gatenby, R.A. and E.T. Gawlinski, Mathematical models of tumour invasion mediated by transformation-induced alteration of microenvironmental pH. *Novartis Found Symp*, 2001. 240: p. 85-96; discussion 96-9.

[222] Gatenby, R.A. and T.L. Vincent, An evolutionary model of carcinogenesis. *Cancer Res*, 2003. 63(19): p. 6212-20.

[223] Gatignol, P., et al., Double dissociation between picture naming and comprehension: an electrostimulation study. *Neuroreport*, 2004. 15(1): p. 191-5.

[224] Germano, I.M., et al., Correlation of histopathological features and proliferative potential of gliomas. *J Neurosurg*, 1989. 70(5): p. 701-6.

[225] Giese, A., Glioma invasion--pattern of dissemination by mechanisms of invasion and surgical intervention, pattern of gene expression and its regulatory control by tumorsuppressor p53 and proto-oncogene ETS-1. *Acta Neurochir Suppl*, 2003. 88: p. 153-62.

[226] Giese, A., et al., Cost of migration: invasion of malignant gliomas and implications for treatment. *J Clin Oncol*, 2003. 21(8): p. 1624-36.

[227] Giese, A., et al., Migration of human glioma cells on myelin. *Neurosurgery*, 1996. 38(4): p. 755-64.

[228] Giese, A., et al., Substrates for astrocytoma invasion. *Neurosurgery*, 1995. 37(2): p. 294-301; discussion 301-2.

[229] Giese, A., et al., Dichotomy of astrocytoma migration and proliferation. *Int J Cancer*, 1996. 67(2): p. 275-82.

[230] Giese, A. and M. Westphal, Glioma invasion in the central nervous system. *Neurosurgery*, 1996. 39(2): p. 235-50; discussion 250-2.

[231] Gil Robles, S., et al., The role of dominant striatum in language: a study using intraoperative electrical stimulations. *J Neurol Neurosurg Psychiatry*, 2005. 76(7): p. 940-6.

[232] Ginsberg, L.E., et al., The significance of lack of MR contrast enhancement of supratentorial brain tumors in adults: histopathological evaluation of a series. *Surg Neurol*, 1998. 49(4): p. 436-40.

[233] Gladson, C.L., The extracellular matrix of gliomas: modulation of cell function. *J Neuropathol Exp Neurol*, 1999. 58(10): p. 1029-40.

[234] Glantz, M.J., et al., Identification of early recurrence of primary central nervous system tumors by [18F]fluorodeoxyglucose positron emission tomography. *Ann Neurol*, 1991. 29(4): p. 347-55.

[235] Godard, S., et al., Classification of human astrocytic gliomas on the basis of gene expression: a correlated group of genes with angiogenic activity emerges as a strong predictor of subtypes. *Cancer Res*, 2003. 63(20): p. 6613-25.

[236] Godfraind, C., et al., Tumour necrosis and microvascular proliferation are associated with 9p deletion and CDKN2A alterations in 1p/19q-deleted oligodendrogliomas. *Neuropathol Appl Neurobiol*, 2003. 29(5): p. 462-71.

[237] Goldbrunner, R.H., J.J. Bernstein, and J.C. Tonn, Cell-extracellular matrix interaction in glioma invasion. *Acta Neurochir (Wien)*, 1999. 141(3): p. 295-305; discussion 304-5.

[238] Goldbrunner, R.H., et al., Models for assessment of angiogenesis in gliomas. *J Neurooncol*, 2000. 50(1-2): p. 53-62.

[239] Goldman, C.K., et al., Epidermal growth factor stimulates vascular endothelial growth factor production by human malignant glioma cells: a model of glioblastoma multiforme pathophysiology. *Mol Biol Cell*, 1993. 4(1): p. 121-33.

[240] Goldstein, B., et al., The impact of low-grade brain tumors on verbal fluency performance. *J Clin Exp Neuropsychol*, 2004. 26: p. 750-8. [240b]. Goldstein, B., et al., The impact of left and right intracranial tumors on picture and word recognition memory. *Brain Cogn*, 2004. 54: p. 1-6. [240c]. Goldstein, B., et al., Attention in adult intracranial tumors patients. *J Clin Exp Neuropsychol*, 2003. 25: p. 66-78. [240d]. Goldstein, B, et al., The impact of frontal and non-frontal brain tumor lesions on Wisconsin Card Sorting Test performance. *Brain Cogn*, 2004. 54: p. 110-6.

[241] Graves, E.E., et al., Serial proton MR spectroscopic imaging of recurrent malignant gliomas after gamma knife radiosurgery. *AJNR Am J Neuroradiol*, 2001. 22(4): p. 613-24.

[242] Grobben, B., P.P. De Deyn, and H. Slegers, Rat C6 glioma as experimental model system for the study of glioblastoma growth and invasion. *Cell Tissue Res*, 2002. 310(3): p. 257-70.

[243] Gross, C.G., Neurogenesis in the adult brain: death of a dogma. *Nat Rev Neurosci*, 2000. 1(1): p. 67-73.

[244] Gutmann, D.H., et al., Mouse models of human cancer consortium symposium on nervous system tumors. *Cancer Res*, 2003. 63(11): p. 3001-4.

[245] Hagel, C., et al., Demonstration of p53 protein and TP53 gene mutations in oligodendrogliomas. *Eur J Cancer*, 1996. 32A(13): p. 2242-8.

[246] Haglund, M.M. and M.S. Berger, Functional mapping of motor, sensory, and language pathways during low-grade glioma removal. *Tech Neurosurg*, 1996. 2: p. 141-9.

[247] Hallett, M., Plasticity of the human motor cortex and recovery from stroke. *Brain Res Brain Res Rev*, 2001. 36(2-3): p. 169-74.

[248] Hamamoto, T., et al., Differences in effects of oncogenes on sensitivity to anticancer drugs. *J Radiat Res (Tokyo)*, 2005. 46(2): p. 197-203.

[249] Hanahan, D. and J. Folkman, Patterns and emerging mechanisms of the angiogenic switch during tumorigenesis. *Cell*, 1996. 86(3): p. 353-64.

[250] Hanahan, D. and R.A. Weinberg, The hallmarks of cancer. *Cell*, 2000. 100(1): p. 57-70.

[251] Hanzely, Z., et al., Role of early radiotherapy in the treatment of supratentorial WHO Grade II astrocytomas: long-term results of 97 patients. *J Neurooncol*, 2003. 63(3): p. 305-12.

[252] Hara, T., et al., Use of 18F-choline and 11C-choline as contrast agents in positron emission tomography imaging-guided stereotactic biopsy sampling of gliomas. *J Neurosurg*, 2003. 99(3): p. 474-9.

[253] Hart, M.N., C.K. Petito, and K.M. Earle, Mixed gliomas. *Cancer*, 1974. 33(1): p. 134-40.

[254] Hatten, M.E., Central nervous system neuronal migration. *Annu Rev Neurosci*, 1999. 22: p. 511-39.

[255] Heesters, M.A., et al., Proliferation and apoptosis in long-term surviving low grade gliomas in relation to radiotherapy. *J Neurooncol*, 2002. 58(2): p. 157-65.

[256] Hegi, M.E., et al., MGMT gene silencing and benefit from temozolomide in glioblastoma. *N Engl J Med*, 2005. 352(10): p. 997-1003.

[257] Heimans, J.J. and M.J. Taphoorn, Impact of brain tumour treatment on quality of life. *J Neurol*, 2002. 249(8): p. 955-60.

[258] Heiss, W.D., et al., Disturbance and recovery of language function: correlates in PET activation studies. *Neuroimage*, 2003. 20 Suppl 1: p. S42-9.

[259] Hemm, S., et al., Thallium SPECT-based stereotactic targeting for brain tumor biopsies. A technical note. *Stereotact Funct Neurosurg*, 2004. 82(2-3): p. 70-6.

[260] Henderson, K.H. and E.G. Shaw, Randomized trials of radiation therapy in adult low-grade gliomas. *Semin Radiat Oncol*, 2001. 11(2): p. 145-51.

[261] Herholz, K., et al., 11C-methionine PET for differential diagnosis of low-grade gliomas. *Neurology*, 1998. 50(5): p. 1316-22.

[262] Hermanson, M., et al., Association of loss of heterozygosity on chromosome 17p with high platelet-derived growth factor alpha receptor expression in human malignant gliomas. *Cancer Res*, 1996. 56(1): p. 164-71.

[263] Herminghaus, S., et al., Determination of histopathological tumor grade in neuroepithelial brain tumors by using spectral pattern analysis of in vivo spectroscopic data. *J Neurosurg*, 2003. 98(1): p. 74-81.

[264] Herminghaus, S., et al., Increased choline levels coincide with enhanced proliferative activity of human neuroepithelial brain tumors. *NMR Biomed*, 2002. 15(6): p. 385-92.

[265] Herschman, H.R., Molecular imaging: looking at problems, seeing solutions. *Science*, 2003. 302(5645): p. 605-8.

[266] Heshmat, M.Y., et al., Neoplasms of the central nervous system. incidence and population selectivity in the Washington DC, metropolitan area. *Cancer*, 1976. 38(5): p. 2135-42.

[267] Hilton, D.A., et al., Accumulation of p53 and Ki-67 expression do not predict survival in patients with fibrillary astrocytomas or the response of these tumors to radiotherapy. *Neurosurgery*, 1998. 42(4): p. 724-9.

[268] Hoang-Xuan, K., et al., Temozolomide as initial treatment for adults with low-grade oligodendrogliomas or oligoastrocytomas and correlation with chromosome 1p deletions. *J Clin Oncol*, 2004. 22(15): p. 3133-8.

[269] Hoang-Xuan, K., et al., Molecular heterogeneity of oligodendrogliomas suggests alternative pathways in tumor progression. *Neurology*, 2001. 57(7): p. 1278-81.

[270] Hoffman, R.M., Orthotopic metastatic mouse models for anticancer drug discovery and evaluation: a bridge to the clinic. *Invest New Drugs*, 1999. 17(4): p. 343-59.

[271] Holland, E.C., A mouse model for glioma: biology, pathology, and therapeutic opportunities. *Toxicol Pathol*, 2000. 28(1): p. 171-7.

[272] Holland, E.C., Animal models of cell cycle dysregulation and the pathogenesis of gliomas. *J Neurooncol*, 2001. 51(3): p. 265-76.

[273] Holland, E.C., Gliomagenesis: genetic alterations and mouse models. *Nat Rev Genet*, 2001. 2(2): p. 120-9.

[274] Holland, E.C., et al., A constitutively active epidermal growth factor receptor cooperates with disruption of G1 cell-cycle arrest pathways to induce glioma-like lesions in mice. *Genes Dev*, 1998. 12(23): p. 3675-85.

[275] Holland, E.C., et al., Modeling mutations in the G1 arrest pathway in human gliomas: overexpression of CDK4 but not loss of INK4a-ARF induces hyperploidy in cultured mouse astrocytes. *Genes Dev*, 1998. 12(23): p. 3644-9.

[276] Holodny, A.I., et al., Translocation of Broca's area to the contralateral hemisphere as the result of the growth of a left inferior frontal glioma. *J Comput Assist Tomogr*, 2002. 26(6): p. 941-3.

[277] Holzer, T., et al., FDG-PET as a prognostic indicator in radiochemotherapy of glioblastoma. *J Comput Assist Tomogr*, 1993. 17(5): p. 681-7.

[278] Horstmann, G.A., et al., Microstereometrically guided cortical stimulation for the intraoperative identification of the central motor strip. *Stereotact Funct Neurosurg*, 1995. 65(1-4): p. 130-5.

[279] Hoshi, M., et al., Correlation between MIB-1 staining indices and recurrence in low-grade astrocytomas. *Brain Tumor Pathol*, 1997. 14(1): p. 47-51.

[280] Hoshino, T., et al., Prognostic significance of the proliferative potential of intracranial gliomas measured by bromodeoxyuridine labeling. *Int J Cancer*, 1993. 53(4): p. 550-5.

[281] Hoshino, T., et al., Prognostic implications of the bromodeoxyuridine labeling index of human gliomas. *J Neurosurg*, 1989. 71(3): p. 335-41.

[282] Hoshino, T., B.C. Wilson, and W.G. Ellis, Gemistocytic astrocytes in gliomas. An autoradiographic study. *J Neuropathol Exp Neurol*, 1975. 34(3): p. 263-81.

[283] Howe, F.A., et al., Metabolic profiles of human brain tumors using quantitative in vivo 1H magnetic resonance spectroscopy. *Magn Reson Med*, 2003. 49(2): p. 223-32.

[284] Howe, F.A. and K.S. Opstad, 1H MR spectroscopy of brain tumours and masses. *NMR Biomed*, 2003. 16(3): p. 123-31.

[285] Hsu, D.W., et al., Use of MIB-1 (Ki-67) immunoreactivity in differentiating grade II and grade III gliomas. *J Neuropathol Exp Neurol*, 1997. 56(8): p. 857-65.

[286] Hu, X. and E.C. Holland, Applications of mouse glioma models in preclinical trials. *Mutat Res*, 2005. 576(1-2): p. 54-65.

[287] Hu, X., et al., mTOR promotes survival and astrocytic characteristics induced by Pten/AKT signaling in glioblastoma. *Neoplasia*, 2005. 7(4): p. 356-68.

[288] Huang, H., et al., Gene expression profiling of low-grade diffuse astrocytomas by cDNA arrays. *Cancer Res*, 2000. 60(24): p. 6868-74.

[289] Huang, H., et al., Gene expression profiling and subgroup identification of oligodendrogliomas. *Oncogene*, 2004. 23(35): p. 6012-22.

[290] Huang, Q., et al., [Establishment of malignant progression associated gene expression profiles in human brain glioma]. *Zhonghua Zhong Liu Za Zhi*, 2003. 25(5): p. 437-40.

[291] Huang, Q., et al., [Preliminary study on differentiation-inducing associated genes of human brain glioma cells in vitro]. *Ai Zheng*, 2003. 22(7): p. 673-9.

[292] Huang, R., et al., Linking pathway gene expressions to the growth inhibition response from the National Cancer Institute's anticancer screen and drug mechanism of action. *Pharmacogenomics J*, 2005. 5(6): p. 381-99.

[293] Huang, Y., et al., Membrane transporters and channels: role of the transportome in cancer chemosensitivity and chemoresistance. *Cancer Res*, 2004. 64(12): p. 4294-301.

[294] Hulleman, E. and K. Helin, Molecular mechanisms in gliomagenesis. Adv *Cancer Res*, 2005. 94: p. 1-27.

[295] Hulsebos, T.J., et al., Dynamics of genetic alterations associated with glioma recurrence. *Genes Chromosomes Cancer*, 1998. 23(2): p. 153-8.

[296] Hwang, S.L., et al., Expression and mutation analysis of the p53 gene in astrocytoma. *J Formos Med Assoc*, 1999. 98(1): p. 31-8.

[297] Ichimura, K., et al., Deregulation of the p14ARF/MDM2/p53 pathway is a prerequisite for human astrocytic gliomas with G1-S transition control gene abnormalities. *Cancer Res*, 2000. 60(2): p. 417-24.

[298] Idbaih, A., et al., Two types of chromosome 1p losses with opposite significance in gliomas. *Ann Neurol*, 2005. 58(3): p. 483-7.

[299] Ikizler, Y., et al., Gliomas in families. *Can J Neurol Sci*, 1992. 19(4): p. 492-7.

[300] Inoue, T., et al., 18F alpha-methyl tyrosine PET studies in patients with brain tumors. *J Nucl Med*, 1999. 40(3): p. 399-405.

[301] Inskip, P.D., et al., Sociodemographic indicators and risk of brain tumours. *Int J Epidemiol*, 2003. 32(2): p. 225-33.

[302] Ishibashi, M., et al., Thallium-201 in brain tumors: relationship between tumor cell activity in astrocytic tumor and proliferating cell nuclear antigen. *J Nucl Med*, 1995. 36(12): p. 2201-6.

[303] Ito, S., et al., Proliferative potential and prognostic evaluation of low-grade astrocytomas. *J Neurooncol*, 1994. 19(1): p. 1-9.

[304] Ivanco, T.L. and W.T. Greenough, Physiological consequences of morphologically detectable synaptic plasticity: potential uses for examining recovery following damage. *Neuropharmacology*, 2000. 39(5): p. 765-76.

[305] Iwadate, Y., et al., Molecular classification and survival prediction in human gliomas based on proteome analysis. *Cancer Res*, 2004. 64(7): p. 2496-501.

[306] Iwadate, Y., et al., Proteome-based identification of molecular markers predicting chemosensitivity to each category of anticancer agents in human gliomas. *Int J Oncol*, 2005. 26(4): p. 993-8.

[307] Jacobs, A., et al., Positron emission tomography-based imaging of transgene expression mediated by replication-conditional, oncolytic herpes simplex virus type 1 mutant vectors in vivo. *Cancer Res*, 2001. 61(7): p. 2983-95.

[308] Jacobs, A.H., et al., Molecular imaging of gliomas. *Mol Imaging*, 2002. 1(4): p. 309-35.

[309] Jacobs, K.M. and J.P. Donoghue, Reshaping the cortical motor map by unmasking latent intracortical connections. *Science*, 1991. 251(4996): p. 944-7.

[310] Jaeckle, K.A., et al., Correlation of tumor O6 methylguanine-DNA methyltransferase levels with survival of malignant astrocytoma patients treated with bis-chloroethylnitrosourea: a Southwest Oncology Group study. *J Clin Oncol*, 1998. 16(10): p. 3310-5.

[311] James, C.D. and J.J. Olson, Molecular genetics and molecular biology advances in brain tumors. *Curr Opin Oncol*, 1996. 8(3): p. 188-95.

[312] Janny, P., et al., Low grade supratentorial astrocytomas. Management and prognostic factors. *Cancer*, 1994. 73(7): p. 1937-45.

[313] Jbabdi, S., et al., Diffusion tensor imaging allows anisotropic growth simulations of low grade gliomas. *Mag Reson Med*, in press.

[314] Jensen, R.L., Growth factor-mediated angiogenesis in the malignant progression of glial tumors: a review. *Surg Neurol*, 1998. 49(2): p. 189-95; discussion 196.

[315] Johannesen, T.B., F. Langmark, and K. Lote, Cause of death and long-term survival in patients with neuro-epithelial brain tumours: a population-based study. *Eur J Cancer*, 2003. 39(16): p. 2355-63.

[316] Johannesen, T.B., F. Langmark, and K. Lote, Progress in long-term survival in adult patients with supratentorial low-grade gliomas: a population-based study of 993

Luc Taillandier, Laurent Capelle and Hughes Duffau

patients in whom tumors were diagnosed between 1970 and 1993. *J Neurosurg*, 2003. 99(5): p. 854-62.

[317] Johnson, J.P. and J.N. Bruce, Angiogenesis in human gliomas: prognostic and therapeutic implications. *Exs*, 1997. 79: p. 29-46.

[318] Johnson, M.H., Development of human brain functions. *Biol Psychiatry*, 2003. 54(12): p. 1312-6.

[319] Jomin, M., et al., [Multifocal glioma. Apropos of 10 cases]. *Neurochirurgie*, 1983. 29(6): p. 411-6.

[320] Kaba, S.E. and A.P. Kyritsis, Recognition and management of gliomas. *Drugs*, 1997. 53(2): p. 235-44.

[321] Kaku, S., et al., [A multicentric glioma presenting different pathological appearances: a case report]. *No Shinkei Geka*, 2004. 32(5): p. 501-6.

[322] Kallio, M., The incidence of intracranial gliomas in southern Finland. *Acta Neurol Scand*, 1988. 78(6): p. 480-3.

[323] Kallio, M., Therapy and survival of adult patients with intracranial glioma in a defined population. *Acta Neurol Scand*, 1990. 81(6): p. 541-9.

[324] Kamiya, M. and Y. Nakazato, The expression of cell cycle regulatory proteins in oligodendroglial tumors. *Clin Neuropathol*, 2002. 21(2): p. 52-65.

[325] Kansal, A.R., et al., Emergence of a subpopulation in a computational model of tumor growth. *J Theor Biol*, 2000. 207(3): p. 431-41.

[326] Kansal, A.R., et al., Simulated brain tumor growth dynamics using a three-dimensional cellular automaton. *J Theor Biol*, 2000. 203(4): p. 367-82.

[327] Karak, A.K., et al., A comparative survival evaluation and assessment of interclassification concordance in adult supratentorial astrocytic tumors. *Pathol Oncol Res*, 2000. 6(1): p. 46-52.

[328] Karamitopoulou, E., et al., Ki-67 immunoreactivity in human central nervous system tumors: a study with MIB 1 monoclonal antibody on archival material. *Acta Neuropathol (Berl)*, 1994. 87(1): p. 47-54.

[329] Karim, A.B., et al., Randomized trial on the efficacy of radiotherapy for cerebral low-grade glioma in the adult: European Organization for Research and Treatment of Cancer Study 22845 with the Medical Research Council study BRO4: an interim analysis. *Int J Radiat Oncol Biol Phys*, 2002. 52(2): p. 316-24.

[330] Karim, A.B., et al., A randomized trial on dose-response in radiation therapy of low-grade cerebral glioma: European Organization for Research and Treatment of Cancer (EORTC) Study 22844. *Int J Radiat Oncol Biol Phys*, 1996. 36(3): p. 549-56.

[331] Karlbom, A.E., et al., Loss of heterozygosity in malignant gliomas involves at least three distinct regions on chromosome 10. *Hum Genet*, 1993. 92(2): p. 169-74.

[332] Karni, A., et al., The acquisition of skilled motor performance: fast and slow experience-driven changes in primary motor cortex. *Proc Natl Acad Sci U S A*, 1998. 95(3): p. 861-8.

[333] Kaschten, B., et al., Preoperative evaluation of 54 gliomas by PET with fluorine-18-fluorodeoxyglucose and/or carbon-11-methionine. *J Nucl Med*, 1998. 39(5): p. 778-85.

[334] Kato, H., et al., Functional evaluation of p53 and PTEN gene mutations in gliomas. *Clin Cancer Res*, 2000. 6(10): p. 3937-43.

[335] Kattar, M.M., et al., Clonal analysis of gliomas. *Hum Pathol*, 1997. 28(10): p. 1166-79.

[336] Kaur, B., et al., Genetic and hypoxic regulation of angiogenesis in gliomas. *J Neurooncol*, 2004. 70(2): p. 229-43.

[337] Kaye, A.H. and D.G. Walker, Low grade astrocytomas: controversies in management. *J Clin Neurosci*, 2000. 7(6): p. 475-83.

[338] Kazner, E. and T. Grumme, [Value and realizability of diagnostic procedures in craniocerebral trauma]. *Chirurg*, 1982. 53(8): p. 477-82.

[339] Keles, G.E., K.R. Lamborn, and M.S. Berger, Low-grade hemispheric gliomas in adults: a critical review of extent of resection as a factor influencing outcome. *J Neurosurg*, 2001. 95(5): p. 735-45.

[340] Keles, G.E., et al., Volume of residual disease as a predictor of outcome in adult patients with recurrent supratentorial glioblastomas multiforme who are undergoing chemotherapy. *J Neurosurg*, 2004. 100(1): p. 41-6.

[341] Keles, G.E., et al., Intraoperative subcortical stimulation mapping for hemispherical perirolandic gliomas located within or adjacent to the descending motor pathways: evaluation of morbidity and assessment of functional outcome in 294 patients. *J Neurosurg*, 2004. 100(3): p. 369-75.

[342] Kemp, G.J., Non-invasive methods for studying brain energy metabolism: what they show and what it means. *Dev Neurosci*, 2000. 22(5-6): p. 418-28.

[343] Kerbel, R.S., Human tumor xenografts as predictive preclinical models for anticancer drug activity in humans: better than commonly perceived-but they can be improved. *Cancer Biol Ther*, 2003. 2(4 Suppl 1): p. S134-9.

[344] Keston, P., A.D. Murray, and A. Jackson, Cerebral perfusion imaging using contrast-enhanced MRI. *Clin Radiol*, 2003. 58(7): p. 505-13.

[345] Khoshyomn, S., et al., Brain tumor invasion rate measured in vitro does not correlate with Ki-67 expression. *J Neurooncol*, 1999. 45(2): p. 111-6.

[346] Kiebert, G.M., et al., Quality of life after radiation therapy of cerebral low-grade gliomas of the adult: results of a randomised phase III trial on dose response (EORTC trial 22844). EORTC Radiotherapy Co-operative Group. *Eur J Cancer*, 1998. 34(12): p. 1902-9.

[347] Kim, C.K., et al., New grading system of cerebral gliomas using positron emission tomography with F-18 fluorodeoxyglucose. *J Neurooncol*, 1991. 10(1): p. 85-91.

[348] Kim, S., et al., Identification of combination gene sets for glioma classification. *Mol Cancer Ther*, 2002. 1(13): p. 1229-36.

[349] Kirkegaard, L.J., et al., Image cytometric measurement of nuclear proliferation markers (MIB-1, PCNA) in astrocytomas. Prognostic significance. *Am J Clin Pathol*, 1998. 109(1): p. 69-74.

[350] Kirkpatrick, J.P. and L.B. Marks, Modeling killing and repopulation kinetics of subclinical cancer: direct calculations from clinical data. *Int J Radiat Oncol Biol Phys*, 2004. 58(2): p. 641-54.

[351] Kitahara, M., et al., [Results of supratentorial low-grade astrocytoma--effects of combined radiochemotherapy]. *No Shinkei Geka*, 1987. 15(6): p. 597-604.

[352] Kitange, G.J., K.L. Templeton, and R.B. Jenkins, Recent advances in the molecular genetics of primary gliomas. *Curr Opin Oncol*, 2003. 15(3): p. 197-203.

[353] Kleihues, P. and W. Cavenee, *Pathology and genetics of tumours of the nervous system.*, ed. P. Kleihues and W. Cavenee. 2000, Lyon: International Agency for Research on Cancer Press.

[354] Klein, M., et al., [Impaired cognitive functioning in low-grade glioma patients: relationship to tumor localisation, radiotherapy and the use of anticonvulsants]. *Ned Tijdschr Geneeskd*, 2004. 148(44): p. 2175-80. [354b]. Klein, M., et al., Epilepsy in low-grade gliomas: the impact on cognitive function and quality of life. *Ann Neurol*, 2003. 54: p. 514-20.

[355] Klein, M., et al., Effect of radiotherapy and other treatment-related factors on mid-term to long-term cognitive sequelae in low-grade gliomas: a comparative study. *Lancet*, 2002. 360(9343): p. 1361-8.

[356] Knisely, J.P. et al., Early vs. delayed radiotherapy in a small cohort of patients with supratentorial low grade gliomas. *J Neurooncol*, 1997. 34(1): p. 23-9

[357] Knopp, E.A., et al., Glial neoplasms: dynamic contrast-enhanced T2*-weighted MR imaging. *Radiology*, 1999. 211(3): p. 791-8.

[358] Ko, L.J. and C. Prives, p53: puzzle and paradigm. *Genes Dev*, 1996. 10(9): p. 1054-72.

[359] Kolb, B., Overview of cortical plasticity and recovery from brain injury. *Phys Med Rehabil Clin N Am*, 2003. 14(1 Suppl): p. S7-25, viii.

[360] Kolles, H., I. Niedermayer, and W. Feiden, [Grading of astrocytomas and oligodendrogliomas]. *Pathologe*, 1998. 19(4): p. 259-68.

[361] Kondziolka, D., L.D. Lunsford, and A.J. Martinez, Unreliability of contemporary neurodiagnostic imaging in evaluating suspected adult supratentorial (low-grade) astrocytoma. *J Neurosurg*, 1993. 79(4): p. 533-6.

[362] Kono, K., et al., The role of diffusion-weighted imaging in patients with brain tumors. *AJNR Am J Neuroradiol*, 2001. 22(6): p. 1081-8.

[363] Koochekpour, S. and G.J. Pilkington, Vascular and perivascular GD3 expression in human glioma. *Cancer Lett*, 1996. 104(1): p. 97-102.

[364] Kordek, R., et al., Proliferating cell nuclear antigen (PCNA) and Ki-67 immunopositivity in human astrocytic tumours. *Acta Neurochir (Wien)*, 1996. 138(5): p. 509-12; discussion 513.

[365] Kordek, R., et al., Apoptosis in glial tumors as determined by in situ nonradioactive labeling of DNA breaks. *Acta Neuropathol (Berl)*, 1996. 91(1): p. 112-6.

[366] Korkolopoulou, P., et al., Hypoxia-inducible factor 1alpha/vascular endothelial growth factor axis in astrocytomas. Associations with microvessel morphometry, proliferation and prognosis. *Neuropathol Appl Neurobiol*, 2004. 30(3): p. 267-78.

[367] Korshunov, A. and A. Golanov, The prognostic significance of vascular endothelial growth factor (VEGF C-1) immunoexpression in oligodendroglioma. An analysis of 91 cases. *J Neurooncol*, 2000. 48(1): p. 13-9.

[368] Kortmann, R.D., Radiotherapy in low-grade gliomas: pros. *Semin Oncol*, 2003. 30(6 Suppl 19): p. 29-33.

[369] Kosel, S., B.W. Scheithauer, and M.B. Graeber, Genotype-phenotype correlation in gemistocytic astrocytomas. *Neurosurgery*, 2001. 48(1): p. 187-93; discussion 193-4.

[370] Koutcher, J.A., et al., MRI of mouse models for gliomas shows similarities to humans and can be used to identify mice for preclinical trials. *Neoplasia*, 2002. 4(6): p. 480-5.

[371] Krainik, A., et al., Role of the healthy hemisphere in recovery after resection of the supplementary motor area. *Neurology*, 2004. 62(8): p. 1323-32.

[372] Kraus, J.A., et al., Shared allelic losses on chromosomes 1p and 19q suggest a common origin of oligodendroglioma and oligoastrocytoma. *J Neuropathol Exp Neurol*, 1995. 54(1): p. 91-5.

[373] Kreth, F.W., et al., The risk of interstitial radiotherapy of low-grade gliomas. *Radiother Oncol*, 1997. 43(3): p. 253-60.

[374] Kreth, F.W., et al., Supratentorial World Health Organization Grade 2 astrocytomas and oligoastrocytomas. A new pattern of prognostic factors. *Cancer*, 1997. 79(2): p. 370-9.

[375] Kreth, F.W., et al., Effect of radiotherapy in patients with low-grade gliomas. *Ann Neurol*, 1995. 37(5): p. 682-3.

[376] Kreth, F.W., P.C. Warnke, and C.B. Ostertag, Low grade supratentorial astrocytomas: management and prognostic factors. *Cancer*, 1994. 74(12): p. 3247-8.

[377] Kreuser, E.D., S. Wadler, and E. Thiel, Biochemical modulation of cytotoxic drugs by cytokines: molecular mechanisms in experimental oncology. *Recent Results Cancer Res*, 1995. 139: p. 371-82.

[378] Krombach, G.A., et al., Intraoperative localization of functional regions in the sensorimotor cortex by neuronavigation and cortical mapping. *Comput Aided Surg*, 1998. 3(2): p. 64-73.

[379] Kros, J.M., et al., Expression of p53 in oligodendrogliomas. *J Pathol*, 1993. 171(4): p. 285-90.

[380] Kros, J.M., et al., Prognostic value of the proliferation-related antigen Ki-67 in oligodendrogliomas. *Cancer*, 1996. 78(5): p. 1107-13.

[381] Kros, J.M., et al., Prognostic implications of glial fibrillary acidic protein containing cell types in oligodendrogliomas. *Cancer*, 1990. 66(6): p. 1204-12.

[382] Kros, J.M., et al., Cytogenetic analysis of gemistocytic cells in gliomas. *J Neuropathol Exp Neurol*, 2000. 59(8): p. 679-86.

[383] Krouwer, H.G., et al., Gemistocytic astrocytomas: a reappraisal. *J Neurosurg*, 1991. 74(3): p. 399-406.

[384] Krouwer, H.G., et al., Oligoastrocytomas: a clinicopathological study of 52 cases. *J Neurooncol*, 1997. 33(3): p. 223-38.

[385] Kuesel, A.C., et al., 1H MRS of high grade astrocytomas: mobile lipid accumulation in necrotic tissue. *NMR Biomed*, 1994. 7(3): p. 149-55.

[386] Kuwert, T., et al., Diagnosis of recurrent glioma with SPECT and iodine-123-alpha-methyl tyrosine. *J Nucl Med*, 1998. 39(1): p. 23-7.

[387] Kuznetsov, Y.E., et al., Proton magnetic resonance spectroscopic imaging can predict length of survival in patients with supratentorial gliomas. *Neurosurgery*, 2003. 53(3): p. 565-74; discussion 574-6.

[388] Laack, N.L., et al., Cognitive function after radiotherapy for supratentorial low-grade glioma: a north central cancer treatment group prospective study. *Int J Radiat Oncol Biol Phys*, in press.

[389] Labrousse, F., et al., Histological grading and bromodeoxyuridine labeling index of astrocytomas. Comparative study in a series of 60 cases. *J Neurosurg*, 1991. 75(2): p. 202-5.

[390] Laigle-Donadey, F., et al., Correlations between molecular profile and radiologic pattern in oligodendroglial tumors. *Neurology*, 2004. 63(12): p. 2360-2.

[391] Lam, W.W., et al., Pre-operative grading of intracranial glioma. *Acta Radiol*, 2001. 42(6): p. 548-54.

[392] Lamszus, K., P. Kunkel, and M. Westphal, Invasion as limitation to anti-angiogenic glioma therapy. *Acta Neurochir Suppl*, 2003. 88: p. 169-77.

[393] Lamszus, K., et al., Scatter factor promotes motility of human glioma and neuromicrovascular endothelial cells. *Int J Cancer*, 1998. 75(1): p. 19-28.

[394] Landman, K.A., G.J. Pettet, and D.F. Newgreen, Mathematical models of cell colonization of uniformly growing domains. *Bull Math Biol*, 2003. 65(2): p. 235-62.

[395] Lang, F.F., et al., Pathways leading to glioblastoma multiforme: a molecular analysis of genetic alterations in 65 astrocytic tumors. *J Neurosurg*, 1994. 81(3): p. 427-36.

[396] Lanier, W.L., Brain tumor resection in the awake patient. *Mayo Clin Proc*, 2001. 76(7): p. 670-2.

[397] Laws, E.R., Jr., et al., Neurosurgical management of low-grade astrocytoma of the cerebral hemispheres. *J Neurosurg*, 1984. 61(4): p. 665-73.

[398] Lazareff, J.A., et al., Tumor volume and growth kinetics in hypothalamic-chiasmatic pediatric low grade gliomas. *Pediatr Neurosurg*, 1999. 30(6): p. 312-9.

[399] Lebelt, A., et al., Proliferative activity of chosen central nervous system (CNS) neoplasms. *Rocz Akad Med Bialymst*, 2004. 49 Suppl 1: p. 242-3.

[400] Lebrun, C., et al., (Neoadjuvant chemotherapy for symptomatic non operable grade II fibrillary astrocytoma in adults). *Rev Neurol (Paris)*, 2004. 160(5 Pt1): p. 533-7.

[401] Lee, Y.Y. and P. Van Tassel, Intracranial oligodendrogliomas: imaging findings in 35 untreated cases. *AJR Am J Roentgenol*, 1989. 152(2): p. 361-9.

[402] Leenstra, S., et al., Molecular characterization of areas with low grade tumor or satellitosis in human malignant astrocytomas. *Cancer Res*, 1992. 52(6): p. 1568-72.

[403] Lefournier, V., et al., [Magnetic resonance cerebral blood volume maps. Comparison with histologic findings in different types of brain lesions]. *J Neuroradiol*, 2003. 30(1): p. 3-9.

[404] Leibel, S.A., et al., The role of radiation therapy in the treatment of astrocytomas. *Cancer*, 1975. 35(6): p. 1551-7.

[405] Leighton, C., et al., Supratentorial low-grade glioma in adults: an analysis of prognostic factors and timing of radiation. *J Clin Oncol*, 1997. 15(4): p. 1294-301.

[406] Leon, S.P., R.D. Folkerth, and P.M. Black, Microvessel density is a prognostic indicator for patients with astroglial brain tumors. *Cancer*, 1996. 77(2): p. 362-72.

[407] Leonardi, M.A. and C.B. Lumenta, Oligodendrogliomas in the CT/MR-era. *Acta Neurochir (Wien)*, 2001. 143(12): p. 1195-203.

[408] Leuraud, P., et al., Correlation between genetic alterations and growth of human malignant glioma xenografted in nude mice. *Br J Cancer*, 2003. 89(12): p. 2327-32.

[409] Levicar, N., et al., Lysosomal enzymes, cathepsins in brain tumour invasion. *J Neurooncol*, 2002. 58(1): p. 21-32.

[410] Levivier, M., et al., Diagnostic yield of stereotactic brain biopsy guided by positron emission tomography with [18F]fluorodeoxyglucose. *J Neurosurg*, 1995. 82(3): p. 445-52.

[411] Licata, B. and S. Turazzi, Bleeding cerebral neoplasms with symptomatic hematoma. *J Neurosurg Sci*, 2003. 47(4): p. 201-10; discussion 210.

[412] Liepert, J. and C. Weiller, Mapping plastic brain changes after acute lesions. *Curr Opin Neurol*, 1999. 12(6): p. 709-13.

[413] Lindegaard, K.F., et al., Statistical analysis of clinicopathological features, radiotherapy, and survival in 170 cases of oligodendroglioma. *J Neurosurg*, 1987. 67(2): p. 224-30.

[414] Linskey, M.E., Multi-agent cytostatic treatment of 'low-grade' gliomas. *Curr Oncol Rep*, 2000. 2(5): p. 454-62.

[415] Linskey, M.E. and M.R. Gilbert, Glial differentiation: a review with implications for new directions in Neuro-oncology. *Neurosurgery*, 1995. 36(1): p. 1-21; discussion 21-2.

[416] Litofsky, N.S., D. Hinton, and C. Raffel, The lack of a role for p53 in astrocytomas in pediatric patients. *Neurosurgery*, 1994. 34(6): p. 967-72; discussion 972-3.

[417] Loftus, C.M., B.R. Copeland, and P.W. Carmel, Cystic supratentorial gliomas: natural history and evaluation of modes of surgical therapy. *Neurosurgery*, 1985. 17(1): p. 19-24.

[418] Loiseau, H., et al., [Supra-tentorial low-grade astrocytomas in adults. Prognostic factors and therapeutic indications. Apropos of a series of 141 patients]. *Neurochirurgie*, 1995. 41(1): p. 38-50.

[419] Loiseau, H., J.F. Dartigues, and F. Cohadon, Low-grade astrocytomas: prognosis factors and elements of management. *Surg Neurol*, 1995. 44(3): p. 224-7.

[420] Lopes, M., et al., [Proposing surgical management to a patient with low-grade glioma: controversies and ethical consequences]. *Neurochirurgie*, 2002. 48(2-3 Pt 1): p. 69-74.

[421] Lote, K., et al., Survival, prognostic factors, and therapeutic efficacy in low-grade glioma: a retrospective study in 379 patients. *J Clin Oncol*, 1997. 15(9): p. 3129-40.

[422] Louis, D.N., The p53 gene and protein in human brain tumors. *J Neuropathol Exp Neurol*, 1994. 53(1): p. 11-21.

[423] Louis, D.N., A molecular genetic model of astrocytoma histopathology. *Brain Pathol*, 1997. 7(2): p. 755-64.

[424] Louis, D.N., et al., Molecular genetics of pediatric brain stem gliomas. Application of PCR techniques to small and archival brain tumor specimens. *J Neuropathol Exp Neurol*, 1993. 52(5): p. 507-15.

[425] Lucas, T.H., 2nd, G.M. McKhann, 2nd, and G.A. Ojemann, Functional separation of languages in the bilingual brain: a comparison of electrical stimulation language mapping in 25 bilingual patients and 117 monolingual control patients. *J Neurosurg*, 2004. 101(3): p. 449-57.

[426] Ludemann, L., et al., Comparison of dynamic contrast-enhanced MRI with WHO tumor grading for gliomas. *Eur Radiol*, 2001. 11(7): p. 1231-41.

[427] Lunsford, L.D., et al., Brain astrocytomas: biopsy, then irradiation. *Clin Neurosurg*, 1995. 42: p. 464-79.

[428] Lunsford, L.D., et al., Survival after stereotactic biopsy and irradiation of cerebral nonanaplastic, nonpilocytic astrocytoma. *J Neurosurg*, 1995. 82(4): p. 523-9.

[429] Ma, J., et al., Biochemical changes associated with a multidrug-resistant phenotype of a human glioma cell line with temozolomide-acquired resistance. *Biochem Pharmacol*, 2002. 63(7): p. 1219-28.

[430] Macdonald, D.R., Low-grade gliomas, mixed gliomas, and oligodendrogliomas. *Semin Oncol*, 1994. 21(2): p. 236-48.

[431] MacDonald, D.R., et al., Successful chemotherapy for newly diagnosed aggressive oligodendroglioma. *Ann Neurol*, 1990. 17(5): p. 573-4

[432] Maher, E.A., et al., Malignant glioma: genetics and biology of a grave matter. *Genes Dev*, 2001. 15(11): p. 1311-33.

[433] Maidment, S.L., The cytoskeleton and brain tumour cell migration. *AntiCancer Res*, 1997. 17(6B): p. 4145-9.

[434] Maintz, D., et al., Molecular genetic evidence for subtypes of oligoastrocytomas. *J Neuropathol Exp Neurol*, 1997. 56(10): p. 1098-104.

[435] Mandonnet, E., et al., Continuous growth of mean tumor diameter in a subset of grade II gliomas. *Ann Neurol*, 2003. 53(4): p. 524-8.

[436] Manninen, P.H. and T.K. Tan, Postoperative nausea and vomiting after craniotomy for tumor surgery: a comparison between awake craniotomy and general anesthesia. *J Clin Anesth*, 2002. 14(4): p. 279-83.

[437] Mansury, Y. and T.S. Deisboeck, The impact of "search precision" in an agent-based tumor model. *J Theor Biol*, 2003. 224(3): p. 325-37.

[438] Mansury, Y., M. Diggory, and T.S. Deisboeck, Evolutionary game theory in an agent-based brain tumor model: Exploring the 'Genotype-Phenotype' link. *J Theor Biol*, 2005.

[439] Mansury, Y., et al., Emerging patterns in tumor systems: simulating the dynamics of multicellular clusters with an agent-based spatial agglomeration model. *J Theor Biol*, 2002. 219(3): p. 343-70.

[440] Marks, J.E. and M. Gado, Serial computed tomography of primary brain tumors following surgery, irradiation, and chemotherapy. *Radiology*, 1977. 125(1): p. 119-25.

[441] Marroni, M., et al., Dynamic in vitro model of the blood-brain barrier. Gene profiling using cDNA microarray analysis. *Methods Mol Med*, 2003. 89: p. 419-34.

[442] Marroni, M., et al., Vascular and parenchymal mechanisms in multiple drug resistance: a lesson from human epilepsy. *Curr Drug Targets*, 2003. 4(4): p. 297-304.

[443] Mason, W.P., Oligodendroglioma. *Curr Treat Options Neurol*, 2005. 7(4): p. 305-314.

[444] Mason, W.P., G.S. Krol, and L.M. DeAngelis, Low-grade oligodendroglioma responds to chemotherapy. *Neurology*, 1996. 46(1): p. 203-7.

[445] Massager, N., et al., Combined magnetic resonance imaging- and positron emission tomography-guided stereotactic biopsy in brainstem mass lesions: diagnostic yield in a series of 30 patients. *J Neurosurg*, 2000. 93(6): p. 951-7.

[446] Mattern, J., et al., Human tumor xenografts as model for drug testing. *Cancer Metastasis Rev*, 1988. 7(3): p. 263-84.

[447] McCann, J., Animal models offer insights into human brain tumors. *J Natl Cancer Inst*, 2003. 95(3): p. 188.

[448] McCormack, B.M., et al., Treatment and survival of low-grade astrocytoma in adults--1977-1988. *Neurosurgery*, 1992. 31(4): p. 636-42; discussion 642.

[449] McDermott, M.W., et al., A comparison of CT contrast enhancement and BUDR labeling indices in moderately and highly anaplastic astrocytomas of the cerebral hemispheres. *Can J Neurol Sci*, 1992. 19(1): p. 34-9.

[450] McDonald, J.D. and G.J. Dohrmann, Molecular biology of brain tumors. *Neurosurgery*, 1988. 23(5): p. 537-44.

[451] McDonald, J.D., et al., Successful chemotherapy for newly diagnosed aggressive oligodendroglioma. *Ann Neurol*, 1990. 27(5) : p. 573-4.

[452] McKnight, T.R., et al., An automated technique for the quantitative assessment of 3D-MRSI data from patients with glioma. *J Magn Reson Imaging*, 2001. 13(2): p. 167-77.

[453] McKnight, T.R., et al., Histopathological validation of a three-dimensional magnetic resonance spectroscopy index as a predictor of tumor presence. *J Neurosurg*, 2002. 97(4): p. 794-802.

[454] Medbery, C.A., 3rd, et al., Low-grade astrocytomas: treatment results and prognostic variables. *Int J Radiat Oncol Biol Phys*, 1988. 15(4): p. 837-41.

[455] Menedez, J., A. Nanda, and R.S. Polin, PET scan for brain tumors. *Sem Neurosurg*, 2000. 11: p. 277-86.

[456] Meyer, F.B., et al., Awake craniotomy for aggressive resection of primary gliomas located in eloquent brain. *Mayo Clin Proc*, 2001. 76(7): p. 677-87.

[457] Meyer, P.T., et al., Comparison of visual and ROI-based brain tumour grading using 18F-FDG PET: ROC analyses. Eur *J Nucl Med*, 2001. 28(2): p. 165-74.

[458] Michaelis, T., et al., Absolute concentrations of metabolites in the adult human brain in vivo: quantification of localized proton MR spectra. *Radiology*, 1993. 187(1): p. 219-27.

[459] Milea, D., et al., Intraoperative frontal eye field stimulation elicits ocular deviation and saccade suppression. *Neuroreport*, 2002. 13(10): p. 1359-64.

[460] Mischel, P.S., T.F. Cloughesy, and S.F. Nelson, DNA-microarray analysis of brain cancer: molecular classification for therapy. *Nat Rev Neurosci*, 2004. 5(10): p. 782-92.

[461] Mokhtari, K., et al., Olig2 expression, GFAP, p53 and 1p loss analysis contribute to glioma subclassification. *Neuropathol Appl Neurobiol*, 2005. 31(1): p. 62-9.

[462] Momota, H., E. Nerio, and E.C. Holland, Perifosine inhibits multiple signaling pathways in glial progenitors and cooperates with temozolomide to arrest cell proliferation in gliomas in vivo. *Cancer Res*, 2005. 65(16): p. 7429-35.

[463] Montine, T.J., et al., Prognostic significance of Ki-67 proliferation index in supratentorial fibrillary astrocytic neoplasms. *Neurosurgery*, 1994. 34(4): p. 674-8; discussion 678-9.

[464] Morantz, R.A., Radiation therapy in the treatment of cerebral astrocytoma. *Neurosurgery*, 1987. 20(6): p. 975-82.

[465] Mousseau, M., et al., A study of the expression of four chemoresistance-related genes in human primary and metastatic brain tumours. *Eur J Cancer*, 1993. 29A(5): p. 753-9.

[466] Mueller, M.M., T. Werbowetski, and R.F. Del Maestro, Soluble factors involved in glioma invasion. *Acta Neurochir (Wien)*, 2003. 145(11): p. 999-1008.

[467] Mueller, W., et al., Clonal analysis in glioblastoma with epithelial differentiation. *Brain Pathol*, 2001. 11(1): p. 39-43.

[468] Mukasa, A., et al., Distinction in gene expression profiles of oligodendrogliomas with and without allelic loss of 1p. *Oncogene*, 2002. 21(25): p. 3961-8.

[469] Muller, W., D. Afra, and R. Schroder, Supratentorial recurrences of gliomas. Morphological studies in relation to time intervals with oligodendrogliomas. *Acta Neurochir (Wien)*, 1977. 39(1-2): p. 15-25.

[470] Muller, W., D. Afra, and R. Schroder, Supratentorial recurrences of gliomas. Morphological studies in relation to time intervals with astrocytomas. *Acta Neurochir (Wien)*, 1977. 37(1-2): p. 75-91.

[471] Murphy, P.S., et al., Monitoring temozolomide treatment of low-grade glioma with proton magnetic resonance spectroscopy. *Br J Cancer*, 2004. 90(4): p. 781-6.

[472] Myal, Y., M.R. Del Bigio, and R.H. Rhodes, Age-related differences in 1p and 19q deletions in oligodendrogliomas. *BMC Clin Pathol*, 2003. 3(1): p. 6.

[473] Naef, F. and J. Huelsken, Cell-type-specific transcriptomics in chimeric models using transcriptome-based masks. *Nucleic Acids Res*, 2005. 33(13): p. e111.

[474] Nakada, M., Y. Okada, and J. Yamashita, The role of matrix metalloproteinases in glioma invasion. *Front Biosci*, 2003. 8: p. e261-9.

[475] Nakamura, M., et al., Analysis of prognostic and survival factors related to treatment of low-grade astrocytomas in adults. *Oncology*, 2000. 58(2): p. 108-16.

[476] Nakamura, M., et al., APO2L/TRAIL expression in human brain tumors. *Acta Neuropathol (Berl)*, 2000. 99(1): p. 1-6.

[477] Neder, L., et al., MIB-1 labeling index in astrocytic tumors--a clinicopathologic study. *Clin Neuropathol*, 2004. 23(6): p. 262-70.

[478] Negendank, W.G., et al., Proton magnetic resonance spectroscopy in patients with glial tumors: a multicenter study. *J Neurosurg*, 1996. 84(3): p. 449-58.

[479] Newman, W.I. and J.A. Lazareff, A mathematical model for self-limiting brain tumors. *J Theor Biol*, 2003. 222(3): p. 361-71.

[480] Ng, H.K. and P.Y. Lam, The molecular genetics of central nervous system tumors. *Pathology*, 1998. 30(2): p. 196-202.

[481] Nguyen, D.K. and M.I. Botez, Diaschisis and neurobehavior. *Can J Neurol Sci*, 1998. 25(1): p. 5-12.

[482] Nicolato, A., et al., Prognostic factors in low-grade supratentorial astrocytomas: a uni-multivariate statistical analysis in 76 surgically treated adult patients. *Surg Neurol*, 1995. 44(3): p. 208-21; discussion 221-3.

[483] Nikas, D.C., et al., Neurosurgical considerations in supratentorial low-grade gliomas: experience with 175 patients. *Neurosurg Focus (web journal)*, 1998. 4(4): p. article 4.

[484] Nikas, D.C., R.A. Danks, and P.M. Black, Tumor surgery under local anesthesia, in *Techniques in Neurosurgery*, C.M. Loftus and H.H. Batjer, Editors. 2001, Lippincott Williams & Wilkins: Philadelphia. p. 70-84.

[485] Nishio, S., et al., Glial tumourettes (glial microtumours): their clinical and histopathological manifestations. *Acta Neurochir (Wien)*, 1996. 138(7): p. 818-23.

[486] Nishiyama, Y., et al., Comparison of 99Tcm-MIBI with 201Tl chloride SPET in patients with malignant brain tumours. *Nucl Med Commun*, 2001. 22(6): p. 631-9.

[487] Nomura, M., et al., Possible participation of autocrine and paracrine vascular endothelial growth factors in hypoxia-induced proliferation of endothelial cells and pericytes. *J Biol Chem*, 1995. 270(47): p. 28316-24.

[488] North, C.A., et al., Low-grade cerebral astrocytomas. Survival and quality of life after radiation therapy. *Cancer*, 1990. 66(1): p. 6-14.

[489] Nowell, P.C., The clonal evolution of tumor cell populations. *Science*, 1976. 194(4260): p. 23-8.

[490] Nozaki, M., et al., Roles of the functional loss of p53 and other genes in astrocytoma tumorigenesis and progression. *Neuro-oncol*, 1999. 1(2): p. 124-37.

[491] Nudo, R.J., Functional and structural plasticity in motor cortex: implications for stroke recovery. *Phys Med Rehabil Clin N Am*, 2003. 14(1 Suppl): p. S57-76.

[492] Nutt, C.L., et al., O(6)-methylguanine-DNA methyltransferase activity, p53 gene status and BCNU resistance in mouse astrocytes. *Carcinogenesis*, 1999. 20(12): p. 2361-5.

[493] Nutt, C.L., et al., Gene expression-based classification of malignant gliomas correlates better with survival than histological classification. *Cancer Res*, 2003. 63(7): p. 1602-7.

[494] Nutt, C.L., et al., Differential expression of drug resistance genes and chemosensitivity in glial cell lineages correlate with differential response of oligodendrogliomas and astrocytomas to chemotherapy. *Cancer Res*, 2000. 60(17): p. 4812-8.

[495] O'Connor, P.M., et al., Characterization of the p53 tumor suppressor pathway in cell lines of the National Cancer Institute anticancer drug screen and correlations with the

growth-inhibitory potency of 123 anticancer agents. *Cancer Res*, 1997. 57(19): p. 4285-300.

[496] Ohgaki, H., Kleihues, P. Population-based studies on incidence, survival rates, and gentic alterations in astrocytic and oligodendroglial gliomas. *J Neuropathol Exp Neurol*, 2005. 64(6): p. 479-89

[497] Olson, J.D., E. Riedel, and L.M. DeAngelis, Long-term outcome of low-grade oligodendroglioma and mixed glioma. *Neurology*, 2000. 54(7): p. 1442-8.

[498] Oriuchi, N., et al., Clinical evaluation of thallium-201 SPECT in supratentorial gliomas: relationship to histologic grade, prognosis and proliferative activities. *J Nucl Med*, 1993. 34(12): p. 2085-9.

[499] Ourednik, V., et al., Neural stem cells are uniquely suited for cell replacement and gene therapy in the CNS. *Novartis Found Symp*, 2000. 231: p. 242-62; discussion 262-9, 302-6.

[500] Pace, A., et al., Temozolomide chemotherapy for progressive low-grade glioma: clinical benefits and radiological response. *Ann Oncol*, 2003. 14(12): p. 1722-6.

[501] Palfi, S., et al., Correlation of in vitro infiltration with glioma histological type in organotypic brain slices. *Br J Cancer*, 2004. 91(4): p. 745-52.

[502] Panetta, J.C., A mathematical model of drug resistance: heterogeneous tumors. *Math Biosci*, 1998. 147(1): p. 41-61.

[503] Papagikos, M.A., E.G. Shaw, and V.W. Stieber, Lessons learned from randomised clinical trials in adult low grade glioma. *Lancet Oncol*, 2005. 6(4): p. 240-4.

[504] Park, K.H., et al., Application of p27 gene therapy for human malignant glioma potentiated by using mutant p27. *J Neurosurg*, 2004. 101(3): p. 505-10.

[505] Peles, E., et al., Angiogenic factors in the cerebrospinal fluid of patients with astrocytic brain tumors. *Neurosurgery*, 2004. 55(3): p. 562-7; discussion 567-8.

[506] Peraud, A., et al., Clinical outcome of supratentorial astrocytoma WHO grade II. *Acta Neurochir (Wien)*, 1998. 140(12): p. 1213-22.

[507] Peraud, A., J. Ilmberger, and H.J. Reulen, Surgical resection of gliomas WHO grade II and III located in the opercular region. *Acta Neurochir (Wien)*, 2004. 146(1): p. 9-17; discussion 17-8.

[508] Peraud, A., et al., Prognostic impact of TP53 mutations and P53 protein overexpression in supratentorial WHO grade II astrocytomas and oligoastrocytomas. *Clin Cancer Res*, 2002. 8(5): p. 1117-24.

[509] Peraud, A., et al., Surgical resection of grade II astrocytomas in the superior frontal gyrus. *Neurosurgery*, 2002. 50(5): p. 966-75; discussion 975-7.

[510] Perry, A., et al., Ancillary FISH analysis for 1p and 19q status: preliminary observations in 287 gliomas and oligodendroglioma mimics. *Front Biosci*, 2003. 8: p. a1-9.

[511] Peters, O., et al., Impact of location on outcome in children with low-grade oligodendroglioma. *Pediatr Blood Cancer*, 2004. 43(3): p. 250-6.

[512] Philippon, J.H., et al., Supratentorial low-grade astrocytomas in adults. *Neurosurgery*, 1993. 32(4): p. 554-9.

[513] Piepmeier, J., et al., Variations in the natural history and survival of patients with supratentorial low-grade astrocytomas. *Neurosurgery*, 1996. 38(5): p. 872-8; discussion 878-9.

[514] Piepmeier, J.M., Observations on the current treatment of low-grade astrocytic tumors of the cerebral hemispheres. *J Neurosurg*, 1987. 67(2): p. 177-81.

[515] Piepmeier, J.M. and S. Christopher, Low-grade gliomas: introduction and overview. *J Neurooncol*, 1997. 34(1): p. 1-3.

[516] Pignatti, F., et al., Prognostic factors for survival in adult patients with cerebral low-grade glioma. *J Clin Oncol*, 2002. 20(8): p. 2076-84.

[517] Pilkington, C.J., The role of the extracellular matrix in neoplastic glial invasion of the nervous system. *Braz J Med Biol Res*, 1996. 29(9): p. 1159-72.

[518] Pirotte, B., et al., Combined use of 18F-fluorodeoxyglucose and 11C-methionine in 45 positron emission tomography-guided stereotactic brain biopsies. *J Neurosurg*, 2004. 101(3): p. 476-83.

[519] Pirzkall, A., et al., Metabolic imaging of low-grade gliomas with three-dimensional magnetic resonance spectroscopy. *Int J Radiat Oncol Biol Phys*, 2002. 53(5): p. 1254-64.

[520] Plate, K.H., G. Breier, and W. Risau, Molecular mechanisms of developmental and tumor angiogenesis. *Brain Pathol*, 1994. 4(3): p. 207-18.

[521] Plate, K.H. and W. Risau, Angiogenesis in malignant gliomas. *Glia*, 1995. 15(3): p. 339-47.

[522] Plathow, C., et al., Fractionated stereotactic radiotherapy in low-grade astrocytomas: long-term outcome and prognostic factors. *Int J Radiat Oncol Biol Phys*, 2003. 57(4): p. 996-1003.

[523] Pollack, I.F., et al., Low-grade gliomas of the cerebral hemispheres in children: an analysis of 71 cases. *J Neurosurg*, 1995. 82(4): p. 536-47.

[524] Pollack, I.F., et al., Association between chromosome 1p and 19q loss and outcome in pediatric malignant gliomas: results from the CCG-945 cohort. *Pediatr Neurosurg*, 2003. 39(3): p. 114-21.

[525] Pomper, M.G. and J.D. Port, New techniques in MR imaging of brain tumors. *Magn Reson Imaging Clin N Am*, 2000. 8(4): p. 691-713.

[526] Postma, T.J., et al., Radiotherapy-induced cerebral abnormalities in patients with low-grade glioma. *Neurology*, 2002. 59(1): p. 121-3.

[527] Preston-Martin, S., Epidemiology of primary CNS neoplasms. *Neurol Clin*, 1996. 14(2): p. 273-90.

[528] Pringle, A.M., R. Taylor, and I.R. Whittle, Anxiety and depression in patients with an intracranial neoplasm before and after tumour surgery. *Neuroradiology*, 1999. 13(1): p. 46-51.

[529] Provenzale, J.M., et al., Comparison of permeability in high-grade and low-grade brain tumors using dynamic susceptibility contrast MR imaging. *AJR Am J Roentgenol*, 2002. 178(3): p. 711-6.

[530] Quinn, J.A., et al., Phase II trial of temozolomide in patients with progressive low-grade gliomas. *J Clin Oncol*, 2003. 21(4): p. 646-51.

[531] Rabinov, J.D., et al., In vivo 3-T MR spectroscopy in the distinction of recurrent glioma versus radiation effects: initial experience. *Radiology*, 2002. 225(3): p. 871-9.

[532] Raffel, C., Molecular biology of pediatric gliomas. *J Neurooncol*, 1996. 28(2-3): p. 121-8.

[533] Raghavan, R., et al., Pediatric oligodendrogliomas: a study of molecular alterations on 1p and 19q using fluorescence in situ hybridization. *J Neuropathol Exp Neurol*, 2003. 62(5): p. 530-7.

[534] Rainov, N.G., et al., Prognostic factors in malignant glioma: influence of the overexpression of oncogene and tumor-suppressor gene products on survival. *J Neurooncol*, 1997. 35(1): p. 13-28.

[535] Rajan B. et al., The management of histologically unverified presumed cerebral gliomas with radiotherapy.*Int J Radiat Oncol Biol Phys*, 1994. 28(2): p. 405-13

[536] Ransom, D.T., et al., Correlation of cytogenetic analysis and loss of heterozygosity studies in human diffuse astrocytomas and mixed oligo-astrocytomas. *Genes Chromosomes Cancer*, 1992. 5(4): p. 357-74.

[537] Rao, J.S., Molecular mechanisms of glioma invasiveness: the role of proteases. *Nat Rev Cancer*, 2003. 3(7): p. 489-501.

[538] Rao, R.D. and C.D. James, Altered molecular pathways in gliomas: an overview of clinically relevant issues. *Semin Oncol*, 2004. 31(5): p. 595-604.

[539] Rasheed, B.K., et al., Molecular pathogenesis of malignant gliomas. *Curr Opin Oncol*, 1999. 11(3): p. 162-7.

[540] Recht, L.D. and M. Bernstein, Low-grade gliomas. *Neurol Clin*, 1995. 13(4): p. 847-59.

[541] Recht, L.D., R. Lew, and T.W. Smith, Suspected low-grade glioma: is deferring treatment safe? *Ann Neurol*, 1992. 31(4): p. 431-6.

[542] Rees, J., Advances in magnetic resonance imaging of brain tumours. *Curr Opin Neurol*, 2003. 16(6): p. 643-50.

[543] Regina, A., et al., Differences in multidrug resistance phenotype and matrix metalloproteinases activity between endothelial cells from normal brain and glioma. *J Neurochem*, 2003. 84(2): p. 316-24.

[544] Reifenberger, G., et al., Amplification at 12q13-14 in human malignant gliomas is frequently accompanied by loss of heterozygosity at loci proximal and distal to the amplification site. *Cancer Res*, 1995. 55(4): p. 731-4.

[545] Reifenberger, J., et al., Epidermal growth factor receptor expression in oligodendroglial tumors. *Am J Pathol*, 1996. 149(1): p. 29-35.

[546] Reifenberger, J., et al., Molecular genetic analysis of oligodendroglial tumors shows preferential allelic deletions on 19q and 1p. *Am J Pathol*, 1994. 145(5): p. 1175-90.

[547] Reijneveld, J.C., et al., Cognitive status and quality of life in patients with suspected versus proven low-grade gliomas. *Neurology*, 2001. 56(5): p. 618-23.

[548] Reis, R.M., et al., Genetic evidence of the neoplastic nature of gemistocytes in astrocytomas. *Acta Neuropathol (Berl)*, 2001. 102(5): p. 422-5.

[549] Reis-Filho, J.S., et al., Evaluation of cell proliferation, epidermal growth factor receptor, and bcl-2 immunoexpression as prognostic factors for patients with World Health Organization grade 2 oligodendroglioma. *Cancer*, 2000. 88(4): p. 862-9.

[550] Reithmeier, T., et al., Neuronavigation combined with electrophysiological monitoring for surgery of lesions in eloquent brain areas in 42 cases: a retrospective comparison of the neurological outcome and the quality of resection with a control group with similar lesions. *Minim Invasive Neurosurg*, 2003. 46(2): p. 65-71.

[551] Retsky, M.W., et al., Is Gompertzian or exponential kinetics a valid description of individual human cancer growth? *Med Hypotheses*, 1990. 33(2): p. 95-106.

[552] Reulen, H.J., et al., [Tumor surgery of the speech cortex in local anesthesia. Neuropsychological and neurophysiological monitoring during operations in the dominant hemisphere]. *Nervenarzt*, 1997. 68(10): p. 813-24.

[553] Reya, T., et al., Stem cells, cancer, and cancer stem cells. *Nature*, 2001. 414(6859): p. 105-11.

[554] Rhodes, R.H., Biological evaluation of biopsies from adult cerebral astrocytomas: cell-growth/cell-suicide ratios and their relationship to patient survival. *J Neuropathol Exp Neurol*, 1998. 57(8): p. 746-57.

[555] Ribom, D., et al., [Low malignancy grade glioma in the Uppsala++/Orebro region. Prognostic factors and survival among 119 patients]. *Lakartidningen*, 2000. 97(36): p. 3880-4.

[556] Ribom, D., et al., Prognostic value of platelet derived growth factor alpha receptor expression in grade 2 astrocytomas and oligoastrocytomas. *J Neurol Neurosurg Psychiatry*, 2002. 72(6): p. 782-7.

[557] Ribom, D., et al., Positron emission tomography (11)C-methionine and survival in patients with low-grade gliomas. *Cancer*, 2001. 92(6): p. 1541-9.

[558] Ribom, D., et al., On the issue of early and aggressive treatment in grade 2 gliomas. *J Cancer Res Clin Oncol*, 2003. 129(3): p. 154-60.

[559] Ricco, R., et al., Real-time quantification of the proliferative state in astrocytomas. *Anal Quant Cytol Histol*, 2000. 22(3): p. 213-7.

[560] Rich, J.N., et al., A genetically tractable model of human glioma formation. *Cancer Res*, 2001. 61(9): p. 3556-60.

[561] Rickardson, L., et al., Identification of molecular mechanisms for cellular drug resistance by combining drug activity and gene expression profiles. *Br J Cancer*, 2005. 93(4): p. 483-92.

[562] Rickman, D.S., et al., Distinctive molecular profiles of high-grade and low-grade gliomas based on oligonucleotide microarray analysis. *Cancer Res*, 2001. 61(18): p. 6885-91.

[563] Rijntjes, M. and C. Weiller, Recovery of motor and language abilities after stroke: the contribution of functional imaging. *Prog Neurobiol*, 2002. 66(2): p. 109-22.

[564] Ringertz, N., Grading of gliomas. *Acta Pathol Microbiol Scand*, 1950. 27(1): p. 51-64.

[565] Roberts, H.C., et al., Quantitative measurement of microvascular permeability in human brain tumors achieved using dynamic contrast-enhanced MR imaging: correlation with histologic grade. *AJNR Am J Neuroradiol*, 2000. 21(5): p. 891-9.

[566] Rock, J.P., et al., Correlations between magnetic resonance spectroscopy and image-guided histopathology, with special attention to radiation necrosis. *Neurosurgery*, 2002. 51(4): p. 912-9; discussion 919-20.

[567] Roelcke, U., et al., Operated low grade astrocytomas: a long term PET study on the effect of radiotherapy. *J Neurol Neurosurg Psychiatry*, 1999. 66(5): p. 644-7.

[568] Ross, D.W., Cancer: the emerging molecular biology. *Hosp Pract (Off Ed)*, 2000. 35(1): p. 63-4, 67-74.

[569] Rossini, P.M., et al., Post-stroke plastic reorganisation in the adult brain. *Lancet Neurol*, 2003. 2(8): p. 493-502.

[570] Rostomily, R.C., G.E. Keles, and M.S. Berger, Radical surgery in the management of low-grade and high-grade gliomas. *Baillieres Clin Neurol*, 1996. 5(2): p. 345-69.

[571] Roszman, T., L. Elliott, and W. Brooks, Modulation of T-cell function by gliomas. *Immunol Today*, 1991. 12(10): p. 370-4.

[572] Roux, F.E., et al., Writing, calculating, and finger recognition in the region of the angular gyrus: a cortical stimulation study of Gerstmann syndrome. *J Neurosurg*, 2003. 99(4): p. 716-27.

[573] Roux, F.E., et al., Functional MRI and intraoperative brain mapping to evaluate brain plasticity in patients with brain tumours and hemiparesis. *J Neurol Neurosurg Psychiatry*, 2000. 69(4): p. 453-63.

[574] Roux, F.E., et al., Intra-operative mapping of cortical areas involved in reading in mono- and bilingual patients. *Brain*, 2004. 127(Pt 8): p. 1796-810.

[575] Roux, F.E. and M. Tremoulet, Organization of language areas in bilingual patients: a cortical stimulation study. *J Neurosurg*, 2002. 97(4): p. 857-64.

[576] Rubinstein, L.J., Presidential address. Cytogenesis and differentiation of primitive central neuroepithelial tumors. *J Neuropathol Exp Neurol*, 1972. 31(1): p. 7-26.

[577] Rushmore, T.H. and A.N. Kong, Pharmacogenomics, regulation and signaling pathways of phase I and II drug metabolizing enzymes. *Curr Drug Metab*, 2002. 3(5): p. 481-90.

[578] Sabatier, J., et al., Characterization of choline compounds with in vitro 1H magnetic resonance spectroscopy for the discrimination of primary brain tumors. *Invest Radiol*, 1999. 34(3): p. 230-5.

[579] Salcman, M., Radical surgery for low-grade glioma. *Clin Neurosurg*, 1990. 36: p. 353-66.

[580] Sallinen, P.K., et al., Prognostication of astrocytoma patient survival by Ki-67 (MIB-1), PCNA, and S-phase fraction using archival paraffin-embedded samples. *J Pathol*, 1994. 174(4): p. 275-82.

[581] Sallinen, S.L., et al., Identification of differentially expressed genes in human gliomas by DNA microarray and tissue chip techniques. *Cancer Res*, 2000. 60(23): p. 6617-22.

[582] Salmon, I., et al., Prognostic scoring in adult astrocytic tumors using patient age, histopathological grade, and DNA histogram type. *J Neurosurg*, 1994. 80(5): p. 877-83.

[583] Salmon, I., et al., Histopathologic grading and DNA ploidy in relation to survival among 206 adult astrocytic tumor patients. *Cancer*, 1992. 70(2): p. 538-46.

[584] Salvati, M., et al., A report on radiation-induced gliomas. *Cancer*, 1991. 67(2): p. 392-7.

[585] Samoto, K., et al., Expression of vascular endothelial growth factor and its possible relation with neovascularization in human brain tumors. *Cancer Res*, 1995. 55(5): p. 1189-93.

[586] Sanai, N., A. Alvarez-Buylla, and M.S. Berger, Neural stem cells and the origin of gliomas. *N Engl J Med*, 2005. 353(8): p. 811-22.

[587] Sander, L.M. and T.S. Deisboeck, Growth patterns of microscopic brain tumors. *Phys Rev E Stat Nonlin Soft Matter Phys*, 2002. 66(5 Pt 1): p. 051901.

[588] Sanson, M., J. Thillet, and K. Hoang-Xuan, Molecular changes in gliomas. *Curr Opin Oncol*, 2004. 16(6): p. 607-13.

[589] Sarang, A. and J. Dinsmore, Anaesthesia for awake craniotomy--evolution of a technique that facilitates awake neurological testing. *Br J Anaesth*, 2003. 90(2): p. 161-5.

[590] Sasaki, H., et al., Histopathological-molecular genetic correlations in referral pathologist-diagnosed low-grade "oligodendroglioma". *J Neuropathol Exp Neurol*, 2002. 61(1): p. 58-63.

[591] Scerrati, M., et al., Prognostic factors in low grade (WHO grade II) gliomas of the cerebral hemispheres: the role of surgery. *J Neurol Neurosurg Psychiatry*, 1996. 61(3): p. 291-6.

[592] Schaller, B., Usefulness of positron emission tomography in diagnosis and treatment follow-up of brain tumors. *Neurobiol Dis*, 2004. 15(3): p. 437-48.

[593] Scheibel, R.S., C.A. Meyers, and V.A. Levin, Cognitive dysfunction following surgery for intracerebral glioma: influence of histopathology, lesion location, and treatment. *J Neurooncol*, 1996. 30(1): p. 61-9.

[594] Schiffbauer, H., et al., Functional activity within brain tumors: a magnetic source imaging study. *Neurosurgery*, 2001. 49(6): p. 1313-20; discussion 1320-1.

[595] Schiffer, D., et al., Proliferative activity and prognosis of low-grade astrocytomas. *J Neurooncol*, 1997. 34(1): p. 31-5.

[596] Schiffer, D., et al., Prognostic value of histologic factors in adult cerebral astrocytoma. Cancer, 1988. 61(7): p. 1386-93.

[597] Schiffer, D., et al., Prognostic factors in oligodendroglioma. *Can J Neurol Sci*, 1997. 24(4): p. 313-9.

[598] Schiffer, D., et al., Role of apoptosis in the prognosis of oligodendrogliomas. *Neurochem Int*, 1997. 31(2): p. 245-50.

[599] Schmidt, E.E., et al., Mutational profile of the PTEN gene in primary human astrocytic tumors and cultivated xenografts. *J Neuropathol Exp Neurol*, 1999. 58(11): p. 1170-83.

[600] Schmidt, M.H., et al., Repeated operations for infiltrative low-grade gliomas without intervening therapy. *J Neurosurg*, 2003. 98(6): p. 1165-9

[601] Schroder, R., et al., The relationship between Ki-67 labeling and mitotic index in gliomas and meningiomas: demonstration of the variability of the intermitotic cycle time. *Acta Neuropathol (Berl)*, 1991. 82(5): p. 389-94.

[602] Seitz, R.J., et al., Large-scale plasticity of the human motor cortex. *Neuroreport*, 1995. 6(5): p. 742-4.

[603] Senger, D.L., et al., Suppression of Rac activity induces apoptosis of human glioma cells but not normal human astrocytes. *Cancer Res*, 2002. 62(7): p. 2131-40.

[604] Shackney, S.E., et al., Model for the genetic evolution of human solid tumors. *Cancer Res*, 1989. 49(12): p. 3344-54.

[605] Shai, R., et al., Gene expression profiling identifies molecular subtypes of gliomas. *Oncogene*, 2003. 22(31): p. 4918-23.

[606] Shankar, A. and V. Rajshekhar, Radiological and clinical outcome following stereotactic biopsy and radiotherapy for low-grade insular astrocytomas. *Neurol India*, 2003. 51(4): p. 503-6.

[607] Shaw, E., et al., Prospective randomized trial of low- versus high-dose radiation therapy in adults with supratentorial low-grade glioma: initial report of a North Central Cancer Treatment Group/Radiation Therapy Oncology Group/Eastern Cooperative Oncology Group study. *J Clin Oncol*, 2002. 20(9): p. 2267-76.

[608] Shaw, E.G., Role of radiation therapy in the management of low-grade gliomas. *Ann Neurol*, 1992. 32(6): p. 835.

[609] Shaw, E.G., et al., Radiation therapy in the management of low-grade supratentorial astrocytomas. *J Neurosurg*, 1989. 70(6): p. 853-61.

[610] Shaw, E.G., B.W. Scheithauer, and J.R. O'Fallon, Supratentorial gliomas: a comparative study by grade and histologic type. *J Neurooncol*, 1997. 31(3): p. 273-8.

[611] Shaw, E.G., et al., Mixed oligoastrocytomas: a survival and prognostic factor analysis. *Neurosurgery*, 1994. 34(4): p. 577-82; discussion 582.

[612] Shaw, E.G. and J.H. Wisoff, Prospective clinical trials of intracranial low-grade glioma in adults and children. *Neuro-oncol*, 2003. 5(3): p. 153-60.

[613] Shaw, E., et al., Prospective randomized trial of low- versus high-dose radiation therapy in adults with supratentorial low-grade glioma: initial report of a North Central Cancer Treatment Group/Radiation Therapy Oncology Group/Eastern Cooperative Oncology Group study. *J Clin Oncol*, 2002. 20(9): p. 2267-76

[614] Shibamoto, Y., et al., Supratentorial low-grade astrocytoma. Correlation of computed tomography findings with effect of radiation therapy and prognostic variables. *Cancer*, 1993. 72(1): p. 190-5.

[615] Shibata, T., P.C. Burger, and P. Kleihues, [Cell kinetics of oligodendroglioma and oligo-astrocytoma--Ki-67 PaP study]. *No To Shinkei*, 1988. 40(8): p. 779-85.

[616] Shields, A.F., et al., Imaging proliferation in vivo with [F-18]FLT and positron emission tomography. *Nat Med*, 1998. 4(11): p. 1334-6.

[617] Shimizu, H., et al., Correlation between choline level measured by proton MR spectroscopy and Ki-67 labeling index in gliomas. *AJNR Am J Neuroradiol*, 2000. 21(4): p. 659-65.

[618] Shinoda, J., et al., Prognostic factors in supratentorial WHO grade II astrocytoma in adults. *Neuroradiology*, 1998. 12(4): p. 318-24.

[619] Shinoura, N., et al., Brain tumors: detection with C-11 choline PET. *Radiology*, 1997. 202(2): p. 497-503.

[620] Shiras, A., et al., A unique model system for tumor progression in GBM comprising two developed human neuro-epithelial cell lines with differential transforming potential and coexpressing neuronal and glial markers. *Neoplasia*, 2003. 5(6): p. 520-32.

[621] Shuman, W.P., et al., The utility of MR in planning the radiation therapy of oligodendroglioma. *AJR Am J Roentgenol*, 1987. 148(3): p. 595-600.

[622] Shweiki, D., et al., Vascular endothelial growth factor induced by hypoxia may mediate hypoxia-initiated angiogenesis. *Nature*, 1992. 359(6398): p. 843-5.

[623] Sidransky, D., et al., Clonal expansion of p53 mutant cells is associated with brain tumour progression. *Nature*, 1992. 355(6363): p. 846-7.

[624] Signorelli, F., The value of cortical stimulation applied to the surgery of malignant gliomas in language areas. *Neurol Sci*, 2001. 22(3): p. 217-8.

[625] Signorelli, F., et al., Intraoperative electrical stimulation mapping as an aid for surgery of intracranial lesions involving motor areas in children. *Childs Nerv Syst*, 2004. 20(6): p. 420-6.

[626] Silber, J.R., et al., O6-methylguanine-DNA methyltransferase activity in adult gliomas: relation to patient and tumor characteristics. *Cancer Res*, 1998. 58(5): p. 1068-73.

[627] Silbergeld, D.L. and M.R. Chicoine, Isolation and characterization of human malignant glioma cells from histologically normal brain. *J Neurosurg*, 1997. 86(3): p. 525-31.

[628] Silverman, C. and J.E. Marks, Prognostic significance of contrast enhancement in low-grade astrocytomas of the adult cerebrum. *Radiology*, 1981. 139(1): p. 211-3.

[629] Simeoni, M., et al., Predictive pharmacokinetic-pharmacodynamic modeling of tumor growth kinetics in xenograft models after administration of anticancer agents. *Cancer Res*, 2004. 64(3): p. 1094-101.

[630] Simon, M., et al., Functional evidence for a role of combined CDKN2A (p16-p14(ARF))/CDKN2B (p15) gene inactivation in malignant gliomas. *Acta Neuropathol (Berl)*, 1999. 98(5): p. 444-52.

[631] Singh, S.K., et al., Cancer stem cells in nervous system tumors. *Oncogene*, 2004. 23(43): p. 7267-73.

[632] Singh, S.K., et al., Identification of a cancer stem cell in human brain tumors. *Cancer Res*, 2003. 63(18): p. 5821-8.

[633] Singh, S.K., et al., Identification of human brain tumour initiating cells. *Nature*, 2004. 432(7015): p. 396-401.

[634] Skirboll, S.S., et al., Functional cortex and subcortical white matter located within gliomas. *Neurosurgery*, 1996. 38(4): p. 678-84; discussion 684-5.

[635] Smith, D.F., et al., The prognosis of primary intracerebral tumours presenting with epilepsy: the outcome of medical and surgical management. *J Neurol Neurosurg Psychiatry*, 1991. 54(10): p. 915-20.

[636] Smith, J.S., et al., Alterations of chromosome arms 1p and 19q as predictors of survival in oligodendrogliomas, astrocytomas, and mixed oligoastrocytomas. *J Clin Oncol*, 2000. 18(3): p. 636-45.

[637] Soffietti, R., et al., Prognostic factors in well-differentiated cerebral astrocytomas in the adult. *Neurosurgery*, 1989. 24(5): p. 686-92.

[638] Soffietti, R., et al., PCV chemotherapy for recurrent oligodendrogliomas and oligoastrocytomas. *Neurosurgery*, 1998. 43(5): p. 1066-73.

[639] Sonoda, Y., et al., Formation of intracranial tumors by genetically modified human astrocytes defines four pathways critical in the development of human anaplastic astrocytoma. *Cancer Res*, 2001. 61(13): p. 4956-60.

[640] Sontheimer, H., Ion channels and amino acid transporters support the growth and invasion of primary brain tumors. *Mol Neurobiol*, 2004. 29(1): p. 61-71.

[641] Soricelli, A., et al., Technetium-99m-tetrofosmin uptake in brain tumors by SPECT: comparison with thallium-201 imaging. *J Nucl Med*, 1998. 39(5): p. 802-6.

[642] St Croix, B. and R.S. Kerbel, Cell adhesion and drug resistance in cancer. *Curr Opin Oncol*, 1997. 9(6): p. 549-56.

[643] Staudenherz, A., et al., Does (99m)Tc-Sestamibi in high-grade malignant brain tumors reflect blood-brain barrier damage only? *Neuroimage*, 2000. 12(1): p. 109-11.

[644] Staunton, J.E., et al., Chemosensitivity prediction by transcriptional profiling. *Proc Natl Acad Sci U S A*, 2001. 98(19): p. 10787-92.

[645] Stege, E.M., et al., Successful treatment of low-grade oligodendroglial tumors with a chemotherapy regimen of procarbazine, lomustine, and vincristine. *Cancer*, 2005. 103(4): p. 802-9.

[646] Stein, W.D., S.E. Bates, and T. Fojo, Intractable cancers: the many faces of multidrug resistance and the many targets it presents for therapeutic attack. *Curr Drug Targets*, 2004. 5(4): p. 333-46.

[647] Stoica, G., et al., Morphology, immunohistochemistry, and genetic alterations in dog astrocytomas. *Vet Pathol*, 2004. 41(1): p. 10-9.

[648] Stosic-Opincal, T., et al., [FLAIR MR sequence in the diagnosis and follow-up of low-grade astrocytomas]. *Vojnosanit Pregl*, 2005. 62(7-8): p. 525-8.

[649] Struikmans, H., et al., Prognostic relevance of MIB-1 immunoreactivity, S-phase fraction, 5-bromo-2'-deoxyuridine labeling indices, and mitotic figures in gliomas. *Radiat Oncol Investig*, 1999. 7(4): p. 243-8.

[650] Struikmans, H., et al., S-phase fraction, 5-bromo-2'-deoxy-uridine labelling index, duration of S-phase, potential doubling time, and DNA index in benign and malignant brain tumors. *Radiat Oncol Investig*, 1997. 5(4): p. 170-9.

[651] Stupp, R., et al., Prognostic factors for low-grade gliomas. *Semin Oncol*, 2003. 30(6 Suppl 19): p. 23-8.

[652] Suess, O., et al., A new cortical electrode for neuronavigation-guided intraoperative neurophysiological monitoring: technical note. *Acta Neurochir (Wien)*, 2000. 142(3): p. 329-32.

[653] Sugahara, T., et al., Correlation of MR imaging-determined cerebral blood volume maps with histologic and angiographic determination of vascularity of gliomas. *AJR Am J Roentgenol*, 1998. 171(6): p. 1479-86.

[654] Sugahara, T., et al., Usefulness of diffusion-weighted MRI with echo-planar technique in the evaluation of cellularity in gliomas. *J Magn Reson Imaging*, 1999. 9(1): p. 53-60.

[655] Sun, J.Y., et al., [Bioinformatic analysis of glioma development relative genes]. *Ai Zheng*, 2003. 22(3): p. 225-9.

[656] Sun, Y.H., et al., [Relationship between the expression of O6-methylguanine-DNA methyltransferase in glioma and the survival time of patients]. *Ai Zheng*, 2004. 23(9): p. 1052-5.

[657] Surawicz, T.S., et al., Descriptive epidemiology of primary brain and CNS tumors: results from the Central Brain Tumor Registry of the United States, 1990-1994. *Neuro-oncol*, 1999. 1(1): p. 14-25.

[658] Surma-aho, O., et al., Adverse long-term effects of brain radiotherapy in adult low-grade glioma patients. *Neurology*, 2001. 56(10): p. 1285-90.

[659] Swanson, K.R., E.C. Alvord, Jr., and J.D. Murray, A quantitative model for differential motility of gliomas in grey and white matter. *Cell Prolif*, 2000. 33(5): p. 317-29.

[660] Swanson, K.R., E.C. Alvord, Jr., and J.D. Murray, Virtual brain tumours (gliomas) enhance the reality of medical imaging and highlight inadequacies of current therapy. *Br J Cancer*, 2002. 86(1): p. 14-8.

[661] Swanson, K.R., E.C. Alvord, Jr., and J.D. Murray, Quantifying efficacy of chemotherapy of brain tumors with homogeneous and heterogeneous drug delivery. *Acta Biotheor*, 2002. 50(4): p. 223-37.

[662] Swanson, K.R., et al., Virtual and real brain tumors: using mathematical modeling to quantify glioma growth and invasion. *J Neurol Sci*, 2003. 216(1): p. 1-10.

[663] Swennen, M.H., et al., Delayed radiation toxicity after focal or whole brain radiotherapy for low-grade glioma. *J Neurooncol*, 2004. 66(3): p. 333-9.

[664] Szybka, M., et al., Microsatellite instability and expression of DNA mismatch repair genes in malignant astrocytic tumors from adult and pediatric patients. *Clin Neuropathol*, 2003. 22(4): p. 180-6.

[665] Tai, I.T., et al., Genome-wide expression analysis of therapy-resistant tumors reveals SPARC as a novel target for cancer therapy. *J Clin Invest*, 2005. 115(6): p. 1492-502.

[666] Taillandier, L., L. Antunes, and K.S. Angioi-Duprez, Models for *Neuro-oncol*ogical preclinical studies: solid orthotopic and heterotopic grafts of human gliomas into nude mice. *J Neurosci Methods*, 2003. 125(1-2): p. 147-57.

[667] Tanaka, S., et al., Drug-resistance gene expression and progression of astrocytic tumors. *Brain Tumor Pathol*, 2001. 18(2): p. 131-7.

[668] Taniguchi, M., et al., Cerebral motor control in patients with gliomas around the central sulcus studied with spatially filtered magnetoencephalography. *J Neurol Neurosurg Psychiatry*, 2004. 75(3): p. 466-71.

[669] Taphoorn, M.J., Neurocognitive sequelae in the treatment of low-grade gliomas. *Semin Oncol*, 2003. 30(6 Suppl 19): p. 45-8.

[670] Taphoorn, M.J., et al., Assessment of quality of life in patients treated for low-grade glioma: a preliminary report. *J Neurol Neurosurg Psychiatry*, 1992. 55(5): p. 372-6.

[671] Taphoorn, M.J. and M. Klein, Cognitive deficits in adult patients with brain tumours. *Lancet Neurol*, 2004. 3(3): p. 159-68.

[672] Taphoorn, M.J., et al., Cognitive functions and quality of life in patients with low-grade gliomas: the impact of radiotherapy. *Ann Neurol*, 1994. 36(1): p. 48-54.

[673] Tate, A.R., et al., Towards a method for automated classification of 1H MRS spectra from brain tumours. *NMR Biomed*, 1998. 11(4-5): p. 177-91.

[674] Taylor, M.D. and M. Bernstein, Awake craniotomy with brain mapping as the routine surgical approach to treating patients with supratentorial intraaxial tumors: a prospective trial of 200 cases. *J Neurosurg*, 1999. 90(1): p. 35-41.

[675] Tedeschi, G., et al., Increased choline signal coinciding with malignant degeneration of cerebral gliomas: a serial proton magnetic resonance spectroscopy imaging study. *J Neurosurg*, 1997. 87(4): p. 516-24.

[676] Thiel, A., et al., Plasticity of language networks in patients with brain tumors: a positron emission tomography activation study. *Ann Neurol*, 2001. 50(5): p. 620-9.

[677] Thirumala, P., D.B. Hier, and P. Patel, Motor recovery after stroke: lessons from functional brain imaging. *Neurol Res*, 2002. 24(5): p. 453-8.

[678] Thomas, L.B., M.A. Gates, and D.A. Steindler, Young neurons from the adult subependymal zone proliferate and migrate along an astrocyte, extracellular matrix-rich pathway. *Glia*, 1996. 17(1): p. 1-14.

[679] Thompson, W.D., et al., Tumours acquire their vasculature by vessel incorporation, not vessel ingrowth. *J Pathol*, 1987. 151(4): p. 323-32.

[680] Thorsen, F. and B.B. Tysnes, Brain tumor cell invasion, anatomical and biological considerations. *AntiCancer Res*, 1997. 17(6B): p. 4121-6.

[681] Tihan, T., et al., Practical value of Ki-67 and p53 labeling indexes in stereotactic biopsies of diffuse and pilocytic astrocytomas. *Arch Pathol Lab Med*, 2000. 124(1): p. 108-13.

[682] Tihan, T., et al., Definition and Diagnostic Implications of Gemistocytic Astrocytomas: a Pathological Perspective. *J Neurooncol*, 2005.

[683] Tong, C.Y., et al., Molecular genetic analysis of non-astrocytic gliomas. *Histopathology*, 1999. 34(4): p. 331-41.

[684] Tonn, J.C. and R. Goldbrunner, Mechanisms of glioma cell invasion. *Acta Neurochir Suppl*, 2003. 88: p. 163-7.

[685] Torp, S.H., Diagnostic and prognostic role of Ki67 immunostaining in human astrocytomas using four different antibodies. *Clin Neuropathol*, 2002. 21(6): p. 252-7.

[686] Torres, I.J., et al., A longitudinal neuropsychological study of partial brain radiation in adults with brain tumors. *Neurology*, 2003. 60(7): p. 1113-8.

[687] Torres-Roca, J.F., et al., Prediction of radiation sensitivity using a gene expression classifier. *Cancer Res*, 2005. 65(16): p. 7169-76.

[688] Touboul, E., et al., Radiation therapy with or without surgery in the management of low-grade brain astrocytomas. A retrospective study of 120 patients. *Bull Cancer Radiother*, 1995. 82(4): p. 388-95.

[689] Tracqui, P., et al., A mathematical model of glioma growth: the effect of chemotherapy on spatio-temporal growth. *Cell Prolif*, 1995. 28(1): p. 17-31.

[690] Trepel, M., et al., Chemosensitivity of human malignant glioma: modulation by p53 gene transfer. *J Neurooncol*, 1998. 39(1): p. 19-32.

[691] Trouillas, P., et al., [Epidemiological study of primary tumors of the neuraxis in the Rhone-Alps region. Quantitative data on the etiology and geographical distribution of 1670 tumors]. *Rev Neurol (Paris)*, 1975. 131(10): p. 691-708.

[692] Tsai, J.C., C.K. Goldman, and G.Y. Gillespie, Vascular endothelial growth factor in human glioma cell lines: induced secretion by EGF, PDGF-BB, and bFGF. *J Neurosurg*, 1995. 82(5): p. 864-73.

[693] Tsatas, D. and A.H. Kaye, The role of the plasminogen activation cascade in glioma cell invasion: a review. *J Clin Neurosci*, 2003. 10(2): p. 139-45.

[694] Tsuboi, K., et al., Regrowth patterns of supratentorial gliomas: estimation from computed tomographic scans. *Neurosurgery*, 1986. 19(6): p. 946-51.

[695] Tubiana, M., [Kinetics of cell proliferation in tumors. Significance of the preclinical period]. Rev Prat, 1980. 30(5): p. 173-8, 183-6.

[696] Tucha, O., et al., Cognitive deficits before treatment among patients with brain tumors. *Neurosurgery*, 2000. 47(2): p. 324-33; discussion 333-4.

[697] Turner, S., et al., From a discrete to a continuous model of biological cell movement. *Phys Rev E Stat Nonlin Soft Matter Phys*, 2004. 69(2 Pt 1): p. 021910.

[698] Ueki, K., et al., Correlation of histology and molecular genetic analysis of 1p, 19q, 10q, TP53, EGFR, CDK4, and CDKN2A in 91 astrocytic and oligodendroglial tumors. *Clin Cancer Res*, 2002. 8(1): p. 196-201.

[699] Uhm, J.H., et al., Mechanisms of glioma invasion: role of matrix-metalloproteinases. *Can J Neurol Sci*, 1997. 24(1): p. 3-15.

[700] Uhrbom, L., et al., Ink4a-Arf loss cooperates with KRas activation in astrocytes and neural progenitors to generate glioblastomas of various morphologies depending on activated Akt. *Cancer Res*, 2002. 62(19): p. 5551-8.

[701] Uhrbom, L. and E.C. Holland, Modeling gliomagenesis with somatic cell gene transfer using retroviral vectors. *J Neurooncol*, 2001. 53(3): p. 297-305.

[702] Ulmer, J.L., et al., Lesion-induced pseudo-dominance at functional magnetic resonance imaging: implications for preoperative assessments. *Neurosurgery*, 2004. 55(3): p. 569-79; discussion 580-1.

[703] Urenjak, J., et al., Proton nuclear magnetic resonance spectroscopy unambiguously identifies different neural cell types. *J Neurosci*, 1993. 13(3): p. 981-9.

[704] Utriainen, M., et al., Evaluation of brain tumor metabolism with [11C]choline PET and 1H-MRS. *J Neurooncol*, 2003. 62(3): p. 329-38.

[705] Van de Kelft, E., Molecular pathogenesis of astrocytoma and glioblastoma multiforme. *Acta Neurochir (Wien)*, 1997. 139(7): p. 589-99.

[706] van den Bent, M.J., et al., Long-term efficacy of early versus delayed radiotherapy for low-grade astrocytoma and oligodendroglioma in adults: the EORTC 22845 randomised trial. *Lancet*, 2005. 366(9490): p. 985-90.

[707] van den Bent, M.J., et al., Chromosomal anomalies in oligodendroglial tumors are correlated with clinical features. *Cancer*, 2003. 97(5): p. 1276-84.

[708] van den Bent, M.J., et al., Current and future trials of the EORTC brain tumor group. *Onkologie*, 2004. 27(3): p. 246-50.

[709] van den Boom, J., et al., Characterization of gene expression profiles associated with glioma progression using oligonucleotide-based microarray analysis and real-time reverse transcription-polymerase chain reaction. *Am J Pathol*, 2003. 163(3): p. 1033-43.

[710] van Kampen, M., et al., Low-grade astrocytoma: treatment with conventionally fractionated stereotactic radiation therapy. *Radiology*, 1996. 201(1): p. 275-8.

[711] Van Meir, E.G., et al., Release of an inhibitor of angiogenesis upon induction of wild type p53 expression in glioblastoma cells. *Nat Genet*, 1994. 8(2): p. 171-6.

[712] van Meyel, D.J., et al., p53 mutation, expression, and DNA ploidy in evolving gliomas: evidence for two pathways of progression. *J Natl Cancer Inst*, 1994. 86(13): p. 1011-7.

[713] van Veelen, M.L., et al., Supratentorial low grade astrocytoma: prognostic factors, dedifferentiation, and the issue of early versus late surgery. *J Neurol Neurosurg Psychiatry*, 1998. 64(5): p. 581-7.

[714] VanMeter, T.E., et al., The role of matrix metalloproteinase genes in glioma invasion: co-dependent and interactive proteolysis. *J Neurooncol*, 2001. 53(2): p. 213-35.

[715] Varela, M., et al., EGF-R and PDGF-R, but not bcl-2, overexpression predict overall survival in patients with low-grade astrocytomas. *J Surg Oncol*, 2004. 86(1): p. 34-40.

[716] Varlet, P., et al., Vascular endothelial growth factor expression in oligodendrogliomas: a correlative study with Sainte-Anne malignancy grade, growth fraction and patient survival. *Neuropathol Appl Neurobiol*, 2000. 26(4): p. 379-89.

[717] Vavruch, L., et al., Prognostic value of flow cytometry and correlation to some conventional prognostic factors: a retrospective study of archival specimens of 134 astrocytomas. *J Neurosurg*, 1996. 85(1): p. 146-51.

[718] Vertosick, F.T., Jr., R.G. Selker, and V.C. Arena, Survival of patients with well-differentiated astrocytomas diagnosed in the era of computed tomography. *Neurosurgery*, 1991. 28(4): p. 496-501.

[719] Vigliani, M.C., et al., A prospective study of cognitive functions following conventional radiotherapy for supratentorial gliomas in young adults: 4-year results. *Int J Radiat Oncol Biol Phys*, 1996. 35(3): p. 527-33.

[720] Viktorsson, K., R. Lewensohn, and B. Zhivotovsky, Apoptotic pathways and therapy resistance in human malignancies. *Adv Cancer Res*, 2005. 94: p. 143-96.

[721] Visted, T., et al., Mechanisms of tumor cell invasion and angiogenesis in the central nervous system. *Front Biosci*, 2003. 8: p. e289-304.

[722] Vogel, T.W., et al., Proteins and protein pattern differences between glioma cell lines and glioblastoma multiforme. *Clin Cancer Res*, 2005. 11(10): p. 3624-32.

[723] Voges, J., et al., 11C-methionine and 18F-2-fluorodeoxyglucose positron emission tomography: a tool for diagnosis of cerebral glioma and monitoring after brachytherapy with 125I seeds. *Stereotact Funct Neurosurg*, 1997. 69(1-4 Pt 2): p. 129-35.

[724] von Deimling, A., et al., Deletions on the long arm of chromosome 17 in pilocytic astrocytoma. *Acta Neuropathol (Berl)*, 1993. 86(1): p. 81-5.

[725] von Deimling, A., et al., Evidence for a tumor suppressor gene on chromosome 19q associated with human astrocytomas, oligodendrogliomas, and mixed gliomas. *Cancer Res*, 1992. 52(15): p. 4277-9.

[726] von Deimling, A., D.N. Louis, and O.D. Wiestler, Molecular pathways in the formation of gliomas. *Glia*, 1995. 15(3): p. 328-38.

[727] Vonofakos, D., H. Marcu, and H. Hacker, Oligodendrogliomas: CT patterns with emphasis on features indicating malignancy. *J Comput Assist Tomogr*, 1979. 3(6): p. 783-8.

[728] Wacker, M.R., et al., The prognostic implications of histologic classification and bromodeoxyuridine labeling index of mixed gliomas. *J Neurooncol*, 1994. 19(2): p. 113-22.

[729] Wagner, W., et al., Infrared-based neuronavigation and cortical motor stimulation in the management of central-region tumors. *Stereotact Funct Neurosurg*, 1997. 68(1-4 Pt 1): p. 112-6.

[730] Walker, C., et al., Phenotype versus genotype in gliomas displaying inter- or intratumoral histological heterogeneity. *Clin Cancer Res*, 2003. 9(13): p. 4841-51.

[731] Walker, C., et al., Characterisation of molecular alterations in microdissected archival gliomas. *Acta Neuropathol (Berl)*, 2001. 101(4): p. 321-33.

[732] Walker, D.G. and A.H. Kaye, Low grade glial neoplasms. *J Clin Neurosci*, 2003. 10(1): p. 1-13.

[733] Wallqvist, A., et al., Establishing connections between microarray expression data and chemotherapeutic cancer pharmacology. *Mol Cancer Ther*, 2002. 1(5): p. 311-20.

[734] Walsh, A.R., R.H. Schmidt, and H.T. Marsh, Cortical mapping and resection under local anaesthetic as an aid to surgery of low and intermediate grade gliomas. *Neuroradiology*, 1990. 4(6): p. 485-91.

[735] Wara, W.M., Radiation therapy for brain tumors. *Cancer*, 1985. 55(9 Suppl): p. 2291-5.

[736] Watanabe, K., et al., p53 and PTEN gene mutations in gemistocytic astrocytomas. *Acta Neuropathol (Berl)*, 1998. 95(6): p. 559-64.

[737] Watanabe, K., et al., Incidence and timing of p53 mutations during astrocytoma progression in patients with multiple biopsies. *Clin Cancer Res*, 1997. 3(4): p. 523-30.

[738] Watanabe, K., et al., Role of gemistocytes in astrocytoma progression. *Lab Invest*, 1997. 76(2): p. 277-84.

[739] Watanabe, T., et al., Phenotype versus genotype correlation in oligodendrogliomas and low-grade diffuse astrocytomas. *Acta Neuropathol (Berl)*, 2002. 103(3): p. 267-75.

[740] Watson, M.A., et al., Gene expression profiling with oligonucleotide microarrays distinguishes World Health Organization grade of oligodendrogliomas. *Cancer Res*, 2001. 61(5): p. 1825-9.

[741] Weber, W.A., et al., Correlation between postoperative 3-[(123)I]iodo-L-alpha-methyltyrosine uptake and survival in patients with gliomas. *J Nucl Med*, 2001. 42(8): p. 1144-50.

[742] Wechsler-Reya, R. and M.P. Scott, The developmental biology of brain tumors. *Annu Rev Neurosci*, 2001. 24: p. 385-428.

[743] Weiss, W.A., et al., Genetic determinants of malignancy in a mouse model for oligodendroglioma. *Cancer Res*, 2003. 63(7): p. 1589-95.

[744] Weller, M. and A. Fontana, The failure of current immunotherapy for malignant glioma. Tumor-derived TGF-beta, T-cell apoptosis, and the immune privilege of the brain. *Brain Res Brain Res Rev*, 1995. 21(2): p. 128-51.

[745] Wesseling, P., D.J. Ruiter, and P.C. Burger, Angiogenesis in brain tumors; pathobiological and clinical aspects. *J Neurooncol*, 1997. 32(3): p. 253-65.

[746] Wesseling, P., et al., Early and extensive contribution of pericytes/vascular smooth muscle cells to microvascular proliferation in glioblastoma multiforme: an immuno-light and immuno-electron microscopic study. *J Neuropathol Exp Neurol*, 1995. 54(3): p. 304-10.

[747] Wessels, P.H., et al., Supratentorial grade II astrocytoma: biological features and clinical course. *Lancet Neurol*, 2003. 2(7): p. 395-403.

[748] Westergaard, L., F. Gjerris, and L. Klinken, Prognostic parameters in benign astrocytomas. *Acta Neurochir (Wien)*, 1993. 123(1-2): p. 1-7.

[749] Whittle, I.R., The dilemma of low grade glioma. *J Neurol Neurosurg Psychiatry*, 2004. 75 Suppl 2: p. ii31-6.

[750] Whittle, I.R. and A. Beaumont, Seizures in patients with supratentorial oligodendroglial tumours. Clinicopathological features and management considerations. *Acta Neurochir (Wien)*, 1995. 135(1-2): p. 19-24.

[751] Whittle, I.R., S. Borthwick, and N. Haq, Brain dysfunction following 'awake' craniotomy, brain mapping and resection of glioma. *Neuroradiology*, 2003. 17(2): p. 130-7.

[752] Whitton, A.C. and H.J. Bloom, Low grade glioma of the cerebral hemispheres in adults: a retrospective analysis of 88 cases. *Int J Radiat Oncol Biol Phys*, 1990. 18(4): p. 783-6.

[753] Winger, M.J., D.R. Macdonald, and J.G. Cairncross, Supratentorial anaplastic gliomas in adults. The prognostic importance of extent of resection and prior low-grade glioma. *J Neurosurg*, 1989. 71(4): p. 487-93.

[754] Woodward, D.E., et al., A mathematical model of glioma growth: the effect of extent of surgical resection. *Cell Prolif*, 1996. 29(6): p. 269-88.

[755] Wunderlich, G., et al., Precentral glioma location determines the displacement of cortical hand representation. *Neurosurgery*, 1998. 42(1): p. 18-26; discussion 26-7.

[756] Xu, X.L. and Y.B. Ling, A study on the expectational model for tumor growth. *Int J Biomed Comput*, 1988. 22(2): p. 135-41.

[757] Xue, D. and R.E. Albright, Jr., Preoperative anaplastic glioma tumor volume effects on patient survival. *J Surg Oncol*, 1999. 72(4): p. 199-205.

[758] Xue, D. and R.E. Albright, Jr., Microcomputer-based technique for 3-D reconstruction and volume measurement of computed tomographic images. Comparison of geometric and planimetry post-operative tumor volume effects on patient survival. *Comput Biol Med*, 1999. 29(6): p. 377-92.

[759] Yamamoto, M., et al., The role of proteolysis in tumor invasiveness in glioblastoma and metastatic brain tumors. *AntiCancer Res*, 2002. 22(6C): p. 4265-8.

[760] Yamashita, T. and T. Kuwabara, Estimation of rate of growth of malignant brain tumors by computed tomography scanning. *Surg Neurol*, 1983. 20(6): p. 464-70.

[761] Yamori, T., Panel of human cancer cell lines provides valuable database for drug discovery and bioinformatics. *Cancer Chemother Pharmacol*, 2003. 52 Suppl 1: p. S74-9.

[762] Yang, D., et al., Cerebral gliomas: prospective comparison of multivoxel 2D chemical-shift imaging proton MR spectroscopy, echoplanar perfusion and diffusion-weighted MRI. *Neuroradiology*, 2002. 44(8): p. 656-66.

[763] Yang, H.J., et al., The significance of gemistocytes in astrocytoma. *Acta Neurochir (Wien)*, 2003. 145(12): p. 1097-103; discussion 1103.

[764] Yeh, S.A., et al., Treatment outcomes and prognostic factors in patients with supratentorial low-grade gliomas. *Br J Radiol*, 2005. 78(927): p. 230-5.

[765] Yingling, C.D., et al., Identification of motor pathways during tumor surgery facilitated by multichannel electromyographic recording. *J Neurosurg*, 1999. 91(6): p. 922-7.

[766] Yokogami, K., et al., Application of SPET using technetium-99m sestamibi in brain tumours and comparison with expression of the MDR-1 gene: is it possible to predict the response to chemotherapy in patients with gliomas by means of 99mTc-sestamibi SPET? *Eur J Nucl Med*, 1998. 25(4): p. 401-9.

[767] Zagzag, D., et al., Vascular apoptosis and involution in gliomas precede neovascularization: a novel concept for glioma growth and angiogenesis. *Lab Invest*, 2000. 80(6): p. 837-49.

[768] Zagzag, D., et al., Molecular events implicated in brain tumor angiogenesis and invasion. *Pediatr Neurosurg*, 2000. 33(1): p. 49-55.

[769] Zembutsu, H., et al., Genome-wide cDNA microarray screening to correlate gene expression profiles with sensitivity of 85 human cancer xenografts to anticancer drugs. *Cancer Res*, 2002. 62(2): p. 518-27.

[770] Zheng, X., S.M. Wise, and V. Cristini, Nonlinear simulation of tumor necrosis, neovascularization and tissue invasion via an adaptive finite-element/level-set method. *Bull Math Biol*, 2005. 67(2): p. 211-59.

[771] Zlatescu, M.C., et al., Tumor location and growth pattern correlate with genetic signature in oligodendroglial neoplasms. *Cancer Res*, 2001. 61(18): p. 6713-5.

ABOUT THE AUTHORS

Luc Taillandier, M.D., Ph.D.
Department of Neurology, CHU Nancy, Hôpital Central
C.O. N°34, 54035 Nancy Cedex, France

Laurent Capelle, M.D. and **Hugues Duffau**, M.D., Ph.D.
Department of Neurosurgery, INSERM U678, Hôpital Salpêtrière,
47-83 Bd de l'hôpital, 75013, Paris, France
Phone : 33 1 42 16 34 28
Fax : 33 1 42 16 34 16
Email : hugues.duffau@psl.ap-hop-paris.fr

INDEX

F

E

G

H

I

Get the eBook FREE!

(PDF, ePub, Kindle, and liveBook all included)

We believe that once you buy a book from us, you should be able to read it in any format we have available. To get electronic versions of this book at no additional cost to you, purchase and then register this book at the Manning website.

Go to https://www.manning.com/freebook and follow the instructions to complete your pBook registration.

That's it!
Thanks from Manning!

Shipping Go

Shipping Go

DEVELOP, DELIVER, DISCUSS, DESIGN, AND GO AGAIN

JOEL HOLMES

MANNING
SHELTER ISLAND

For online information and ordering of this and other Manning books, please visit www.manning.com. The publisher offers discounts on this book when ordered in quantity. For more information, please contact

Special Sales Department
Manning Publications Co.
20 Baldwin Road
PO Box 761
Shelter Island, NY 11964
Email: orders@manning.com

 Manning Publications Co.
20 Baldwin Road
PO Box 761
Shelter Island, NY 11964

Development editor:	Becky Whitney
Technical development editor:	Arthur Zubarev
Review editor:	Adriana Sabo
Production editor:	Andy Marinkovich
Copy editor:	Michele Mitchell
Proofreader:	Melody Dolab
Technical proofreader:	Alex Rios
Typesetter and cover designer:	Marija Tudor

ISBN 9781617299506
Printed in the United States of America

To my wife, Chelsea,
who encourages me to follow my dreams;
and to my sons, Eli and Abel,
for whom all of my dreams exist.

brief contents

contents

vii

preface

I've been thinking for a very long time about writing this book. At the beginning of my software engineering career, I could not have cared less about processes and procedures for getting things done. It all seemed so boring. But given some inspiration from my managers, I started diving into API development, Agile processes, unit testing, continuous delivery, and integration, and I soon found myself drowning in resources, guides, and conference talks.

It wasn't until I read *The Phoenix Project* by Gene Kim, George Spafford, and Kevin Behr that it all clicked. Here was a story about a company struggling to develop and ship quality software products. Where was this book when I started out?! I paired *The Phoenix Project* with *The Pragmatic Programmer,* by Andy Hunt and Dave Thomas, and felt like I had gained a brand-new perspective on my career.

Like all young idealists, I annoyed my colleagues with my newfound knowledge and sense of superiority, only to be brought back to earth by others who showed me where we had already implemented some of the concepts I learned. I interviewed coworkers and those who'd worked in the industry for many years and then used this information, along with books by Martin Fowler and Kent Beck, to help me understand areas where my company could improve.

Soon, I sent write-ups and documents to my bosses and made suggestions during meetings—but there were too many ideas and too little time. Frustrated at my lack of progress internally and with a mountain of research material and sample code piling up, I decided to move onward in my career journey.

It took me landing three additional positions to put many of these ideas into practice and experiment with others. As you'll find out in this book, we developers need to not only deliver on ideas but also reflect on how we can make them better. I found this theme of the continuous feedback loop throughout all the books I read about writing,

testing, and deploying software but never all in one book with examples. When Manning approached me to write this book, it was originally about a completely different topic, and then, over the course of various forms of feedback by editors, reviewers, early purchasers, and industry professionals, we arrived at the book you are now reading. The embodiment of the process described in this book went into making the book (deployments and CI were even used). Even the title was changed several times to nail down the one that best describes what the book is about!

You'll find that I've structured the book in a way that mirrors the complexity that arises with growth. Startups and preliminary projects need to be fast and light to find their market, whereas in the later stages, they need to consider code, architecture, and testing more broadly and at scale, so I focus on describing easy and inexpensive solutions at the beginning and introduce more advanced and complex solutions at the end. I also hope you see that the material I present here is modular. Languages, platforms, and deployment patterns don't matter. What does matter is building a process. To emphasize this, I use many languages and deployment patterns throughout the book.

I chose Go as the primary language because it is what I write code in daily. But I've worked in many languages, and many concepts described in this book are language agnostic, so we've selected a few other popular languages as examples in the appendices. Additionally, at the end of the book, I discuss a split in patterns in the industry, using infrastructure as code, as compared to container-based deployment strategies.

In the spirit of *The Phoenix Project* (and its inspiration, *The Goal,* by Eliyahu Goldratt), this book is told in a semi-narrative format. My hope here is to have you, the reader, draw on your own experiences and struggles so that you can compare it to the ones I'm writing about. Did you encounter the same problem? How did you fix it? Would this strategy have helped? Or could it be adapted to help in the future?

This book does not have to end when you close it.

acknowledgments

When I started writing this book, I didn't realize how many people would be involved. First and foremost, I would like to thank my wife, Chelsea, who supported me in this endeavor and all the other endeavors I've participated in. It wasn't the best plan on paper to start a new job and write a book with two children to manage, but she helped me stick with it and push the book over the finish line.

I'd also like to thank my two sons, Eli and Abel, who inspire and challenge me in all the best ways. Their curiosity and interest forced me to think about concepts that seemed self-explanatory and to find a way of explaining them, which is, in a technical sense, what most programming books try to do for people!

This book could not have been written without the immense support of Manning's publishing team. Thank you, Andy Waldron, for working with me on finding a theme (and the right title!) for this book, which I am truly proud to have written. Thank you also to Aliénor Latour, who advised me on the technical aspects of the content and on the overall tone and direction of the book.

As a reviewer of many Manning books myself, I especially appreciate all those who provided feedback in the book reviews. To Alain Lompo, Alex Harrington, Alex Lucas, Amit Lamba, Arun Saha, Bhagvan Kommadi, Borko Đurković, Camal Cakar, Clifford Thurber, Diego Stamigni, Eldon Alameda, Jorge Ezequiel Bo, Katia Patkin, Kent Spillner, Laud Bentil, Manoj Reddy, Marleny Núñez Alba, Mattia Di Gangi, Michele Di Pede, Mihaela Barbu, Muneeb Shaikh, Nathan B Crocker, Philippe Vialatte, Roman Zhuzha, Ryan Quinn, Sergio Britos Arévalo, Sudeep Batra, Tiklu Ganguly, Tymoteusz Wolodzko, and Walter Alexander Mata López, your suggestions helped make this a better book. And I appreciate those who purchased this book early via MEAP and provided feedback and support.

I am very grateful for all the help, guidance, patience, and laughs that Becky Whitney provided. She was an amazing guide throughout the entire writing process and eased my mind about many of my decisions. Writing this book would have been overwhelming to me without her guidance and, instead, it was a well-organized journey.

To Thoro.ai for giving me the freedom and encouragement to write this book.

To Frank, who took me under his wing and received talks, papers, and a repository of experience in return.

To Mike L., who discussed process and improvement first thing in the morning with me to come up with ideas for this book.

To John M. and Verone, who gave me my first job and encouraged me to grow.

To my parents, who encouraged me to grow and reach for new goals.

To my high school English teachers, who encouraged my writing and helped me establish my voice.

To Otto, who, with every walk we took, led me one step closer to the end of this book.

about this book

Shipping Go is intended to walk you through building a product. Experimenting and hacking will require process and automation to help turn an idea into something other people use. Placing this book into a single category is difficult because it intentionally moves you into areas of testing and infrastructure along with creating process and automation. You'll find yourself moving between Development, QA, and Ops worlds in developing an experimental project. Putting all these elements together is an automated pipeline that provides a feedback cycle that we enhance as we progress throughout.

Who should read this book?

This book, which is intended for anyone who has a solid grasp on any programming language, was conceived and written as the first book you should read after you've learned Go, JavaScript, Python, or whatever other fun language you're excited to build something in. Given this knowledge, you will be given a crash course in the software development process, continuous integration and deployment, and various infrastructure elements. This book was written using examples in a particular language and cloud infrastructure that is transferable to other languages, as demonstrated in the appendices.

Managers and architects may find the concepts useful to help design teams around new projects. These concepts can be slowly introduced to existing development environments as well as new ones. Considering the advancements in both languages and architecture, you may fear that the book content will become outdated, yet the concepts should project forward toward new languages and infrastructure elements. What is written here is only a subset of what can be done but should serve as a solid foundation for you and your team to build on.

How this book is organized: A roadmap

This book is organized into three parts, consisting of a chapter apiece on process, testing, and infrastructure that progress in complexity in each part. This way, you can hop into the book at the pertinent chapter or part related to your area of expertise (or lack thereof). Each concept should be transferable to other languages and pieces of infrastructure. Throughout this book, it was mentioned that the code and examples can be applied to different languages and frameworks. The appendices address common languages that can demonstrate similar techniques. Each attempts to produce a similar API that was built with various testing techniques and other analysis tools.

About the code

The code is basic-level Go code with the CI engine using GitHub actions. These actions use YAML as the primary language, which is easily transferable to other systems, though the libraries will be different. I chose (for no particular reason) Google Cloud as the cloud host throughout this book; you can swap it out with similar products in other cloud offerings. Additionally, I chose the route of container-based deployments rather than standing up individual servers as a matter of preference, as many greenfield projects tend to move in this direction. However, appendix D provides some basic infrastructure examples.

This book contains many examples of source code both in numbered listings and inline with normal text. In both cases, source code is formatted in a `fixed-width font like this` to separate it from ordinary text. Sometimes code is also **in bold** to highlight code that has changed from previous steps in the chapter, such as when a new feature adds to an existing line of code.

In many cases, the original source code has been reformatted; we've added line breaks and reworked indentation to accommodate the available page space in the book. In rare cases, even this was not enough, and listings include line-continuation markers (➡). Additionally, comments in the source code have often been removed from the listings when the code is described in the text. Code annotations accompany many of the listings, highlighting important concepts.

You can get executable snippets of code from the liveBook (online) version of this book at https://livebook.manning.com/book/shipping-go. The complete code for the examples in the book is available for download from the Manning website at www.manning.com and from GitHub at https://github.com/holmes89/hello-api.

liveBook discussion forum

Purchase of *Shipping Go* includes free access to liveBook, Manning's online reading platform. Using liveBook's exclusive discussion features, you can attach comments to the book globally or to specific sections or paragraphs. It's a snap to make notes for yourself, ask and answer technical questions, and receive help from the author and other users. To access the forum, go to https://livebook.manning.com/book/shipping-go/discussion. You can also learn more about Manning's forums and the rules of conduct at https://livebook.manning.com/discussion.

Manning's commitment to our readers is to provide a venue where a meaningful dialogue between individual readers and between readers and the author can take place. It is not a commitment to any specific amount of participation on the part of the author, whose contribution to the forum remains voluntary (and unpaid). We suggest you try asking the author some challenging questions lest their interest stray! The forum and the archives of previous discussions will be accessible from the publisher's website for as long as the book is in print.

about the author

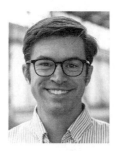

JOEL HOLMES is a software developer who has focused on building cloud native applications. He has worked at several startups and has helped to architect, design, and develop new products and services to help those companies develop and grow. Along the way, he has been able to help establish tools and processes that have helped development and increased quality. He lives in Pittsburgh with his family and currently works at Thoro.ai building cloud applications in the growing robotics industry.

The technical editor on this book is **ALIÉNOR LATOUR**, a Golang tech lead focused on quality and simplicity in her team's software, and an advocate for diversity in development roles. Outside of work hours, she travels Europe for Scottish dance events, knits, sews skirts with pockets, and reads about linguistics and sociology.

about the cover illustration

The figure on the cover of *Shipping Go* is captioned "Femme de Martavan en Sirie," or "Woman of Martavan in Syria," taken from a collection by Jacques Grasset de Saint-Sauveur, published in 1797. Each illustration is finely drawn and colored by hand.

In those days, it was easy to identify where people lived and what their trade or station in life was just by their dress. Manning celebrates the inventiveness and initiative of the computer business with book covers based on the rich diversity of regional culture centuries ago, brought back to life by pictures from collections such as this one.

Part 1

Startup

The beginning of a new project is extremely exciting and at times a bit daunting. You aren't encumbered by old code or bugs, but you are starting from scratch on an idea that you aren't sure will work. You don't know if the market will like it or if it will stand up to high loads of traffic. You definitely don't want to paint yourself into a corner too quickly, nor do you want to make things so broad that it becomes impossible to reason about. This is the difference between having a narrow, unstable base and an expansive, cumbersome base.

The goal is to be flexible at this stage. Build your product so that it can change and grow comfortably for both you and your team. In this section, we discuss how to start a project with documentation and a plan in chapter 2. We establish a simple and flexible way of writing tests in chapter 3 early on to help find bugs quickly. We release a product to production that will cost nothing until it is heavily used in chapter 4. Throughout this process, we build tools that automate a good portion of the process of moving your code through testing and delivery.

Delivering value 1

This chapter covers

- Using small chunks of work to increase workflow
- Establishing feedback loops for product and process improvement
- Outlining phases of product growth and development
- Iterating between various feedback cycles

What you will find in this book has been gathered from past practices in Agile software development, lean startup ideals, and DevOps culture. This book is intended for those who want to take the language they've learned and build something with it. You know how to write code, and you want to ship it. The concepts and processes taught here should be agnostic to the technology or language you use, but I provide concrete examples using Go and GitHub Actions. By using their terminology, you should be able to easily adapt what I write here to Python and GitLab or JavaScript and CircleCI, but in this book, we will ship Go code.

The book follows a semi-narrative format wherein I put you in the shoes of a developer at a company that wants to rapidly develop an enhanced product. While

this project is simple, the intention is to give you an idea of the process of developing a product. Many of these elements are drawn in part from my personal experiences and hindsight. This pattern may also not fit your company's culture or process, but hopefully you can find some elements that help your team move forward. The focus here is the process and mentality rather than the technology.

Finally, each section is broken down so that you deliver a product at the end. Each chapter will build off of the existing chapters, but you can stop at any point if you are satisfied with the process. Each section brings your product to scale in different ways, such as by expanding teams or higher resource utilization. We explore integration with legacy systems and different deployment options based on cost.

1.1 Simple concepts

This book brings together concepts and processes from across various industries to help with the quick creation of quality software. Some of these concepts predate the development of computers and the software development industry. Over the past few decades, software companies have looked to other industries to help them build products more efficiently to meet the demands of their customers. What they found were processes that created fast feedback from their customers. Based on that feedback, they were able to adapt their product. Adapting their products allowed them to grow into the Googles, Apples, and Facebooks of today, yet they are rooted in the assembly lines of the industrial revolution and the lean manufacturing techniques created in Japan.

Let's assume you are reading this book so that you can build a product. You have some idea that you think will change your company (or the world), and you want to see if it works. Is this what customers want? Does this help your company? It is hard to know. Projects may get started and eventually fail. They may pivot or change or just be left to the scrap heap of experience. If a project is almost predestined to change or be thrown out, then how much effort should you put in?

It's curious to think of putting in the least amount of effort as possible into something. It can seem lazy or uninspired. Instead, consider being told you need to build a device that takes someone from one location to another in the fastest way possible. With no additional details, you could spend years creating and designing an airplane only to find out your customer needs to travel 10 miles. Compare the two development processes in figure 1.1.

In software, this happens all of the time. Companies pivot. They start small and evolve. They fail. They make millions. How do they do it? It comes from a notion of developing three key features: people, process, and product. People drive organizations and product development. A process helps us underline how the work should be done. Finally, the product opens us up to feedback from our customers. Once you've established your process, you can automate it as much as possible. This allows your team of people to sit at one end and a product to be delivered at the other end.

Your team will develop features or make changes that your customer wants. These changes will then be delivered to your customers, who in turn will create a discussion about the product or feature. This will trigger a design step, which will start the whole

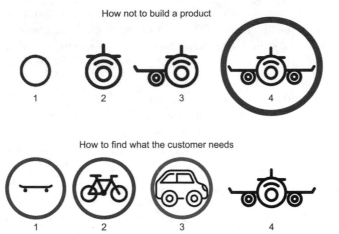

How not to build a product

1   2   3   4

How to find what the customer needs

1   2   3   4

Figure 1.1   Talk with customers to get an accurate idea of which product to build them.

thing over. I like to refer to this loop as the *four Ds*: develop, deliver, discuss, and design. This is a feedback loop and becomes a key part of our *value stream*, as seen in figure 1.2.

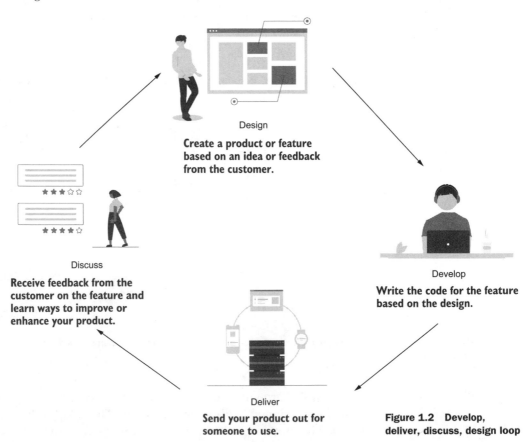

Design

Create a product or feature based on an idea or feedback from the customer.

Discuss

Receive feedback from the customer on the feature and learn ways to improve or enhance your product.

Develop

Write the code for the feature based on the design.

Deliver

Send your product out for someone to use.

Figure 1.2   Develop, deliver, discuss, design loop

The value stream is exactly as it sounds, the flow of work that creates value within the company. This means establishing a relationship with your customers and building a product that you think will be valuable to them. Yet your investment should be as small as possible until you can learn what your customer wants. How do you reduce your investment costs? Through automation. When your source code is committed, it should be treated as a raw resource, and the manufactured product should be delivered at the end.

We can look to another profession for the answers. Industrial engineers have been dealing with how to deliver products for a long time. We can look at innovations such as the assembly line, which showed us the benefits of automated handoffs between workstations. We can look at lean manufacturing techniques to help us understand the importance of reducing work in progress and just-in-time delivery to reduce waste. The technology world has watched and adopted many of these principles to help design and build delivery pipelines, which automate the flow of work from a single idea to a feature in your application. These ideas and features are created when a customer asks for them just in time for development rather than by guessing the customer's desires and spending time and money upfront developing something that may not be what they want. This pipeline can be seen in figure 1.3, wherein a raw resource goes in one end, a product is shipped, and customer feedback is given to design a new feature. This cycle is pivotal to the success of companies and is a concept we will explore throughout this book.

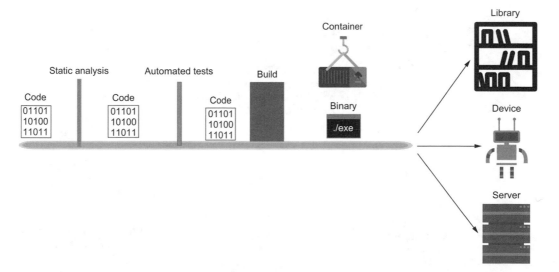

Figure 1.3   Code is moved along a pipeline where it is analyzed, built, and then shipped as a library to a device or a server.

We can see that the code goes through a series of automated steps to verify quality before a product is built and shipped to the end customer. This can be through a library package that is used in another project, a device out in the field for an update,

or a server running in the cloud. All move along with little to no human interaction, making the timeline dependable between when the code is written and when the customer gets to use the product.

1.2 Small pieces

A key theme you will find in this book is creating small, iterative steps to invite feedback into your process. So, as we build our product, we will take small, iterative steps so that you can see how a product grows. You may find the steps in section 1 too simple for your needs and choose to skip them. Or you may find that you only need up to the end of part 2 to take your product to market.

Imagine you have spent three weeks developing a feature that hasn't been looked at or tested by anyone. How long do you think it will take for someone to test all of the different pieces of your feature? How many bugs do you think they'll find? How quickly can you turn around on those bugs? How much change has accrued while you developed this feature?

Creating small pieces of work allows us to decrease our work in progress (WIP) and speed up delivery. In Eliyah Goldratt's book *The Goal* (Routledge, 2014), the author points out that WIP ties up revenue. You invest time and money in something that is not getting to the customer. This is a loss of value until it is delivered. Creating smaller amounts of work ties up less revenue in your value stream, so we will focus on smaller chunks of work to deliver value early and often.

While each chapter is important to building a complete pipeline, in the end you will find that your pipeline will be different because each product and company is different. What stays the same is the process. Ideas go in, code gets written, and products ship out. Figure 1.4 demonstrates this loop.

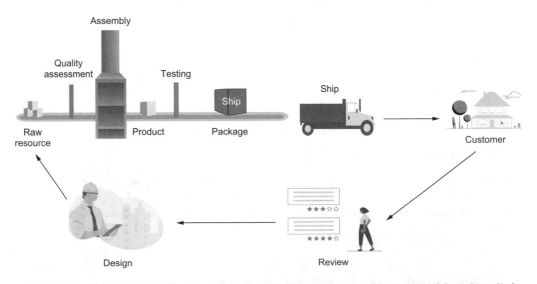

Figure 1.4 Product development goes through a life cycle that starts with raw materials and results in a product that customers provide feedback on, resulting in improvements and changes to the product.

Collaboration becomes key in this step because you are tearing down the walls between different groups. It used to be that tribes existed in companies that were constantly at war with each other. Testers blamed developers for poor-quality code. Developers blamed operations for slow deployments. Operations blamed testers for the number of deployments that happened because of missed bugs. This is unhealthy and harmful to our customers, so instead of putting up walls, we tear them down, put lines of communication between them, and collaborate on building a tool that takes in ideas and delivers value.

You will be given a holistic view of product development so that you can turn your ideas into products. What does this view look like from a distance? What steps do we need to build our pipeline? Let's take a look.

1.2.1 Continuous

There are so many continuous things: continuous integration, continuous testing, continuous delivery, continuous improvement. What do they all have in common? They are . . . continuous—a cycle, a full rotation, a circle. All of these "continuous" things tell us that they all need to connect at the beginning. Toyota incorporated this model to build its famous Toyota Production System (TPS). The company is constantly evaluating each phase of its development process, from the way the assembly line runs, to manual assembly, to experimentation. Each phase has a feedback cycle where any employee can seek ways of improving the company.

From a development perspective, being continuous allows you to write code without much concern about doing a lot of manual work after that. If a pipeline is assembled correctly, checking in a piece of code should trigger a list of automated processes that will give you feedback about the code. It may fail a quality assessment or not compile, but the developer is notified and can fix it, creating a loop. If the deployment was successful, the developer can move on to the next task, continuing the process of improvement.

This book is written in a way that tries to follow this pattern. The TPS has many steps and hits a very broad market, so it would be too theoretical for this book. What we will do instead is break it down into three broad categories: process, quality, and delivery.

Each phase can be simple or complicated depending on your needs and where you are in your product development. What is provided is not a prescription but guidelines to help you implement these various techniques.

1.2.2 Process

Humans are still an essential element of software engineering. They come up with designs. They write the code. They verify the results. But humans aren't needed for everything. In fact, the more you can invest in less human time, the greater benefits you will get from your team.

This isn't to say that you automate away your development team. Instead, consider this: Would you rather spend an hour deploying an application or developing a new feature? We adopt an approach that is found in TPS: "automation with a human touch." This means we try to automate as much as possible, which increases how efficiently we

work. But this is not a black box or a set of corporate commands. Instead, the developers create and add the necessary tools to help them in their development.

What does this look like? Well, it becomes a set of documents, scripts, and tools that help make development go quickly. What format should my code be in? Use a formatter tool. How do I create a new feature? Use a code generator. How can we improve our deployment process? Use a pipeline.

This process is going to be fragile at first but will evolve into something essential to your team. You will find that the flow of work through your company will become easier and you will be able to meet demands quickly and efficiently.

1.2.3   *Quality*

Quality is a tricky word and the basis for some philosophical discussion. Robert Pirsig, in his book *Zen and the Art of Motorcycle Maintenance* (Mariner Books, 2005), put it this way:

> *"Quality . . . you know what it is, yet you don't know what it is. But that's self-contradictory. But some things are better than others, that is, they have more quality. But when you try to say what the quality is, apart from the things that have it, it all goes poof! There's nothing to talk about. But if you can't say what Quality is, how do you know what it is, or how do you know that it even exists? If no one knows what it is, then for all practical purposes it doesn't exist at all. But for all practical purposes it really does exist."*

So when people say "delivering a quality product," what does that mean? For our purposes, we'll say that first and foremost *quality does not mean perfect.* No code or product will ever be perfect. Quality, therefore, becomes an approximation of perfection.

Perfection can be approximated by putting additional quality measurements into your development process. What you, your team, and your company must do is determine your definition of quality for your customers. Your code may be beautiful, but in most cases, it gets compiled and is never seen by a customer. If that beautiful code has bugs, is it quality code? Or if you have code that works and has worked for years but is difficult to read or debug, is that quality code?

Our quality checks will mostly be through various types of test code. Different patterns and strategies will be used to ensure that our product is functioning as expected by the developer and the customer. This step reduces waste in our system, which occurs through rework (bugs) and delays (missed requirements). We use tests in a variety of ways to give ourselves confidence that our product works before we ship it. This will not address everything we need for quality code. Things such as code clarity and maintainability also help with the quality of our code and will be additional steps we add. In the end, though, it is the writers and maintainers of the code who are the stewards of quality.

1.2.4   *Delivery*

Delivery is the last step needed before we can loop back to the beginning. This is where the value comes into our pipeline. After the code has been written and pushed,

we validate what we wrote by how our customers react to it. Changes may be requested, or the user may be satisfied or dissatisfied. This feedback loop only happens once a product is delivered.

Delivery is the act of shipping an artifact. An *artifact* can be a version of a library, an executable binary, a container image, or something else that can be used by another person. Artifacts can be delivered privately and publicly. In some cases, a company will build what's called a *release candidate*, which is a product that is almost ready to be given out to the general public. This candidate can be run through another set of automated tests to check for performance problems (load testing), usability problems (UI testing), or if it even works (smoke testing). The manual tests can be run to explore the product, get a stamp of approval, and be released to the public, as shown in figure 1.5.

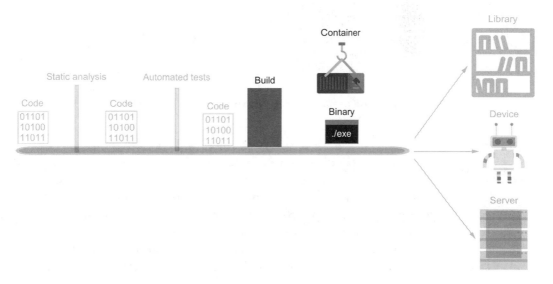

Figure 1.5   Code is built into an executable file or wrapped in a universal runtime, such as a container.

The process of making an artifact run is known as a *deployment*. In some cases, this can range from installing an application on a server, setting up a new function on a server-less environment, running a new container on a container-run engine, or simply doing an over-the-air update to the customer's machine (e.g., operating system updates). It is at this point that we begin to see the full value in what we have built, as shown in figure 1.6.

Throughout this process, we continue to learn what customers want and need and how they use the product, which provides information back to our development team. If an application doesn't start, we know we broke something that needs to be repaired. If it falls over when too many people use it, we know something needs to be changed.

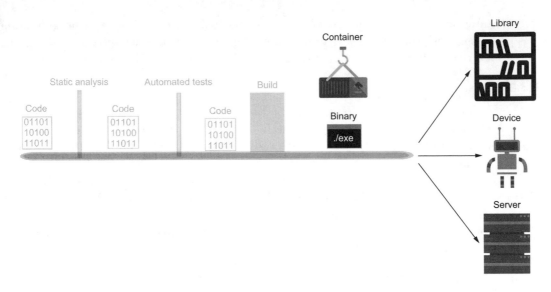

Figure 1.6   The output is shipped to a customer as a library onto an embedded device or a server.

If only a small set of users finds the feature unhelpful or not of value, we may need to go back to the drawing board.

1.3   Building your product

What happens in the product development cycle is very similar to the scientific method. You have a hypothesis, and you do experiments to see if your hypothesis is correct. Sometimes you may need to change the parameters of your experiments or explore a different direction. Products can be similar. Your idea (hypothesis) may not meet the market needs, so you make a change (experiment) and ultimately find if it is successful. In either case, you learn something.

As part of building your product, there will be various stages. As you progress, each part can become more complicated and will outline the mature stages of a product.

1.3.1   Initial setup

What goes into starting a new project? Is it just a great idea, or is it more? When you are starting a project, as we do in chapter 2, you need to gather information about what the system is supposed to do and how you expect it to work. As you progress, you need instructions and scripts to set up the project for others. When working in an organization or on a larger project, you will not be the only one doing the work. Someone at some point will want to contribute, and it's easier to document the steps now than worry about it later.

Documentation and scripts will help you scale team members and contributors. Building a basic pipeline also becomes important at the onset because retrofitting one can often be tricky. In this section, we start down our path toward industrial program-

ming instead of hacking. There is a time and place for both types of programming, but in this instance, we worry about building a product and not vetting an idea. Once we've established some basic installation and a process, we will add to it as we go.

1.3.2   *Basic validation*

Validating that your code works as expected is another step along the path to developing a great product. Teams often push items like testing toward the bottom of their priority lists because they feel their product is too volatile at the beginning, but tests are more than just security blankets for developers. Instead, they tell developers about the business rules they are writing and steer the product toward their intended goal. These guard rails can help developers in the long term, and establishing them as basic validation in a pipeline helps accelerate the growth of a product and gives autonomy to developers by documenting the business expectations through code. We explore this process in chapter 3 by setting up a basic unit testing process.

1.3.3   *Zero-cost deployment*

Without shipping, you have a product that sits on a shelf. Deployment is taking your product and putting it out there on a server so that someone can use it. Yet when you look at all of the options, there are tons of things to consider. The biggest of these is cost. That is why there is such a large focus on low-cost technologies to get products deployed.

Starting in chapter 4, we will walk through various options that are free and scale with your company as your user base grows. I like to call this "zero cost" because early on, it should not cost you anything to run a product to get market validation. To do this, we will explore serverless technologies such as deployed functions and hosted platforms.

1.3.4   *Code confidence*

The standardization of work is a core tenant of industrialized production. In the same way, developers have created techniques to standardize how software is written. As a team grows, coding standards and formatting will become important. By using these techniques, we can catch bugs earlier and continue to check the quality of the product automatically before it even gets tested.

Additionally, in chapter 5, we will explore a code review process and see how this can aid in creating a quality product and how it can be used as a teaching mechanism for team members. We will also use documentation to help our team understand the code we write and work toward creating code that is easy to understand.

1.3.5   *Integrations*

Systems rarely work in a vacuum. They either interact with a database, a file system, or another application. This is known as integration, which becomes a critical part of testing our systems. In chapter 6, we will explore different techniques for testing integrations with other systems. We will interact with simple stubbed systems as well as more advanced mocking techniques. To do this, we will need to create a layer that

allows us to invert the dependencies so that we develop against an abstraction instead of a concrete system. In doing this, we will give ourselves higher flexibility.

1.3.6 *Portability*

"It worked on my machine" is a trope that occurs often in software development circles. You spend months creating a system, and you know all of the ins and outs of it. Suddenly, someone else wants to run it and it won't work. They follow your setup, but you missed a dependency. You developed it on Linux, but they are using Windows.

How do we resolve this? In chapter 7, we will explore abstraction tools that help us with virtualization and packaging our product so that it can run on a universal runtime. This will be done using Buildpacks and containers. Ultimately, we will integrate this into a system that is portable for everyone, including our various cloud deployment options.

1.3.7 *Adaptability*

As you ship your product, you will find yourself building incomplete features or turning features off. Typically, companies create a separate product to test before releasing it to a customer "once it is stable," but this has been found to reduce teams' productivity and can often cause delays in shipping. Instead, the industry has moved toward changing the way our applications work through the use of configuration. By configuring our applications, as we will do in chapter 8, we can change the functionality without changing the code itself. This means that experimental features can be tested by setting a variable or changing an endpoint by changing a flag. Configuration means you can adapt your applications so that they can move as quickly as you do.

1.3.8 *User acceptance*

Simple tests are great at testing how functions and methods work within your application. They help you hone in on the technical aspects but do little to tie your work to what the user wants. A user may want an API that expects a specific format or a business rule that has specific expectations. In this instance, our testing shifts from technical to something a little more "squishy." In chapter 9, we explore other techniques. We are not interested in how it is done but rather whether we are meeting the specifications set out for us. "If my balance is less than the amount to withdrawal, then I should get an error" is an example of a specification we would want to test.

1.3.9 *Scaled product*

Using various abstractions in our deployment environments will help us build a customer base. Over time, these abstractions will cost you and your company either money or performance, so you start ripping apart these abstractions, which requires more technical expertise about the servers and systems you are building, for a reduced cost and the ability to scale servers as you see fit. In chapter 10, we will explore creating and delivering products on visualized server instances and how to maintain these products through code.

1.3.10 *End to end*

The final step in any product, once it has reached a critical mass, is to test it for quality. By this point, we will have created several ways of testing quality through testing and linting. But as the product rolls to production, we will want to assert what the customer will experience. Often this is done through a quality assurance team, but we want to automate as much of this as possible so that our team can explore more nuanced bugs or search for areas of improvement. In chapter 11, we will add our final capstone to our pipeline, which will give us a sense of whether our entire system works as expected from the stance of a customer. We focus on pushing the quality checks throughout the system, but we should, in the end, have a final check to see if everything works as a whole. Since this is an expensive operation (in terms of time and upkeep), we save it for last, as it is often the last piece to be implemented once a product has matured. In chapter 11, we will demonstrate some tests to allow your team to explore other areas of improvement.

1.4 *Feedback loop*

I guess it's easy to ask what the point of all of this is. The answer is simply to allow you to create fast and tight feedback loops throughout the growth of your product, team, and company. These principles are also easily transferable to other businesses and projects.

Agility is a term thrown around a lot in software development, and it aims to capture the idea of being nimble and quick to change direction. Yet I feel that this is an inadequate term because it can often feel like you are playing a game of dodgeball trying to deflect or dodge feedback rather than embrace it. Instead, our development process should be like driving a race car where you need to make split-second decisions to keep moving toward the finish line. As we move through this book, I hope you can find some guidance for your project and your team on how to move forward and win the race.

Summary

- Product development is a process that constantly changes.
- Focusing on feedback loops will help guide areas of improvement.
- Automation is key to establishing faster feedback loops.

Introducing continuous integration 2

This chapter covers

- Documenting requirements in your source code
- Establishing a central code repository as the starting point for your pipeline
- Automating the steps needed to build your product by using a continuous integration system
- Creating a basic application to start development

It's Monday, and you've been drinking your morning coffee and scrolling through emails when you see an invitation to a meeting titled "Kickoff." You check the time and realize you are going to be late. Grabbing your laptop, you run to the conference room and see just one person sitting there, a product manager. As you close the door and walk to a seat, they say, "Glad you could make it; sorry about the last-minute invite, but we need to get something built this week. Our company would like to explore creating a new hello translation service that is cheaper and faster than our legacy system. In the future, we want to expand beyond just translating 'hello,' but our system will not scale. The conversation has been going on too long

15

at this point, and I want to prove to them we can get something done quickly and still meet their targets. Do you think we can do it?"

A new service to replicate the functionality of an old service in less than a week, with better performance and at a cheaper cost? Sure, why not? What do you have to lose?

"What I want is for you to do this in pieces and write it so that we can get feedback quickly. Also, I want to demo this tomorrow from a live server. It doesn't need to be perfect; it just needs to show what we were able to do in a day. I also want it so that we can have others join you once this demo is over. And we need to be sure it works as we expect and that we can prove why it does."

As they're talking, you quickly open a terminal and type `mkdir hello-api &&` `touch hello-api/README.md`. You open your `README.md` file and write the code in the following listing.

Listing 2.1 `README.md`

```
# Hello API

## Release Milestones

### V0 (1 day)
- [ ] Onboarding Documentation
- [ ] Simple API response (hello world!)
- [ ] Unit tests
- [ ] Running somewhere other than the dev machine

### V1 (7 days)
- [ ] Create translation endpoint
- [ ] Store translations in short-term storage
- [ ] Call existing service for translation
- [ ] Move towards long-term storage
```

"Great, once you are done, let me know, and we can chat about the next steps. I appreciate you doing this. I think it will be great for us to show our company how rapid product development can work and make us a success."

You leave the room with your laptop and go get some more coffee. When you get back to your desk, you look at the time: 9:15. It's time to start coding.

2.1   *Where to start?*

Beginning a project based on an idea can be a little overwhelming. What language do you write it in? How should it be structured? What are the various use cases?

Interestingly, none of that matters. If you are asked to create something in a day, you will go with the language you are most comfortable with. You will write the code in the simplest way possible. You will never know all of the use cases, so it is best to just get something in the hands of the customers. With this project, you have the benefit of knowing some business requirements because there is a legacy system, but in most cases, you will never know.

As you start, it is a great idea to create a document to write down your setup process, milestones, testing process, and so forth. You already started the documentation in your

meeting when you started a `README.md`. Most developers will open this file first, and it is a great way of communicating asynchronously. The README file is not a new concept and has been a fixture of software development for decades. Its purpose is to give the user relevant information to configure, install, run, or use a piece of software. What goes into your README depends on your team, but often it will hold the following:

- Instructions on how to run the software
- Configurations in your environment to run the software
- Known dependencies
- Troubleshooting information
- Common use cases and examples of using the software
- Software milestones

Figure 2.1 shows how a document acts as a map for new team members.

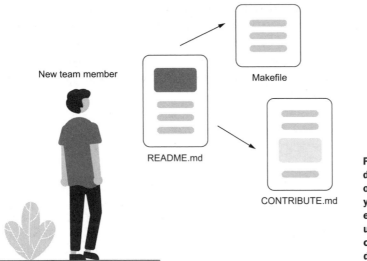

Figure 2.1   The README document is a pointer to all other documents within your product. This will help enhance the developers' understanding of how to contribute, run, build, or debug your product.

You have already added one of these items from the list: software milestones. Now you want to add a description of what the software does, what it needs, and how to start working on it. The README has now become a lab notebook in which you tell others what you are doing and how to replicate the experiment. It should also have a thesis or a purpose that tells the reader what this product does. If you find it hard to write a thesis, you may not have a great idea of what you are building. Let's write this out:

```
# Hello API
```

This is an improved version of the current `hello-api` we use in production. It will use less memory and be cheaper to run in production, and it will scale, expand to additional words, and be more stable:

```
## Dependencies

- Go version 1.18

## Setup

## Release Milestones
...
```

Great! You've used this to make your first decision. Choosing Go was natural for you because it is a fun, newer language you've been using in your spare time. It will be a great way to introduce this to your company and has a reputation for using little memory, being scalable, and being stable. Notice that you left `Setup` blank. This is intentional. This is a living document that should be updated when infrastructure changes are implemented. This will help us throughout the chapter by guiding us to the logical step that we should take next.

2.2   *A greenfield project*

For this book, we use a Unix-based development environment. Why? Because most of the deployment services we will use are Linux based. Windows even has this neat feature available to run Ubuntu Linux inside Windows. Between Linux and Windows, we have a pretty large share of users. macOS will work for most things, so we need to indicate when it won't. This is very important to note, so we should probably add this to our `README.md` file:

```
...
## Setup

...
```

Development expects to run in a Unix-like system. If you are running Windows, please consider following these directions (http://mng.bz/VpQr).

Now we need to install Go. It would be easy to simply paste a link to a download and tell users to follow the instructions. However, you might be on version 1.7.2 and the next person on 1.7.3, and the person after that on a different version. Soon everyone is on a different version, which seems benign but could become a problem when you're helping a colleague solve a problem, because it works on your machine and not theirs.

It's at times like this when we want to use standardized tools to help create repeatable tasks. To do this, we will create a Makefile—a standard in the developing world, which can become very complex. Our Makefile will just house some small commands that we can reference in the documentation and aid us in development. Open a new Makefile in your code editor, and add the code in the following listing.

Listing 2.2   Makefile

```
GO_VERSION :=1.18

.PHONY: install-go init-go        ◁──┐   .PHONY is used to define some of
                                          our methods in advance so that we
                                          can use them in the setup phase.

setup: install-go init-go         ◁───────────────────────────────
```

.PHONY is used to define some of our methods in advance so that we can use them in the setup phase.

Runs commands to install Go and setup environment

```
#TODO add MacOS support              Downloads a specific version
install-go:                          of Go and installs it
  wget "https://golang.org/dl/go$(GO_VERSION).linux-amd64.tar.gz"
  sudo tar -C /usr/local -xzf go$(GO_VERSION).linux-amd64.tar.gz
  rm go$(GO_VERSION).linux-amd64.tar.gz
                                          Adds Go location to your
init-go:                                  local environment
  echo 'export PATH=$$PATH:/usr/local/go/bin' >> $${HOME}/.bashrc
  echo 'export PATH=$$PATH:$${HOME}/go/bin' >> $${HOME}/.bashrc
```

> **Alternatives**
>
> The following code is in Make because it is used fairly often by the DevOps commu-
> nity and developers:
>
> - TaskFile[https://taskfile.dev/] - Modern Make alternative using YAML
>
> > **NOTE** If you are not using Bash as your shell, you will have to modify these
> > steps to add Go to your system path.

Notice the TODO comment here. This is okay. Remember that we are trying to move
fast but also be helpful. What is important is to document what is missing so that others will know when they join your codebase. TODO items are a great way for people to
start contributing! Add the code in the following listing to your README.

Listing 2.3   README.md

```
...
## Setup

### Install Go        <─┐
`sudo make setup`       │  macOS is not supported
                        │  by this Makefile yet.
### Upgrade Go        <─┘
`sudo make install-go`
...
```

By using standardization and documentation, you establish a guide on how to work on
this product. This is almost like pulling out a set of building instructions for a table
from Ikea. Anyone who picks it up should be able to follow the directions and have a
running application. Standardizing our system allows others to contribute. Given our
tools and our documentation, the next step in the evolution of product development
is automation. For factories, this came in the form of the assembly line. For software, it
came from the continuous integration pipeline.

2.3   *The assembly line*

Once producers were able to standardize the way they did their work in their homes,
they started moving to centralized factories. These factories still had each worker

sitting at their workbench assembling items by themselves. One worker's job may have been to cut the leather for a shoe and then deliver the stack of cut pieces to another worker, who attached it to a bottom piece, and so on. Today, assembly lines are much different. Some people stand and do repetitive tasks, but with the advent of more advanced automation, these stations have become more skilled and nuanced, requiring special training and knowledge, much like today's software developers.

In software, we can imagine this as a developer sitting at their machine, writing code, compiling it, and then deploying it. While many people produce code this way, it does not scale well. Artisans will produce custom furniture, and in the same way, many programmers will sit at home hacking away at a project on their own. But this isn't industrial development. These are solo projects. Most companies do not need artisanal software; they need predictability and reliability.

What is needed is a way of automating the flow of items through a factory so that workers aren't doing everything themselves or spending time handing things off. In factories, this was called the assembly line; in software development, it is called a *continuous integration pipeline*.

A continuous integration pipeline, or CI system, is just an application that moves code along a set of predefined processes. A CI system can be as simple as copying a file to a different location to as complicated as handling multiple deployments and quality checks. In this book, we will move from the former to the latter using GitHub Actions. Table 2.1 outlines some of the most common CI systems.

Table 2.1   Continuous integration servers have also evolved over the years and often have a cloud-based hosting solution so you don't need to run them yourself.

Continuous integration system	Year	Hosted service
Azure DevOps	2005	Yes
TeamCity	2006	Yes
Circle CI	2011	Yes
Jenkins	2011	No
Travis CI	2012	Yes
GitLab	2014	Yes
GitHub Actions	2020	Yes

GitHub Actions is a fairly new technology to help create integration pipelines for developers' source code. It uses a special YAML file to help us define the various stages that we want our code to go through, when to run the stages, and what to do if something doesn't work. The pipeline is broken down into a set of jobs. Each job can have a series of steps involved and can depend on other jobs. Each step can either run a command directly on the underlying system (bash commands, scripts, etc.) or use libraries to help do repetitive tasks (set up Go, check out code, etc.). When you look at some definitions,

you will see things like `actions/setup-go@v2`, which means we will use the `Github-Action` command to set up our Go environment with the proper version.

Additionally, we want to understand the first pipeline we are building. At first, all we want to do is create a binary and upload it as an artifact to our GitHub repository. You should see the following steps:

1 Set up Go.
2 Check out the code.
3 Build a binary.
4 Copy the file to the upload directory.
5 Upload the artifact to GitHub.

To show how simple it is, we will create our pipeline now before we have written any code. In your terminal, type `mkdir -p .github/workflows && touch .github/workflows/pipeline.yml`, and open the file. In it, we will add the code in the following listing.

Listing 2.4 `pipeline.yml`

```
name: CI Checks

on:
  push:
    branches:            ◁──┐ We will only run this CI
      - main                │ process when a change is
                            ┘ made to the main branch.
jobs:                   ◁──┐ These are the various stages
  build:                   ┘ that are run in our pipeline.
    name: Build App
    runs-on: ubuntu-latest    ◁──┐ Run this on a
    steps:                        ┘ Linux-based machine.

    - name: Set up Go 1.x      ◁──┐ Ensures that our image
      uses: actions/setup-go@v2    ┘ has Go 1.18 or higher
      with:
        go-version: ^1.18

    - name: Check out code into the Go module directory    ◁──┐ Pulls code from
      uses: actions/checkout@v2                                ┘ a local repository

    - name: Build             ◁──┐ Tells our build command
      run: make build             ┘ to build a binary

    - name: Copy Files     ◁──┐ Copies the resulting binary
      run: |                    ┘ to a directory to upload
          mkdir  artifacts
          cp api artifacts/.          ◁──┐ Creates an archive to be attached
    - name: Archive                       ┘ to the workflow with the binary
      uses: actions/upload-artifact@v2
      with:
          name: api        ◁──┐ Names the binary directory something
          path: artifacts      ┘ you will be able to identify it with
```

Hopefully, some of you will have caught that we have a new make target listed. Here, we are standardizing our build using make build. Why? Well, Go allows us to configure our builds using flags and various other features, and we want to make sure that we have it standardized. For now, we will use the simple Go build, but in future chapters, we will have alternative configurations that we will want to use. Let's add our build command to our Makefile using the code in the following listing.

Listing 2.5   \.gitignore

```
GO_VERSION := 1.18

setup:
    ...

build:
    go build -o api cmd/main.go
```
The build command will compile the main application into a binary named api.

You may be wondering where the code is built. Trust me, we'll get there. For now, you can see how we can tie in the standardized build system to our assembly line. Our developers can use the same commands that we use on the assembly line to ensure they work locally but will be triggered automatically on our pipeline. If we need to change the process, it can then be reflected across both local and production environments.

NOTE   You changed a process. Did you update the documentation?

The assembly line is often mistaken as an invention of Henry Ford. However, the concept of an assembly line goes back decades before Ford's use of it on his famous Model T. Clothing, machines, bicycles, and boats were all applications of the concept of moving pieces between divided pieces of labor as far back as the industrial revolution. Automated tracks of materials would move around assembly or unit production. You can compare the two in figure 2.2.

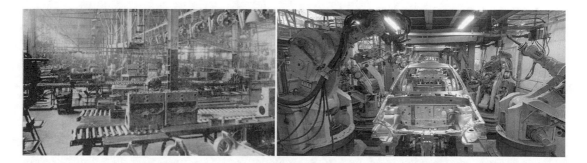

Figure 2.2   Assembly lines have evolved over the years in what they can do. Automation enhances the worker's ability to create higher-quality products more efficiently.

Henry Ford didn't even create the *automated* assembly line. What he is famous for is his application of the assembly line by creating core principles that efficiently delivered his product from start to finish.

His principles were simple:

- Place the tools and people in the order of operation.
- Optimize the flow for each station of work.
- Automate the line to move the product being assembled.

These principles boil down to grouping tools and workers: create a system that is easy to assemble and requires pieces to move automatically from each stage. Today, assembly lines are more sophisticated and have higher levels of automation, but the principles remain the same: make your tools easy to use, use the tools efficiently, and automate the flow to the next step.

We have just created our assembly line, moving our artisan development into industrial development. What we need to do now is find a way of moving materials into factories and moving products out.

2.4 *Warehouses*

I live in Pittsburgh, the Steel City. It got that name because of the large steel industry that was built here in the late 1800s. Throughout the outskirts of the city today, you will still see functioning steel mills and abandoned ones. What caused the steel industry to be so big here? Was it the climate? The population? The technology? No. The success was its proximity to the materials needed to create steel and its proximity to the distribution networks of the time. Coal, iron, and limestone would come down from the mountains surrounding the city and nearby areas into the factories. The factories would then produce steel and ship it out on the railroad or on barges down one of the rivers.

The *proximity of resources* and *distribution networks* are essential to modern production as well. Instead of relying on the location of natural resources, now companies will build warehouses to store their materials until they can get around to processing them. When a product is completed, it then goes to another warehouse until it is needed by a customer. These warehouses also go by another, more generic name: repositories.

Repositories are locations to store things. In software, we have code repositories that store our code. As with manufacturing, we want our source code to have close proximity to our factory to make product development more efficient. In our case, we want our software code to be close to our pipeline code as it gets assembled. Code repositories come in many shapes and sizes, but we will use Git for our code repository hosted on GitHub.

We will build a project to use throughout the book. The source code can be found at https://github.com/holmes89/hello-api. In each chapter, we add new tasks and procedures to our repository to show how we can test, build, and deploy multiple products from a single repository.

First, if you haven't already signed up for a GitHub Account, go to https://github.com/join and then http://mng.bz/xdxq (SSH access to your account).

Then navigate to the upper right-hand corner, click the plus sign, and select New Repository. Then you will be on a setup page. Pick a name and add a description if you'd like. Follow the setup in figure 2.3.

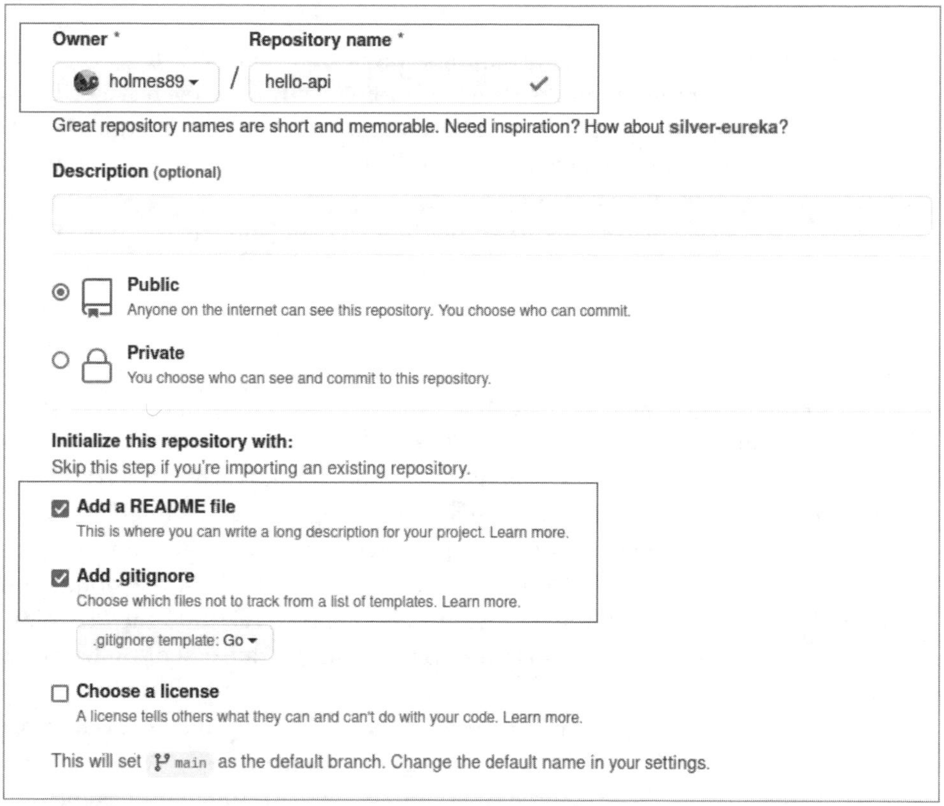

Figure 2.3   Provide a name, and create a `.gitignore` file using a Go template.

Then click Create Repository. Congratulations! You've created a repo. Please make sure that you have Git installed (http://mng.bz/AlXE). Then we will configure our local directory to use this repository. In your directory, run the following code:

```
git init
git remote add origin git@github.com:holmes89/hello-api.git
```

We now can store our code in a central location, and our actions will produce a binary that is also shared here with others. This repository is essential for the growth of our product. Once we share our code, others can start contributing and sharing as well. Our code is the material used by our system to build, test, and ship our products.

This means that our product code, testing code, and infrastructure code all reside in the same repository, where they can be processed and used to ship the product. Not only does our product code get checked for quality, but so does our test code and infrastructure code. We will see this as we move throughout this book. It is visualized in figure 2.4, where you see that material that is used for a product is shipped to a single assembly, and a product is then shipped.

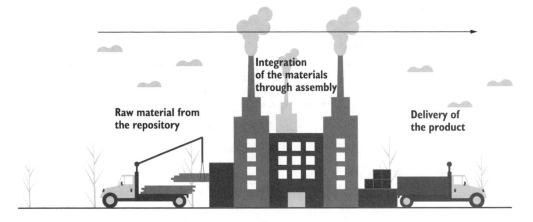

Figure 2.4 In manufacturing, materials are delivered from a repository of raw resources and are then assembled into a finished product, which is delivered to a customer.

The repository will need to hold everything that goes into making our product. This includes product code, deployment code, infrastructure definitions, testing plans, automated testing frameworks, and so forth. This may seem radical to some people, but it is core to the idea of continuous integration. This is the single source of truth for how to build our product and creates a sense of ownership for everyone working on it. You may find that a project may require more than one repository or rely on external systems. These fall into different patterns of development and deployment. We focus on a single project repository in this instance to keep our work simple and organized. What we want is code going in and a product going out, as illustrated in figure 2.5.

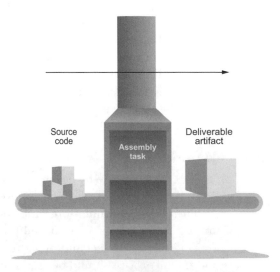

Figure 2.5 Similar to the manufacturing process, we can assemble our source code into a product through an integration layer to then be shipped to a customer.

With a single repository, you can solve a lot of organizational problems. For example, by having your test code in the same repository as your product code, you can have your assembly line easily run integration tests after a build before the artifact is deployed. Otherwise, a trigger may need to happen on the testing repository to start tests after the build has been completed. Or you may find that you have a chicken or egg problem when it comes to releasing a new feature or schema change. As I mentioned before, this will need to be based on how you and your team want to structure it.

Some items may not be required to check into your repository. Specifically, things like compiled binaries and external libraries aren't typically checked in but are scraps left over from your development that you don't want to add to the repository. To handle this, we can create a special file called `.gitignore`. Create one, open it, and add the following:

```
# Binaries for programs and plugins
*.exe
*.exe~
*.dll
*.so
*.dylib

# Test binary, built with `go test -c`
*.test

# Output of the go coverage tool, specifically when used with LiteIDE
*.out

# Dependency directories (remove the comment below to include it)
# vendor/
                    ┌─ We do not want to save the
api          ◁──────┘  binary to our source control.
```

This should prevent us from adding these files to our repository so that it stays clean. You may not need all of these files, but they are standard files you wouldn't want to check into your repository.

We now have standardization with a Makefile, documentation in a README, process in the form of a pipeline, storage in the form of a repository, and shipping in the form of a release. All we are missing is the material to produce our product.

2.5   *Material*

Where is the code? Why haven't we written a single line of Go yet? Why are we going through all of this setup before we even have a product?

These are good questions, and to be honest, it does seem a little backward to be putting in all of this work to build a pipeline and document it without anyone else working on the project and no code written. This was intentional, though, to prove a point. Our process should be agnostic of the code we have written. I chose Go for this book for a variety of reasons, but you may be a JavaScript or Python developer, and these principles still apply. We can imagine that our project changes from a

hello-service to a good-bye-service, and all of the work we did will not change. The code does not matter!

To demonstrate this magic, let's write our code. Type `mkdir cmd && touch cmd/main.go`, open the file, and add the code in the following listing.

Listing 2.6 `main.go`

```go
package main

import (
    "encoding/json"
    "log"
    "net/http"
)

func main() {

    addr := ":8080"          ◁──  Hardcoding system port; for
                                  now, we will be able to
                                  configure it in the future.

    mux := http.NewServeMux()

    mux.HandleFunc("/hello",                            Creates a single handler, for
      func(w http.ResponseWriter, r *http.Request) {  ◁── now, to meet the minimum
        enc := json.NewEncoder(w)                       requirements of our system
        w.Header().
        Set("Content-Type",
        "application/json; charset=utf-8")    ◁──  Sets the default header type
        resp := Resp{                              since this will be a REST API
            Language:    "English",
            Translation: "Hello",
        }
        if err := enc.Encode(resp); err != nil {
            panic("unable to encode response", err)
        }                                          Additional logging information for
    })                                             the server port; this information is
                                                   often helpful for running multiple
    log.Printf("listening on %s\n", addr)    ◁──  servers on a single machine.

    log.Fatal(http.ListenAndServe(addr, mux))  ◁─  Runs
}                                                   the server

type Resp struct {                      ◁────────  Common structure to store
    Language    string `json:"language"`           translation information
    Translation string `json:"translation"`
}
```

We will use the internal HTTP `mux` library and Gorilla Mux in this book, but there are other options as well:

- Gin
- kit
- beego

Let's also package our code so that others will know which libraries it depends on. To do this, we will initialize a Go module. For more information on Go modules, please visit https://go.dev/blog/using-go-modules.

Type `make build` and then `./api`, and see your server run. Test it by running it in a separate terminal:

```
curl localhost:8080/hello
{"language":"English","translation":"Hello"}
```

Just like magic. Now, for my next trick, we will let our pipeline produce a binary. In your terminal type

```
git add .
git commit -am "Initial creation"
git push origin main
```

Navigate to GitHub, click on the Actions tab, and see your pipeline run. Hopefully, everything turns green. Click on the run, and you will see a binary called `api`. Download it and run it, and you will see that it works the same as the local instance. You can play around with the code and change the output to see the pipeline run and deliver new binaries.

This code is pretty dumb, but this is intentional. Think about the level of effort put in and what this opens up for others. If a coworker is waiting on this to work to build a UI, they don't need the fully developed system to start integrating. Or, if we aren't sure exactly what our customer wants quite yet, we can just get this out there for a demo. It's not perfect, but it works. And this is the essence of continuous integration and deployment: small slices of work that can keep you moving forward. Now that we have the basic code written, we need to put it on the conveyor belt for assembly and delivery.

We can now deliver a product for someone to use as we go back and improve the code we wrote. Breaking down tasks into small pieces is essential to creating a high-quality product that meets customers' demands. It also reduces the risk of introducing more code and features than what we need or can support.

Our project manager wanted a demo by tomorrow to show that this will work, and you have just done that. It isn't dynamic, and that's okay. That is a complexity we will add along the way, but it will be easy now that we have an automated way to do it.

You look at your clock and realize that it is time for lunch. You stand up and see the head of the QA department walking right toward your desk. Your eyes lock, and they wave, yelling, "Hey, do you have a quick minute?" You nod and sit back down.

Summary

- The code repository is the start of your pipeline where all code lives.
- Use scripts and tools to make environments uniform for all developers and systems.
- Document everything in your code base to make developers productive from day one.
- Automate all tasks associated with your code.

Introducing continuous testing

3

This chapter covers

- Creating a process of writing tests as you write code
- Establishing testing boundaries for sections of code
- Creating a quality gate using tests in our pipeline
- Using code coverage as a guide for refactoring and testing

The head of QA comes by your desk and grabs the chair next to you. They look a little frustrated, which makes sense because the QA team has been under immense pressure to get a new release out the door. It always seems like they are hammered with a ton of bugs, problems, and misinterpreted features. The development and QA teams always seem to be butting heads instead of working together to solve problems. The QA team feels that they are the gateway of a quality project, while development feels that QA gets in the way. Developers keep releasing buggy code and are engaged in a sadistic version of Whack-a-Mole with bugs. This relationship is so strained that

it is unhealthy. When you saw QA coming toward your desk, you knew that this wasn't going to be an easy conversation.

"Look, I'm sure you know that we are underwater at this point with the weekend release coming up. But I just got word that you are writing a new project to replace our existing translation service. We've been debugging that product for years, and at this point it is stable, so I'm not sure I'm comfortable replacing it. Yet our PM insists that this is something we need to do to grow as a company. I know you are still in the early stages of development, but I want there to be some sort of assurance that this product will work and that my team won't have to spend hours finding the same bugs we encountered years ago. Our time shouldn't be wasted dealing with these little bugs. We need to be focusing on our product being the best possible one for the customer. Do you understand?"

You nod your head and take some notes. No one likes to write bad software. No one feels good after they are blamed for a bug. No one likes to create more work for anyone else. QA stands for quality assurance, but this is a misnomer. A single person or group will never be able to assure quality, so having a special team be responsible for quality seems dubious. Quality should be the focus of everyone in the company, and various groups should test the product in different ways to make sure it's the best product you can release. You decide to sketch this out and explain your plan to the head of QA.

"What you are proposing is moving testing closer to the source code and using it as a way of documenting various test cases," the QA lead comments. "I know we have some unit tests in other areas, but they don't ever seem to catch the bugs we need. Our problem is that these tests seem to be written after the code, and they don't meet our business requirements. They are also never run, so we don't use them. It would be nice if we could have these tests run before anyone needs to test them. Do you think that's something you would be able to do?"

Sure, why not? You take some notes, find the bugs and feature requests for the old system, and get to work.

3.1   What to test

Where do you start? This is a great question, especially if you are somewhat new to development. Programming books will show you the language, and many will go as far as to show you the modern testing frameworks or libraries, but they won't show you how to write tests. They also won't show you what to test. Determining what to test and how to test it is a skill that develops over time and is something for which your team should have set standards.

For example, the head of QA is concerned about repeated bugs and wasted time. Developers are also concerned about bugs because they waste time. QA has been trained to think about various use cases, while developers have a clearer understanding of how the system works. When you are given a task to develop, it doesn't hurt to sketch out some use cases and test cases ahead of time. Once this list has been written, bounce it off of someone to see if you missed anything. Let's look at our code in the following listing.

Listing 3.1 `Main.go`

```go
package main

import (
    "encoding/json"
    "fmt"
    "log"
    "net/http"
)

func main() {

    addr := ":8080"

    mux := http.NewServeMux()

    mux.HandleFunc("/hello",
      func(w http.ResponseWriter, r *http.Request) {
        enc := json.NewEncoder(w)
        w.Header().
        Set("Content-Type",
        "application/json; charset=utf-8")
        resp := Resp{
            Language:    "English",
            Translation: "Hello",
        }
        if err := enc.Encode(resp); err != nil {
            panic("unable to encode response")
        }
    })

    log.Printf("listening on %s\n", addr)

    log.Fatal(http.ListenAndServe(addr, mux))
}

type Resp struct {
    Language    string `json:"language"`
    Translation string `json:"translation"`
}
```

What was our code supposed to do? Translate a given word into another language. Does our code do that? No. Remember, we did a minimal amount of work in the last chapter to get our pipeline working. Now we are going to focus on what the business or customers want from our code. If we look at our current implementation, we'll notice that there are three parts: the translation service, the translation handler, and the server. The service may be the least clear because it is the hardcoded value in the Resp struct. But in the future, this will be the core piece of our product and will not be hardcoded. The handler will be in charge of taking the requests and converting them so that they can be passed to the service and return the results. The server will then run the handler to tie the whole thing together.

The best way to start testing is to break our work into easily testable units. These are called *systems under test*, or SUT. The SUT has a clear boundary on what you are testing and should be treated as a *black box*, meaning that you are mostly testing the inputs and asserting the outputs are correct. We will break our SUTs into the following categories: service, handler, and server.

Right now, our code is one giant main method that makes it difficult to test, so let's break it down. First, let's tackle the service that houses all of our business logic. Remember that our service is a translation service, so the main business functions could be defined as taking a word plus a language and returning the translated word. The definition would look something like this:

```
func Translate(word string, language string) string
```

Let's create the file:

```
mkdir translation
touch translation/translator.go
```

Great; this gives us something to start with. Let's create a package called `translation`. In it, we will create a file called `translator.go`. Open `translator.go`, and add the code in the following listing.

Listing 3.2   `translator.go`

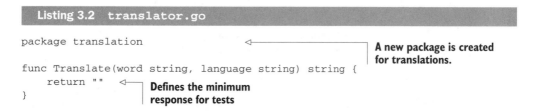

```
package translation                                          ◁───────   A new package is created
                                                                         for translations.
func Translate(word string, language string) string {
    return ""   ◁───┐   Defines the minimum
}                   │   response for tests
```

Now that we've established our initial package, we need to come up with an idea of what we should be testing. We have established the least amount of code needed to write a test. Let's now take a moment and think about what would need to be tested. Sometimes a great primer for writing tests can be to follow a given-when-then format. This format is derived from behavior-driven development and gives us a general format for how we want to structure our tests. For example, "Given a word when it is to be translated into English should then return the word."

Here, we have broken down the business need. Let's write out some more to complete our unit testing list:

- Given a word when it is to be translated into English should then return the word.
- Given a capitalized word or language when translating should then return the same answer as an uncapitalized word or language.
- Given a word or language with extra spaces when translating should then return the same answer as a word or language without spaces.
- Give a word or language when translating that is not supported should then return an empty string.

Here is where you can involve your testers or team. Send them this list to make sure you didn't miss anything and that it meets the business requirements. Remember, this is just a starting point. You may find that this list expands as you write more tests. This list is crucial in writing solid and consistent tests that help instill confidence in your code.

3.2 Writing unit tests

We have our approved list of tests; now we can start writing them. For that, we will use Go's built-in testing library and focus on writing the least amount of code possible to satisfy that test. Let's do that using our first item on the list. Open your test file, and add the code in the following listing.

Listing 3.3 `translator_test.go`

```
package translation_test          ◁─── Uses a separate package to
                                        provide black box testing
import (
    "testing"
    "github.com/holmes89/hello-api/translation"
)

func TestTranslate(t *testing.T) {
    // Arrange                     ◁─── Adds all variables to be used in
    word := "hello"                     tests for clearer organization
    language := "english"

    // Act                                    Calls the function to be tested
    res := translation.Translate(word, language)   ◁─── and captures the result

    // Assert                      Checks the
    if res != "hello" {            expected value
        t.Errorf(`expected "hello" but received "%s"`, res)    ◁─────
    }
}                                              Provides clear error responses
                                                for easier debugging of tests
```

Here is our first test. You will notice a few interesting things about this code. The first is the `Arrange`, `Act`, `Assert` pattern that we have established. Do you notice how they translate from the Given, When, Then sentences from our business needs list? This is to help us focus on what we are testing and point back to a list of testable items. We'll incorporate this back into the tests shortly so that the cases that we have covered are more clear.

You will also notice the use of the *black box* testing approach. This refers to code packages in which tests cannot see inside the code to see how it works. This allows us to write tests that assert behavior and not implementation. Remember that the system under test should be tested on its inputs and outputs and not how it works internally. This also requires you to think of an appropriate *interface*, or exposed definition for your application and code. The unit you are developing is an abstraction for others to use. Writing good tests helps drive a good interface. Having a good interface is

important because once an interface is exposed, you will need to support it in the future, and it will become hard to change.

Run all of your tests by typing the Go test command `go test  ./...`. You should see a failure. Now we need to fix it. Again, we will try to write the least amount of code possible to satisfy this test. We can handle that in our code by just returning the `word`, as in the following listing.

Listing 3.4 `translator.go`

```
package translation

func Translate(word string, language string) string {      Provides the minimum
    return word                                         ◁─┘ effort in fixing the test
}
```

After running this test, you will see that it passes! This is what in *test-driven development* is called the *red, green, refactor*. First, the test fails the first expectation, giving you a red error; then you fix the test, which makes it go green; then you add to the test or change the underlying code to make it simpler, which is refactoring. This limits the amount of work you are doing for the given feature.

Test-driven development is a design practice that many developers follow and was popularized by Kent Beck. In his book, *Test-Driven Development By Example* (Addison-Wesley Professional, 2002), Beck outlines a pattern of writing a failing test, making it pass, and then changing the code to make it fail again by taking an item off of the test list that we wrote earlier.

Why not just write all of the tests at once and be done with them? This is a great question and one that we should consider in a larger context. Test-driven development is a development pattern. It influences how you do something. By following this pattern, you are forcing developers to think through the code they are writing in the context of the requirements. It moves the development stage to a secondary operation by forcing the developer to first consider the requirements, prove that the requirements are satisfied, and then actually implement them.

To think of this another way, you can view each test as an experiment you wish to do to *prove* that your code works. In the scientific method, there are three main steps you complete: question, test, and results. With your test code, you can wonder what the result of input *x* should be based on the expected business logic. Testing will call the method, and the results will be asserted in your code.

A developer, Ian Cooper, put it another way when he advocated for developers to be "duct tape programmers." With a basic test and interface defined, the developers should just move forward and make it work. Then they can use tests to help refine their implementation, revisit it, and be confident that it works as expected. This drive helps developers meet the requirements without over-engineering a solution. Code is supposed to be dynamic, not static, so developers should be revisiting their code, refactoring it to be better, and constantly improving.

We've now satisfied this test. To verify it, run your `go test ./...` command again, and see things passing. Now let's add some more languages.

3.3 *Refactor, refactor, refactor*

For our demo, we want to support some other languages. Let's add German and Finnish to our requirements, and while we are at it, we can cross off one of our test cases:

- Given a word when it is to be translated into English should then return the word.
- Given a capitalized word or language when translating should then return the same answer as an uncapitalized word or language.
- Given a word or language with extra spaces when translating should then return the same answer as a word or language without spaces.
- Given a word or language when translating that is not supported should then return an empty string.
- Given the word *hello* when translating should then be translated into "hallo" and "hei" for languages German and Finnish.

We crossed off the first item because we have a satisfied test case. This does not mean that this test will never fail. It will fail eventually, but we have in place a test to protect us from having the business case missed.

NOTE If you find yourself changing a test instead of changing the implementation, you should consider the business effect of the change. Tests align with business requirements.

Let's add some language support. We will update our tests to include the code in the following listing.

Listing 3.5 `translator_test.go`

```go
package translate_test

import (
    "testing"
    "github.com/holmes89/hello-api/translation"
)

func TestTranslate(t *testing.T) {
    res := translation.Translate("hello", "english")      // Tests to see if translation works for English
    if res != "hello" {
        t.Errorf(`expected "hello" but recieved "%s"`, res)
    }
    res = translation.Translate("hello", "german")        // Tests to see if translation works for German
    if res != "hallo" {
        t.Errorf(`expected "hallo" but recieved "%s"`, res)
    }
    res = translation.Translate("hello", "finnish")       // Tests to see if translation works for Finnish
    if res != "hei" {
```

```
        t.Errorf(`expected "hei" but received "%s"`, res)
    }

    res = translation.Translate("hello", "dutch")      ◁─┐  Tests to see that Dutch
    if res != "" {                                        └─ returns an empty string
        t.Errorf(`expected "" but received "%s"`, res)
    }

}
```

Run it, and see that the test fails.

That means that we have different features to add to our service. Switch back to our `translator.go` file, and modify it so that we can handle these new test cases. Again, our tests are helping to drive the functionality of our code. Here we see that we are supporting translations in both German and Finnish but not Dutch, and that if a translation is not found, we return an empty string.

In this case, we are not just testing the "happy path" but also a negative one. Asserting the behavior of positive results is important, but more often than not, errors or edge cases are going to occur. *Edge cases* are rare or extreme conditions that can happen on a system and that you aren't expecting. An example of this is inputting strange characters as input or very large or small numbers. Here we can say that we need to handle the case when we don't have a translation for a language. The following listing outlines what the code would look like.

Listing 3.6 `translator.go`

```
package translation

func Translate(word string, language string) string {
    switch language {                  ◁─┐  Checks the language being passed
    case "english":                      └─ and returns the translated word
        return "hello"
    case "finnish":
        return "hei"
    case "german":
        return "hallo"
    default:
        return ""      ◁─┐  If unknown, returns
    }                    └─ an empty string
}
```

You should be able to see your test pass now. This cycle can continue for a long time. In some cases, you can head off some of the minor things right away. Keep in mind that you shouldn't leap too far ahead in your development at the risk of over-design. Try to anticipate some different use cases, as we will see in the next section. For now, we have established a pattern for working on this function.

Can you see some other edge cases in our code? Did we capture them on our list?

Tests will also need to be refactored to help make things clearer and easy to expand. I'm sure some of you who are familiar with writing software cringed a little at

the repetitive code in our tests. We can alter our structure slightly to make it easier to add tests through the use of table tests. The following listing provides an example of how we can refactor our tests to be concise.

Listing 3.7   `translator_test.go`

```go
package translation_test

import (
    "testing"
    "github.com/holmes89/hello-api/translation"
)

func TestTranslate(t *testing.T) {
    // Arrange
    tt := []struct {                          Creates an array of anonymous
        Word        string                    structs containing all test cases
        Language    string
        Translation string
    }{
        {                                     Each case houses input
            Word:        "hello",             and output results for tests.
            Language:    "english",
            Translation: "hello",
        },
        {
            Word:        "hello",
            Language:    "german",
            Translation: "hallo",
        },
        {
            Word:        "hello",
            Language:    "finnish",
            Translation: "hei",
        },
        {
            Word:        "hello",
            Language:    "dutch",
            Translation: "",
        },
    }
                                              Iterates over sets
    for _, test := range tt {                 of test cases                Runs the test and
        // Act                                                             captures the results
        res := translation.Translate(test.Word, test.Language)

        // Assert                             Checks results and responds
        if res != test.Translation {          with proper errors
            t.Errorf(
                `expected "%s" to be "%s" from "%s" but received "%s"`,
                test.Word, test.Language, test.Translation, res)
        }
    }
}
```

This pattern of testing is common in Go and other languages because it puts all of your test scenarios in one place and again pushes for a cleaner interface to our test code.

Now our assertion area is very small and is no longer repeated, and our tests are organized in such a way that we can quickly add more results. Run your tests to make sure the refactoring worked. Everything should pass. Now let's add a case that we may have not been expecting. Remember that our system is supposed to just handle "hello" for the time being. What happens if we input a word other than "hello"? Let's see what happens when we add the code in the following listing.

Listing 3.8 `translator_test.go`

```
package translate_test

import (
    "testing"
    "translation"
    "github.com/holmes89/hello-api/translation"
)

func TestTranslate(t *testing.T) {
    tt := []struct{
        Word string
        Language string
        Translation string
    }{
...
        {                          Negative case of an untranslatable
                            ◁┘     word and unsupported language
            Word: "bye",
            Language: "dutch",
            Translation: "",
        },
    }
...
}
```

Run your test. It passes. Was this what you were expecting? Did you cover all of the other cases? Remember earlier when I asked about other edge cases? This is where you need to put on your user hat and not your developer hat to start seeing where your code can go wrong. Often, we rely on other team members to find these cases (often in QA), but if it has reached that point in testing, then you are wasting valuable cycles and potentially sending out bugs in your code.

> **NOTE** The closer the quality checks are to the implementation, the less chance there is for rework, which translates into higher levels of work in progress, which translates to lost money.

Alan Perlis, a famous computer scientist, once said, "A software system can best be designed if the testing is interlaced with the designing instead of being used after the design." This sums up why we are focusing on unit tests at the moment. Unit tests can

be integrated into our development process to create leaner and more well-defined code. The corresponding tests will help guard us against making business-level logic changes that would affect the system. This does not mean that more tests are better. What is needed are quality tests that assert functionality and not fragile tests that fail constantly.

Now that we can start thinking more from a user perspective, we can focus on adding more edge cases to our unit tests to ensure that things are working as expected. Let's add another test (see the following code listing).

Listing 3.9 `translator_test.go`

```go
package translate_test

import (
    "testing"
    "translation"
    "github.com/holmes89/hello-api/translation"
)

func TestTranslate(t *testing.T) {
    // Arrange
    tt := []struct{
        Word string
        Language string
        Translation string
    }{
...
        {                          ◁──┐ Negative case of an untranslatable
            Word: "bye",                │ word with a supported language
            Language: "german",
            Translation: "",
        },
    }
...
}
```

Run your test. Now you should see a failure! We get "hallo" back when we are looking for an empty string since we are only translating "hello." How can we solve this? Go to our service again and add the code in the following listing.

Listing 3.10 `translator.go`

```go
package translation

func Translate(word string, language string) string {
    if word != "hello" {        ◁──┐ Adds check for
        return ""                    │ supported word
    }

    switch language {
    case "english":
```

```
            return "hello"
    case "finnish":
            return "hei"
    case "german":
            return "hallo"
    default:
            return ""
    }
}
```

Run your test again; now it passes! There is one final case we should possibly consider at this point. All too often developers will forget about *input sanitation*, or the process of making input uniform. This can range from white space being used, to negative numbers, invalid parameters, and uppercase or lowercase letters, just to name a few. How robust would our service be right now if we were to add uppercase letters? Let's find out by adding the code in the following listing.

Listing 3.11   `translator_test.go`

```
package translate_test

import (
    "testing"
    "github.com/holmes89/hello-api/translation"
)

func TestTranslate(t *testing.T) {
    // Arrange
    tt := []struct{
        Word string
        Language string
        Translation string
    }{
...
        {
            Word: "hello",
            Language: "German",         ◁──┐  Edge case of
            Translation: "hallo",          │  capitalized language
        },
        {
            Word: "Hello",              ◁──┐  Edge case of the
            Language: "german",            │  capitalized word
            Translation: "hallo",
        },
        {
            Word: "hello ",             ◁──┐  Edge case of
            Language: "german",            │  space in word
            Translation: "hallo",
        },
    }
...
}
```

I know I said one final case, but here are three different test cases! Can you guess what the fixes need to be?

Often it is the job of the service to implement "input sanitation" to ensure that the service is durable and flexible enough to handle most incoming messages. This is often a favorite verification technique that many QA members will attempt to do as soon as you create a service or a web page and should be handled at various levels just in case. In this instance, we can add a method that cleans the input for both the language and the word, using the code in the following listing.

Listing 3.12 `translator.go`

```
package translation

import "strings"

func Translate(word string, language string) string {        Sanitizes
    word = sanitizeInput(word)                                incoming word
    language = sanitizeInput(language)              Sanitizes incoming
                                                    language
    if word != "hello" {
        return ""
    }

    switch language {
    case "english":
        return "hello"
    case "finnish":
        return "hei"
    case "german":
        return "hallo"
    default:
        return ""
    }

}

func sanitizeInput(w string) string {           Creates a function
    w = strings.ToLower(w)                      to sanitize input
    return strings.TrimSpace(w)
}
```

Tests should pass now, but this is just the tip of the iceberg. We still have a lot of additional testing to do. We've only tackled the service layer, and it is still pretty fragile. Now we need to examine how the values get to the service in the first place, and this is through our handler.

3.4 Testing pyramid

Earlier we identified three distinct pieces of our system to be tested: service, handler, and server. Each portion can be tested in different ways. Broadly, these tests are separated into two categories:

- *Unit-level tests*—Small, contained tests that run portions of code in isolation. These can be viewed as testing individual boards and screws that are building a bridge. If one is rotten or rusted, you don't want to use it. In isolation, these tests become easier to write and manage and are the foundation of any automated test platform.
- *System-level tests*—Require interactions between various code segments or systems. This category envelops a large number of testing types and practices that become complicated to manage and therefore become less reliable or more expensive (in time and resources) to run.

Figure 3.1 demonstrates this difference.

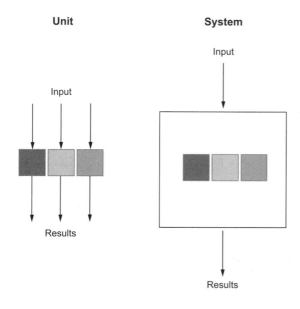

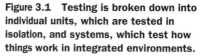

Figure 3.1   Testing is broken down into individual units, which are tested in isolation, and systems, which test how things work in integrated environments.

Unit tests are the fastest tests to run and should encompass all of the building blocks (or units) of our system. In figure 3.2, we can see testing as a pyramid wherein the unit tests form the base because of the number of tests. If the unit tests do not pass, we should not move up the testing pyramid to more extensive tests. This saves us time, as unit tests should be fast to run, easy to understand, and simple to debug. As we move up the pyramid, we see *integration* tests that verify the functionality between units of work, often including the integration with an external dependency such as a database. Finally, you have a layer of testing that verifies the system as a whole or tests it from end to end to see that the system works completely as expected. Additional types of end-to-end testing are available, such as *load testing*, which tests how the system functions with a large number of users. The inverted pyramid in figure 3.2 is an unstable pattern, while the regular pyramid supports itself.

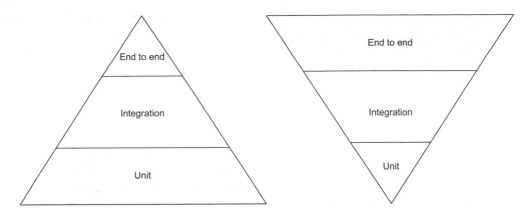

Figure 3.2 End-to-end tests are smaller at the top because they are more expensive and not as dependable. They should be supported by larger suites of integration and unit tests. Each layer should run on its own. Start with unit tests and progress up the pyramid in different phases.

Moving up the pyramid on the left, each layer becomes smaller. This is because as we move up, the ability to run these tests become more expensive because they may require dependencies or more resources. They may also not be consistent in how they run, and therefore the results may not be *deterministic*, or predictable. If we were to flip the pyramid into a "snow cone" on the right, we can imagine the world we would be in. End-to-end tests constantly change because of the ever-evolving nature of our application. If we spend so much time expanding that level of testing, we will have an immense amount of rework with no ability to verify if the underlying modules are working. If a failure occurs, you untangle all of the inner workings of the system to verify the results, whereas if you have an extensive unit test suite, you can verify bugs or changes at the module level.

You will find where you will need to expand or contract to test based on your team's needs. We have already established unit tests at the service level, establishing our base. Now we want to expand it to include some other automated tests to ensure our system works as expected.

3.5 *System testing*

Now that we've established a separate service for translation, we can call this service with a REST handler. In Go and many programming languages or frameworks, the implementation of the HTTP protocol is agnostic to the output: HTML, plain text, GraphQL syntax, and almost anything that can be returned. We try to organize our Handler files by the type of response they send. In this case, we send a REST API response.

REST stands for *Representational State Transfer*, which is a generic name for a generic style of API writing. Though most will associate it with JSON (JavaScript Object Notation), it can also be used with files or the XML format. The design is extremely flexible using the basic HTTP calls (POST, PUT, DELETE, etc.) and using HTTP headers

to send the information to the user to help decode the information. For right now, we will use JSON for our format.

To do this, we create a new package called `handlers/rest`. In it, we will create a file called `translate.go`:

```
mkdir -p handlers/rest
touch handlers/rest/translate.go
touch handlers/rest/translate_test.go
```

For now, we know that our service only handles a single word, "hello," so we are only going to support that request; otherwise, we will return a "not found," or 404 error. By default, the translation will be English unless the user passes `?language=` parameter. Let's use the code in the following listing to build an empty handler to get our tests started.

Listing 3.13   `translator.go`

```
package rest                          ◁─┐ New rest package
                                         │ for API work
import (
    "encoding/json"
    "net/http"
)
                                         ┌ Builds a struct to house
type Resp struct {                    ◁─┘ the response structure
    Language    string `json:"language"`
    Translation string `json:"translation"`
}

func TranslateHandler(w http.ResponseWriter, r *http.Request) {
    enc := json.NewEncoder(w)
    w.Header().Set("Content-Type", "application/json; charset=utf-8")
    resp := Resp{                     ◁─┐ Hardcoded response
        Language:    "English",          │ for initial work
        Translation: "Hello",
    }
    if err := enc.Encode(resp); err != nil {
        panic("unable to encode response")
    }
}
```

I'm sure you realize that this is the content from our `main` function. However, we will replace this with the actual business logic shortly. This process allows us to iterate and test as we go. We have also pulled our handler out of the main function so that it can be easily tested. Like our unit test, we want to test just an individual portion of the code, but unlike our unit test, we depend on an external part of the same system to test. A change in the `translate` library would affect this test, so it is not considered a unit test but a system test. In future chapters, we will refactor this to work in isolation, but for now, we'll have it integrate directly with the service (see the following listing).

Listing 3.14 `translator_test.go`

```go
package rest_test                          ◁─── Creates a new testing package
                                                to use black box testing
import (
    "encoding/json"
    "net/http"
    "net/http/httptest"
    "testing"
                                                            Imports a rest
    "github.com/holmes89/hello-api/handlers/rest"   ◁─── package for testing
)

func TestTranslateAPI(t *testing.T) {
                                        Creates an HTTP
    // Arrange                          recorder that will be    Creates a new request
    rr := httptest.NewRecorder()    ◁── used for assertion       against a given endpoint
    req, _ := http.NewRequest("GET", "/hello", nil)   ◁──       with no body content

    handler := http.HandlerFunc(rest.TranslateHandler)   ◁─── Registers a handler
                                                               to test against
    // Act
    handler.ServeHTTP(rr, req)   ◁──  Serves the content to pass
                                      through the handler for a
    // Assert                         response based on the request
    if rr.Code != http.StatusOK {
        t.Errorf(`expected status 200 but received %d`, rr.Code)
    }
                                            Decodes the body of the response
    var resp rest.Resp                 ◁── into a struct to be asserted
    json.Unmarshal(rr.Body.Bytes(), &resp)

    if resp.Language != "english" {
        t.Errorf(`expected language "english" but received %s`,
            resp.Language)
    }

    if resp.Translation != "hello" {
        t.Errorf(`expected Translation "hello" but received %s`,
            resp.Translation)
    }
}
```

Checks the status code from the response

Run the tests, and you should get a failure! This is because we are not using the service to lowercase our messages. Let's change our handler to now use the service instead of the hardcoded values we wrote. We will find that our tests in the handler and the service will be "tightly coupled," meaning that changes in one affect the other and that the series of tests will look similar. But remember what we are testing here is not the logic of the service but rather the handling and transformation of the request and response process.

You will also notice that we are not only asserting the body of the response message but also the status code. HTTP status codes help convey additional information to the end user by telling them what happened at a system level. 200 OK is one of the most

common and tells us that everything went fine. Table 3.1 lists common codes to use to help send messages.

Table 3.1   Common HTTP messages that most APIs utilize

Code	Message	Common Uses
200	OK	Everything went as expected.
201	Created	New entity was added to the system.
401	Unauthorized	Missing credentials.
403	Forbidden	Not allowed to access to endpoint or resource.
404	Not Found	Cannot find resource or endpoint.
500	Internal Server Error	System failed for some unknown reason.
503	Service Unavailable	System isn't working and is known.

In general, these codes are broken into several broader categories, as spelled out in table 3.2.

Table 3.2   General grouping of HTTP messages

Code	Type	Common Uses
1xx	Informational	Information about the system.
2xx	Successful	Everything went as expected.
3xx	Redirect	Something has moved and needs to change the request.
4xx	Client error	Client has something wrong.
5xx	Server error	Server failed to process request.

Our response code should reflect the type of message we are returning. The proper message in the body of our response should provide the necessary information. We do this by adding the code in the following listing.

Listing 3.15   `translator.go`

```
const defaultLanguage = "english"

func TranslateHandler(w http.ResponseWriter, r *http.Request) {
    enc := json.NewEncoder(w)
    w.Header().Set("Content-Type", "application/json; charset=utf-8")

    language := defaultLanguage
    word := strings.ReplaceAll(r.URL.Path, "/", "")
    translation := translation.Translate(language, word)
    resp := Resp{
        Language:     language,
```

Sets the header for the content type to be a JSON specification

Gets word from the URL path

Default language to English for now

Translates the word

```
        Translation: translation,
    }
    if err := enc.Encode(resp); err != nil {
        panic("unable to encode response")
    }
}
```

We will now add some additional functionality. But, as before, let's restructure these tests to be table tests so that we can rapidly refactor what we are writing. We'll rewrite it using the code in the following listing.

Listing 3.16 `translator_test.go`

```
func TestTranslateAPI(t *testing.T) {
    tt := []struct {                          ◁─┐  Defines test cases to be an endpoint,
        Endpoint            string              │  status, translation, and language
        StatusCode          int
        ExpectedLanguage    string
        ExpectedTranslation string
    }{
        {
            Endpoint:            "/hello",
            StatusCode:          http.StatusOK,
            ExpectedLanguage:    "english",
            ExpectedTranslation: "hello",
        },
        {
            Endpoint:            "/hello?language=german",
            StatusCode:          http.StatusOK,
            ExpectedLanguage:    "german",
            ExpectedTranslation: "hallo",
        },
    }
                                                          ┌─  Registers
    handler := http.HandlerFunc(rest.TranslateHandler)  ◁─┘  Handler

    for _, test := range tt {                  ◁─────────────  Iterates through
        rr := httptest.NewRecorder()                          all test scenarios
        req, _ := http.NewRequest("GET", test.Endpoint, nil)

        handler.ServeHTTP(rr, req)

        if rr.Code != test.StatusCode {
            t.Errorf(`expected status %d but received %d`,
                test.StatusCode, rr.Code)
        }

        var resp rest.Resp
        json.Unmarshal(rr.Body.Bytes(), &resp)

        if resp.Language != test.ExpectedLanguage {
            t.Errorf(`expected language "%s" but received %s`,
                test.ExpectedLanguage, resp.Language)
        }
```

```
        if resp.Translation != test.ExpectedTranslation {
            t.Errorf(`expected Translation "%s" but received %s`,
                test.ExpectedTranslation, resp.Translation)
        }
    }
}
```

Run your tests, and you'll see a new failure. Let's fix the test (see the following code listing).

Listing 3.17 `translator.go`

```go
func TranslateHandler(w http.ResponseWriter, r *http.Request) {
    enc := json.NewEncoder(w)
    w.Header().Set("Content-Type", "application/json; charset=utf-8")

    language := r.URL.Query().Get("language")      ◁┐ Retrieves language
    if language == "" {                            │ from query parameters
        language = defaultLanguage
    }
    word := strings.ReplaceAll(r.URL.Path, "/", "")
    translation := translation.Translate(word, language)
    resp := Resp{
        Language:    language,
        Translation: translation,
    }
    if err := enc.Encode(resp); err != nil {
        panic("unable to encode response")
    }
}
```

Run your tests, and add one more case, where if a translation is missing, the response should be 404 Not Found with no values. Let's add it (see the following listing).

Listing 3.18 `translator_test.go`

```go
func TestTranslateAPI(t *testing.T) {
    tt := []struct{
        Endpoint string
        StatusCode int
        ExpectedLanguage string
        ExpectedTranslation string
    }{
        {
            Endpoint: "/hello",
            StatusCode: 200,
            ExpectedLanguage: "english",
            ExpectedTranslation: "hello",
        },
        {
            Endpoint: "/hello?language=german",
            StatusCode: 200,
            ExpectedLanguage: "german",
            ExpectedTranslation: "hallo",
```

```
        },
        {
            Endpoint: "/hello?language=dutch",          On a missing language or
            StatusCode: http.StatusNotFound,            translation, we should
            ExpectedLanguage: "",                       get a 404 error code.
            ExpectedTranslation: "",
        },
    }
    ...
}
```

See the failures, and fix the code (see the following listing).

Listing 3.19 `translator.go`

```go
func TranslateHandler(w http.ResponseWriter, r *http.Request) {
    enc := json.NewEncoder(w)
    w.Header().Set("Content-Type", "application/json; charset=utf-8")

    language := r.URL.Query().Get("language")
    if language == "" {
        language = "english"
    }
    word := strings.ReplaceAll(r.URL.Path, "/", "")
    translation := translation.Translate(word, language)
    if translation == "" {
        language = ""
        w.WriteHeader(http.StatusNotFound)
        return
    }
    resp := Resp{
        Language:    language,
        Translation: translation,
    }
    if err := enc.Encode(resp); err != nil {
        panic("unable to encode response")
    }
}
```

We should have success!

3.6 Adding it to the pipeline

Now that we've refactored our services, we should update our function and add the
tests to the pipeline. First, let's update our `main.go` file to use our new handler and
service (see the following listing).

Listing 3.20 `main.go`

```go
package main

import (
    "log"
```

```
        "net/http"
)

func main() {

    addr := ":8080"                                    Sets the port
                                                         to listen on
    mux := http.NewServeMux()
                                                                        Registers the
    mux.HandleFunc("/hello", rest.TranslateHandler)                      translation Handler

    log.Printf("listening on %s\n", addr)               Logs the listening port

    log.Fatal(http.ListenAndServe(addr, mux))            Runs the server
}                                                         and logs if it fails
```

Ah, that looks so much cleaner! We have successfully pulled out a good portion of our application into smaller pieces that can be tested on their own, making the system easier to reason about. We've spent all of this time writing these tests so that we can use them to help verify functionality when we check our code. Once we add this to our pipeline it will be just like the build step in that it protects us from pushing broken changes out, yet testing becomes our first "gate" in the system.

A *quality gate* is a term used in industrial engineering in which a product is checked for quality before various stages along the assembly line. You want to protect each stage from wasting time. In our little program, the build step runs fairly quickly, but on larger, more complicated systems, build times can take much longer, so we want to make sure we don't waste time trying to build something that is broken or shipping code that doesn't work as intended.

Suppose that you are planning on cooking a meal. You mix a bunch of ingredients for a recipe to get to a step and realize that the main ingredient has gone bad. Now you either need to run to the store quickly or scrap the whole thing, wasting either time or money. But if you had checked the quality of all of the ingredients ahead of time, you would have been able to save yourself some trouble.

We will structure our pipeline to do the same. By adding a testing step before the build step, we can make sure that our code is running before we build. Most CI systems allow you to create a dependency graph between various steps in order to chain these steps together to save time and effort on the system as a whole. We will extend this in the future to add additional guards, builds, and deployments that can be run in parallel.

For now, let's add the test check to the pipeline from the code in the following listing.

Listing 3.21 **pipeline.yml**

```
name: CI Checks

on:
  push:                           Only runs on
    branches:                     the main branch
        - main
jobs:
```

```
test:
  name: Test Application
  runs-on: ubuntu-latest          ◁──┐  Defines base
  steps:                                  operating system
  - name: Set up Go 1.x          ◁──┐  Sets up the Go
    uses: actions/setup-go@v2            environment
    with:
      go-version: ^1.18
  - name: Check out code into the Go module directory    ◁──┐  Checks out
    uses: actions/checkout@v2                                    the code
  - name: Downloads
    run: go get -t ./...
  - name: Run Test
    run: go test ./...           ◁──┐  Runs tests
build:
  name: Build  App
  runs-on: ubuntu-latest
  needs: test                     ◁──┐  Waits for tests to pass before
  steps:                                  moving onto the build step

  - name: Set up Go 1.x
    uses: actions/setup-go@v2
    with:
      go-version: ^1.18

...
```

Commit your changes, and push your branch! Go to your repository, and watch the tests run. Now you can see the results.

3.7   Code coverage

Writing tests to see if the code works is helpful. We added several tests to poke and prod various parts of our system and added functionality as we went. But did we get it all? Do we need to test *everything*?

Many languages, including Go, provide the ability to see the "code coverage" of your tests, which means they will highlight a percentage of the code that has been tested and highlight areas that may have been missed. As your code grows, you will have branches of logic that you may need to test or additional error conditions that may occur, and it is always helpful to make sure you can extend the testing so you hit all of the areas you need. Let's see how much we have already tested:

```
go test ./... -cover
```

Figure 3.3 shows the coverage.

```
jholmes:hello-api (main) $ go test ./... -cover
?       github.com/holmes89/hello-api   [no test files]
ok      github.com/holmes89/hello-api/handlers/rest    0.003s  coverage: 92.3% of statements
ok      github.com/holmes89/hello-api/translation      0.002s  coverage: 100.0% of statements
```

Figure 3.3   Output reflects the coverage of lines in a package.

You should see a chart showing all of the tested files and the coverage amounts, along with a total at the bottom. The percentage tells us that we haven't hit all of our code and should perhaps consider adding more testing. You may be wondering how much coverage is needed. Over time, your code coverage should increase due to the addition of more tests. This ensures that you are improving your system over time. This can mean writing more tests in areas that are lacking or even deleting unused code.

Code coverage can be a hot topic in some development groups. Some people say you need to cover every line of code and test every possible way a portion of code can be executed to ensure the highest quality. While this is a worthwhile endeavor, it won't mean that your code is working as intended. Attempting to reach total code coverage can lead to poorly written tests that are difficult to maintain over time. Often arbitrary goals like this, while well intended, lead toward blocking the overall goal of the company: delivering a product.

What we want to do is enforce a certain level of testing, say 80%, and we also want to provide our developers an easy way to see if there are any branches or areas they are missing that they can easily add tests to. We will add some tools to our Makefile to make this easier.

Go has a built-in tool that allows you to output a coverage profile and then use tools that help you manipulate it so that you can see the coverage and generate a report. First, let's open our Makefile and add the code in the following listing.

Listing 3.22   Makefile

```
test:
    go test ./... -coverprofile=coverage.out

coverage:
    go tool cover -func coverage.out | grep "total:" | \
    awk '{print ((int($$3) > 80) != 1) }'
```

← **Generates the output coverage from the test**

← **Uses the code coverage tool to find the total line count and check the value to make sure it meets coverage expectations**

This script will help ensure that the coverage profile is created instead of just running go test. Remember, we want to provide the same tools to our developers that the pipeline will use to help keep the two in sync. The second line provides a bit of "Unix magic" that pipes the results from the coverage tool into a grep command to look for the total and then checks the result to make sure it is higher than our minimum testing threshold. The result of this will return an error code if the condition does not pass, meaning that our pipeline will fail.

Now we can use this same coverage profile to generate a coverage report, which we will add as an artifact to our pipeline. It will help guide our current and future testing efforts to see where we are lacking. This can also help leaders on the team determine if they should do a testing day where developers take a day to clean up code and add tests. We'll discuss more activities like this in later chapters, but what you should

understand now is that communication is key to building a successful team. Reports that come from the pipeline are great in helping steer the overall developer experience and product development as time goes on.

NOTE Communication is key to building a successful team.

To generate a report, we will add another tool to the Makefile:

```
report:
    go tool cover -html=coverage.out -o cover.html
```

In the report in figure 3.4, you will see lines that you have been able to test and those that have been missed. Do you see any areas that we could have tested? Can we refactor our code so that it is easier to get to these missing sections? Try it yourself to see if you can get to a higher level, and time yourself to see how long that takes and if it helps to solve a possible bug.

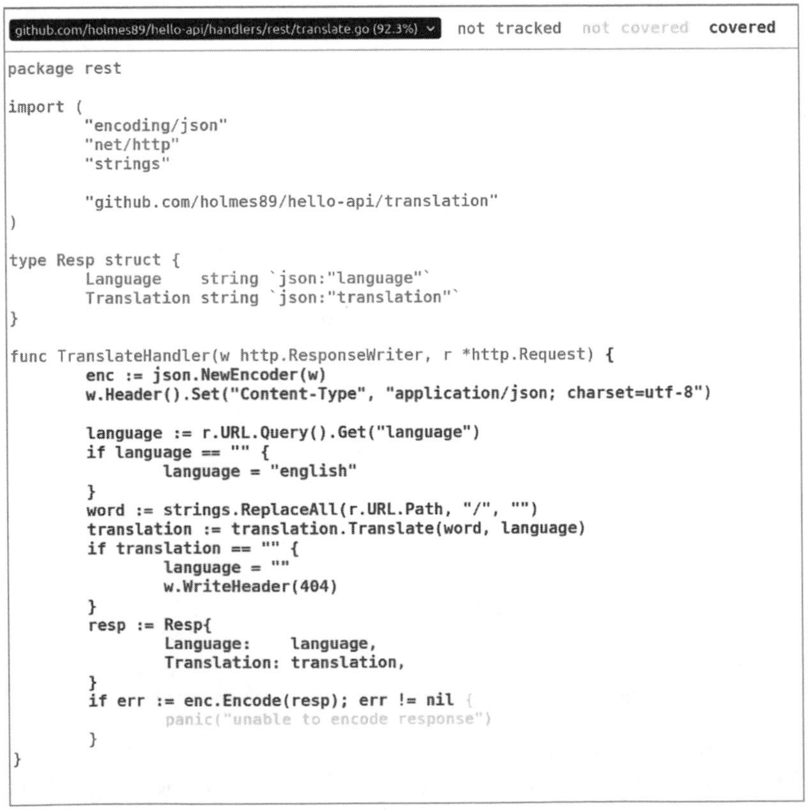

```
github.com/holmes89/hello-api/handlers/rest/translate.go (92.3%) ⌄     not tracked   not covered   covered

package rest

import (
        "encoding/json"
        "net/http"
        "strings"

        "github.com/holmes89/hello-api/translation"
)

type Resp struct {
        Language    string `json:"language"`
        Translation string `json:"translation"`
}

func TranslateHandler(w http.ResponseWriter, r *http.Request) {
        enc := json.NewEncoder(w)
        w.Header().Set("Content-Type", "application/json; charset=utf-8")

        language := r.URL.Query().Get("language")
        if language == "" {
                language = "english"
        }
        word := strings.ReplaceAll(r.URL.Path, "/", "")
        translation := translation.Translate(word, language)
        if translation == "" {
                language = ""
                w.WriteHeader(404)
        }
        resp := Resp{
                Language:    language,
                Translation: translation,
        }
        if err := enc.Encode(resp); err != nil {
                panic("unable to encode response")
        }
}
```

Figure 3.4 Lines are highlighted in green if the test code has covered that code, while lines in red have not. If you are unable to differentiate the color, please note that the error section is the only untested area of the code.

These output files should be stored locally and should not be checked into our source control. Open your `.gitignore`, and add the following:

```
coverage.out
cover.html
```

Now we can update our CI code to run a coverage check and upload a report. Your team could do some additional steps post-processing to allow for publishing these results to a team dashboard or a Slack post for others to see easily, but for now, we will allow it to be downloaded along with the binary (see the following listing).

Listing 3.23 `pipeline.yml`

```yaml
name: CI Checks

on:
  push:
    branches:
      - main
jobs:
  test:
    name: Test Application
    runs-on: ubuntu-latest
    steps:
    - name: Set up Go 1.x
      uses: actions/setup-go@v2
      with:
        go-version: ^1.18
    - name: Check out code into the Go module directory
      uses: actions/checkout@v2
    - name: Run Test                      Uses the test
      run: make test                      make command
    - name: Coverage Check
      run: make coverage                  Checks coverage
    - name: Generate Report               for the tests
      run: make report          Generates a report
    - name: Copy Files        based on coverage
      run: |
          mkdir reports
          cp cover.html reports/.      Uploads reports
    - name: Archive                       to an archive
      uses: actions/upload-artifact@v2
      with:
          name: reports
          path: reports
```

We have now successfully added the first check on our system. Testing can seem cumbersome at first to some, and others may need convincing of its benefits, but it is an easy way to make sure you are moving forward with quality code. In the future, you will find a test that saves you from making a mistake. Even while writing this book, I've found that the tests that I've written have fixed bugs in my sample code. Stopping to think and work through the problems at hand helps you become a better developer as well.

Testing is a very sensitive area for some development teams. Some members will have a higher level of passion for it than others. It becomes important that you and your team establish the testing patterns and practices you'd like to accomplish and standardize them if possible. Testing should not become dogmatic, nor should it hinder the development of your product. It is a tool to tell your company and your customers that you are meeting their expectations.

You look up and see people leaving the office. It's the end of the day, and you've committed and pushed your code. When you navigate to the repository, you see a nice little green check mark, and you smile. In a day, you've written a proof of concept with tests to go along with it. Tomorrow you will need to find a way to get it live before your demo at noon. Luckily, you have a plan in mind.

Summary

- Automated testing helps validate that the system works as expected.
- Unit tests are small, independently run tests that focus on a small portion of code.
- System tests integrate into multiple modules that assert the overall behavior of the system.
- Focus on testing the interface to the code and not the code itself.
- Strive for high test coverage, but it's okay for it to be less than 100%.

Introducing
continuous deployment

You get to work early. After dropping your stuff off at your desk, you migrate to the coffee machine. As you arrive, you see a group of operations people talking. You'd like to say this is a coincidence, but it's not. You know that the operations team gets in early and that this is the best time to talk to them.

Greeting them, you casually mention the demo you have been working on. Someone groans: "I can't see how they can expect us to keep doing this. We just don't have the resources to keep funding and running these little projects. We have a backlog of work to be done: new projects, deployments, system upgrades, and performance tuning. On top of that, we are constantly being pulled off because of emergencies. I'm not blaming you, but it's just a nightmare sometimes."

It is a nightmare sometimes. You remember completing a feature just a couple of months ago and waiting for it to be deployed. It took over a week for the

scheduled release, and the deployment failed because someone else's configuration change broke the system. What transpired was a whole-day event with people going through all of the changes trying to figure out what broke. The gap between creating the code and the deployment of it was too great and caused so many problems.

"What I'd like to do is have developers own more of the deployment piece. We set up the process and approved services and they own the deployments themselves. We would help update and maintain the machines while they focus on the deployments and problems surrounding them. If we could use some of these new services that don't require us to maintain a server, it would be ideal. But honestly, I don't know what this model would look like and if anyone would go for it. In the long run, it would save us money and time."

That's exactly what you were hoping someone would say. Give the power to the developer. Run the service without the server overhead. Iterate quickly and deliver often. You mention that you could include it as part of your demo.

"Really?" the operations person says, "You'd add that scope to your project for us? That would be great, and I'd love to hear about what you find and what options we could have."

Taking this as permission, you pour your coffee and head back to your desk.

4.1 Delivery

The first thing you realize is that you want to get this into the hands of other people eventually. Yesterday it was the QA team who were interested, and tomorrow it may be the entire development team. You need to put the compiled product out there for others to easily consume. You need to deliver.

> **NOTE** See chapter 2 for a list of pipeline tools to use like Jenkins, GitLab, and CircleCI.

To do this, we can attach a binary to our pipeline, just like we did with the code coverage report in the last chapter. Let's open up our `pipeline.yml` file and add the code in the following listing.

Listing 4.1 `pipeline.yml`

```
name: CI Checks

on:
  push:
    branches:
      - main

jobs:
    test:
        ....
    deliver:              ⟵── Creates a new step in our
        name: Release          pipeline called deliver
```

```
needs: build
runs-on: ubuntu-latest
steps:
- name: Checkout code
    uses: actions/checkout@v2
- name: Download binary
    uses: actions/download-artifact@v2
    with:
        name: api
- name: Create Release
    id: create_release
    uses: actions/create-release@v1
    env:
        GITHUB_TOKEN: ${{ secrets.GITHUB_TOKEN }}
    with:
        tag_name: ${{ github.ref }}
    release_name: Release ${{ github.ref }}
    body: |
        Still in experimentation phase
    draft: true
    prerelease: true
- name: Upload Release Binary
    uses: actions/upload-release-asset@v1
    env:
        GITHUB_TOKEN:
            ${{ secrets.GITHUB_TOKEN }}
    with:
        upload_url:
            ${{ steps.create_release.outputs.upload_url }}
    asset_path: api
    asset_name: api
    asset_content_type: application/octet-stream
```

Downloads the binary from our build step

GitHub Actions provides an internal token for authorization to update your repository.

Names the release using the same mechanism as in the previous step

Tags the release using the changed reference that triggered the build. Now it is just changing to the main branch that will be used later for other deployment triggers. This is a property that is passed to us from the GitHub Action environment.

This is not a finalized release, so we mark it as a draft so that it is not viewable by customers.

Similarly, we aren't finalized, so we mark this as a pre-release.

Uploads the binary file to the release URL created in a previous step

The content type is a binary, so we need to define this as an octet stream so that it can be recognized by GitHub.

We can now push our change to our pipeline and watch it run. Once complete, you should see a new release on the Releases tab on your repository, as shown in figure 4.1.

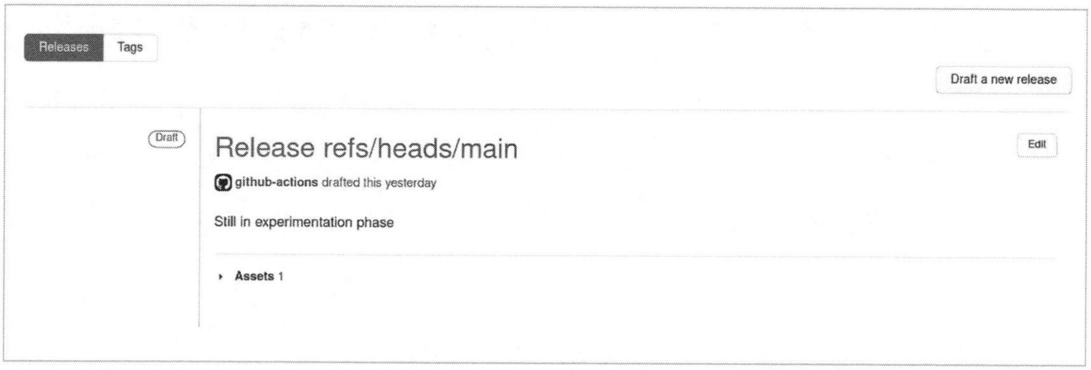

Figure 4.1   The page contains all the information we need right now, along with a downloadable binary.

There you have it! You are delivering a product right away, but this isn't the end of our pipeline. The reason we are focused on just publishing our product is that it is the simplest form of *delivery*—providing a product for someone to use, but that doesn't necessarily mean deployment, which is making the product run. *Deployment* is the final step in a process in which you run and use your product as a service. Not all products get deployed, but all should be delivered. A library is a common product that is not deployed but delivered. Deployments can also get complicated (as we will see) based on their run location. Building and running new servers or software upgrades are additional forms of deployment. In this chapter, we will tackle both.

The only way to know if a product is viable in a marketplace is to get it out there. Once people start using your product, you receive feedback on what they want, what they like, and what they don't like. This feedback drives the development of your product. Thus far, we've written what is known as a *minimal viable product*, or MVP. Though our example is simple, you should be able to see that what you first write doesn't need to be perfect. In fact, it will never be perfect. Many companies wait too long to get feedback on what they are building because they don't put themselves out there fast enough.

Feedback can be in the form of a single person who has a vision, a group of pilot users, investors, or the general public. Getting your product out isn't the only thing you need to worry about. You must also focus on how fast you can get your product released. This is what we've been building toward. Our pipeline will help transform our code into a product and release it. It is this last step that we still need to finish, but once we have done so, we can start iterating on our process to make a better product.

It might seem strange that we are already releasing something this early in the book, but this is the essence of what we are trying to do. Like our product, our pipeline will never be perfect. You and your team need to revise and enhance your pipeline just as you do your product. Manufacturers go through a similar process of not only creating and enhancing the products they make but also increasing the efficiency with which they produce them.

4.2   Developers as operators

To some of you, this process may seem odd. Why am I doing the deployment when I have an entire operations team to handle it? This is a good question. Many companies will structure their teams to be focused on particular areas in which they are specialists. While this allows individuals to focus on being experts in specific areas, it often puts up barriers between teams. This can put teams at odds with one another and prevent positive collaboration. The collaboration breaks down because it becomes easier to play a blame game instead of taking the time to understand the problems and working together toward a solution.

Take the following scenario: A tester finds a bug with an incorrect date on a report and files a ticket assigned to a developer. The developer looks at the bug and writes, "This works fine on my machine; the server must not be configured for the correct time zone" and attaches a screenshot. The ticket then gets punted to the operations

team, and they just reassign the ticket with the comment "`Server is configured properly; will not complete." There the ticket sits for weeks while everyone thinks it isn't their problem.

Who is the victim here? QA? Developers? Operations? Wrong. It's the customer.

When we don't work as a team, we don't understand each other's roles. When we don't understand each other's roles, we don't think of solutions that can help them and ultimately the customer.

In the early days of NASA's space program, there was a realization that mission control was having problems troubleshooting and understanding the technologies they were developing and using. This was all new to everyone because no one had been in space at that time. Gene Kranz, then a procedures officer (he later became the flight director during Apollo 13), realized there was a disconnect and that engineers needed to become operators. Engineers built the systems; they understood them technically but never actually used them as part of a larger system. Operators, on the other hand, did not need to understand the inner workings of the device; they just needed to know how to make it run and what problems it could create.

Today we can look at the same process as asking our software engineers to become operators. This is known as DevOps, which combines software development and IT operations. As Gene Kranz found during the early days of NASA, systems can become complicated very quickly, and there is a loss of knowledge between each line of communication. In space missions, if someone didn't know what caused a blinking red light, the results could have been catastrophic.

DevOps has taken over the industry in so many ways, but often it becomes a misnomer and ends up being operations. Real DevOps comes when a developer has the opportunity to deploy and manage products in production, while operations teams can make changes to code for either deployments or problems with the product. It's a portmanteau for a reason. The teams become blended. In fact, if I had it my way, I would call it DevOpQas and include the testing as part of all of this.

We have already done some DevOps work in our project, but I find that it's good to take a quick aside to tell you why it is important. As a developer, you can have insight into how your code works; as an operations member, you have insight into how it should run. There will be operations members who have a better understanding of how a project should be deployed, and they can guide you through the solution or provide examples or modules for you to use. There will be developers who will be able to help enhance and build deployments and pipelines to make their products run efficiently.

To build effective products, you need to find a way to work as a team. Understanding is the key to success, and that success will make your customers happy.

4.3 Setting up a deployment account

A notification appears in your email. It reads, "Thanks for looking into deploying your project on your own. I have elevated your account on our Google Cloud account for you to experiment with. For your demo, I would suggest looking into some of their 'as a service' products. Try a few out and let me know what you think. We can talk later."

Great! You now have the power to deploy things in production. Use this power wisely!

This is exciting because you've been reading up on various products and ways of deploying them. However, before you can get started, you need to create an account and set up a deployment key. To create the account, we will need to navigate to https://cloud.google.com/free. Click on Get Started for the link. After your account is set up, we will create a deployment key by using a service account.

> **NOTE** We will use Google's Cloud Platform (GCP) for all of the deployments we do here. GCP offers a great free tier that allots a credit for their products, and many of their products run for free under a specific load. We can use GCP to develop and deploy our product without incurring any upfront costs. The principles we adopt here are easily transferable to other platforms such as Amazon Web Services (AWS) and Microsoft Azure.

To do this, go to the right-hand hamburger menu, find APIs & Services, and select Credentials, as shown in figure 4.2.

Once on this page, click the Create Credentials button at the top, and select Service Account.

> **NOTE** A service account is extremely important to have whenever you are building a product on an external system. Your account houses things like credit cards and other personal identifying information and typically has full access to the full range of products on a given platform. It is also locked with specific permissions and privileges that will not compromise your account if for some reason a person outside of your organization gains access to it. The service account setup will look like figure 4.3.

Here, you will choose a name that you feel is appropriate. You should create a service account for a specific product you are building or a specific service you are utilizing. In this case, we will focus on the product itself and call it hello-api.

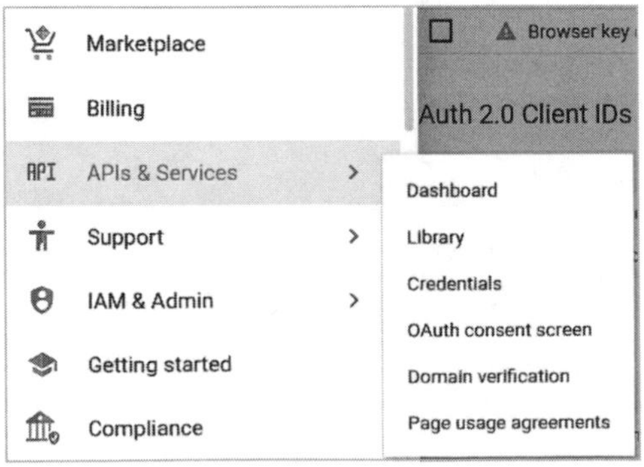

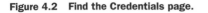

Figure 4.2 Find the Credentials page. 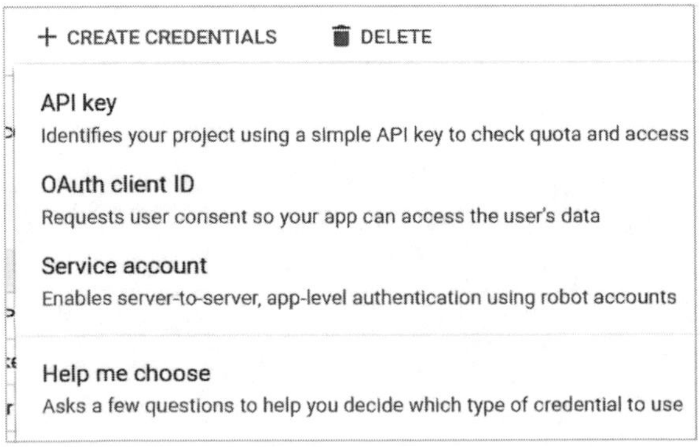   **Figure 4.3 Create a new service account.**

Next, we will be prompted to select specific roles for a service account. We will add additional permissions in the future, but for now, use the search prompt that appears to select the following roles:

- *App Engine admin*—Provides administrator functions for App Engine, such as deleting and calling endpoints
- *App Engine deployer*—Permits deployment of App Engine applications
- *Cloud build editor*—Allows the user to edit cloud functions
- *Cloud functions admin*—Allows the user to create and destroy cloud functions
- *Cloud functions developer*—Allows the creation and editing of cloud functions
- *Storage admin*—Allows files to be stored

Select products from figure 4.4.

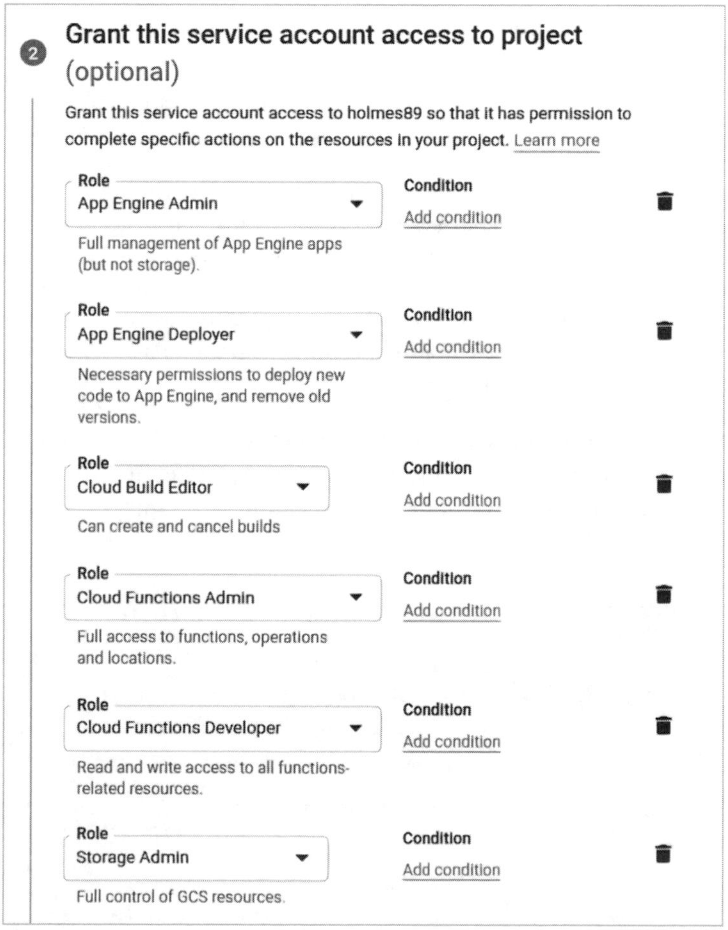

Figure 4.4   Each product will be used for different permissions for different products.

Once all of these are selected, click Continue, and then click Done. Click on your newly created user, and then select Keys at the top.

Click Add Key → Create New Key, select JSON, and download the file. This is a credentials file that we can then add to our GitHub account as a secret for deployments. Keep it safe somewhere. Figure 4.5 shows an example key setup.

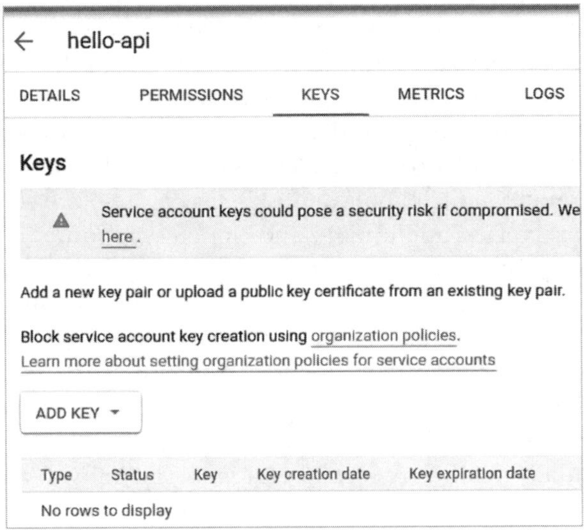

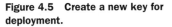

Figure 4.5   Create a new key for deployment.

In the meantime, open a tab, navigate to your GitHub repository, and select Settings → Secrets. There, create a new secret called GCP_CREDENTIALS. Add the contents of your JSON file to this and save it. Now we can add our function to the pipeline as shown in figure 4.6.

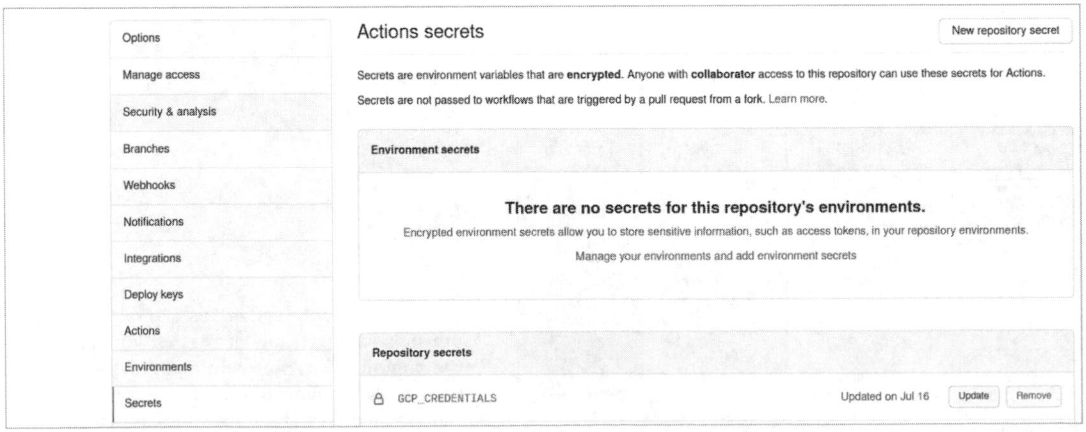

Figure 4.6   Add the contents of the key to a secret in GitHub.

Now we are ready to create a deployment for any product we want to run our application. But which do we choose?

4.4   *As you like it*

Gone are the days when most of us worried about setting up a physical server. AWS launched its compute platform in 2006, and it revolutionized how companies run and maintain their servers. Servers were then virtualized and controlled by a set of unique API commands that allowed for the easy creation and destruction of server instances and provided a great abstraction, known as Infrastructure as a Service (IaaS), for developers to work with. The following year, in 2007, a company called Heroku made the job even easier for developers to get their products deployed. They created what is known as Platform as a Service (PaaS). This platform provided abstractions that allowed developers to quickly create and iterate on their applications. Between these two companies, we have seen a revolution in serverless applications and cloud computing.

Today, other products are labeled "as a service." Each service provides a different layer of abstraction to a developer as it is needed. Abstractions are helpful because they hide certain details about the underlying system from the user. This abstraction comes at two costs. First is the financial cost of using the abstraction because often the higher the abstraction, the higher the overall cost. Over time, if a product takes off, it may become more affordable to start using other services that are cheaper but rely more on developers to maintain them. The second cost is the inability to access certain features hidden by the abstraction. For example, in a Function as a Service, the user is not able to use system libraries to do things such as image processing or video splitting. As with everything, this comes with various trade-offs and is something you and your company will need to decide on. As you can see in figure 4.7, all of these services run on servers, but what you need to worry about varies based on the abstraction. Moving from right to left, your cost often becomes time, while moving from left to right, the cost becomes money.

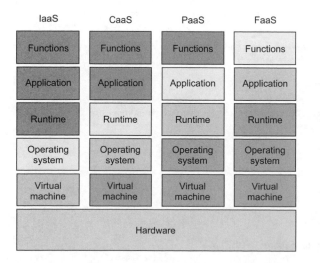

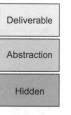

Figure 4.7   Each type of "as a service" product provides various levels of abstraction that you as the customer interact with and provide releasable items based on this abstraction. Below the abstraction are various elements of servers that in the past have been the responsibilities of entire teams to maintain.

The way you develop your code also changes when moving in different directions. Moving to the right provides a lot of abstraction and therefore focuses on a single function that can be run. Moving to the left allows you to utilize more system-level functions such as storage and operating system calls. Table 4.1 outlines the various services.

Table 4.1 "As a service" applications

Abbreviation	Service	Products
IaaS	Infrastructure as a Service	AWS EC2, Google Compute
CaaS	Container as a Service	AWS ECS, Google Cloud Run
PaaS	Platform as a Service	Heroku, Google App Engine, AWS Elastic Beanstalk
FaaS	Function as a Service	AWS Lambda, Google Cloud functions

To create an effective demonstration for your company, you must first outline the cost decisions for what you are doing and show how flexible your product can be in each of these environments as time progresses. An operations member suggested picking one, but you think, "Why not pick two for the demonstration?" The first deployment type will demonstrate rapid development at a low cost through a Function as a Service (FaaS), and the second will demonstrate a scalable application service through a Platform as a Service (PaaS). Most companies will move from right to left in figure 4.7 until they find the one that fits them best. We will use this approach throughout the book so that we can pull back various layers of abstraction.

First, let's create a serverless application due to its low-cost usage. A *serverless* application is another name for a FaaS application because it has a single entry point that is the function, and the developer doesn't need to know or understand anything about the platform or runtime. This abstraction buys your team time as they will not need to focus on doing security updates to systems or library upgrades for a container. Nor do they need to pay for idle time on the system. Most cloud solutions will charge you by the hour to have a service run. FaaS instead focuses on the number of invocations your function encounters. This allows you and your team to experiment with your product while it is in development and incurs little to no costs.

4.5 *Function as a Service (FaaS)*

Unfortunately, there is no universal way to create FaaS applications across different platforms. You define a package and function to run a command from, and that is what is built and deployed on GCP. Go uses a standard http.Handler, so there will be little to change for our product. However, GCP will look only in a designated root folder and will not handle functions in sub-packages.

Open a new `faas.go` file in the root of your project, and put in the code in the following listing.

> **Listing 4.2   Adding a proxy handler to move our calls**

```
package faas

import (
  "net/http"

  "github.com/holmes89/hello-api/handlers/rest"
)

func Translate(w http.ResponseWriter, r *http.Request) {
  rest.TranslateHandler(w, r)
}
```

You can always use an http.Mux here to reroute multiple calls in the future through a single function.

That's all we need to do to get our function working. Now we can create a deployment step to our pipeline. Open your pipeline.yml file, and add the deployment step (see the following listing).

> **Listing 4.3   `pipeline.yml`**

```
jobs:
...
  deploy-function:
    name: Deploy FaaS
    runs-on: ubuntu-latest
    needs: test
    if: ${{ github.event_name == 'push' && github.ref == 'refs/heads/main' }}
    steps:
    - name: Check out code into the Go module directory
      uses: actions/checkout@v2
      with:
        fetch-depth: 0
    - name: Deploy function
      id: deploy
      uses: google-github-actions/deploy-cloud-functions@main
      with:
        name: translate          ◁──┐  Gives the function
        entry_point: Translate   ◁─    a name to reference
        runtime: go116
        credentials: ${{ secrets.gcp_credentials }}   ◁──┐
    - id: test
      run: curl "${{ steps.deploy.outputs.url }}/hello"   ◁──┐
```

Gives the name of the function to call → (points to `entry_point: Translate`)

Uses the secret that is registered for the service account to conduct the deployment

Tests the call to see if it works

When tests pass, the deployment step will occur. From the output from your deployment, you should see an endpoint. Before you can call it, you will need to update the permissions to allow public access to this endpoint. Navigate to your Google Cloud console and search for "functions." You should see your newly created function, as shown in figure 4.8.

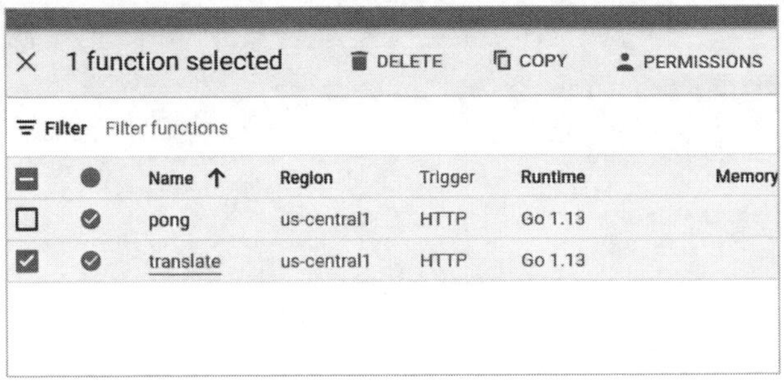

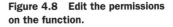

Figure 4.8   Edit the permissions on the function.

NOTE You may need to enable the Cloud functions: http://mng.bz/KlOZ.

Click Add Member, type "allUsers," and give it the Cloud function invoker role. It will give you a prompt telling you that this will make your function public, as seen in figure 4.9.

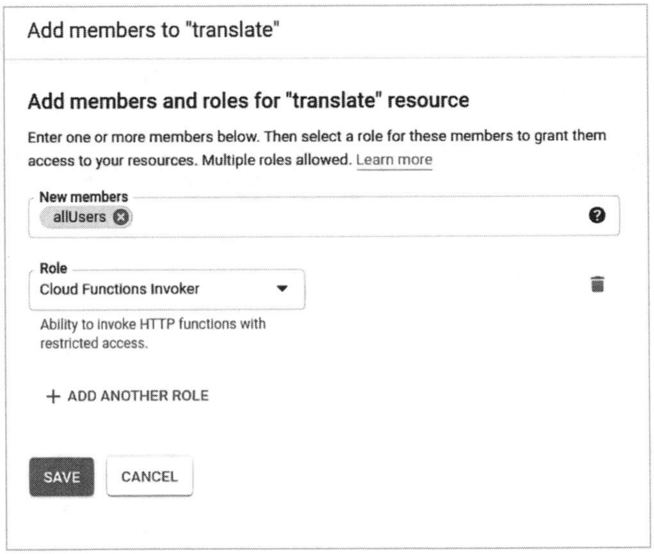

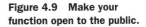

Figure 4.9   Make your function open to the public.

Press the confirmation in the prompt, open up a browser, and type in the URL found in the pipeline output with `/translate/hello?language=german`. You should see the response come back! Change the language. What do you see? Play around with different inputs and see what you can do to make it work (or cause it to break!).

When your trial runs out, you may incur some costs for running these various applications. To prevent this, remove the applications when you are done with this book.

To underline the power of what we just did, let's modify our code by supporting a new language. Open your `translate.go` file, and add a translation for French using the code in the following listing.

Listing 4.4 `translate.go`

```go
func Translate(word string, language string) string {
  word = sanitizeInput(word)
  language = sanitizeInput(language)

  if word != "hello" {
    return ""
  }

  switch language {
  case "english":
    return "hello"
  case "finnish":
    return "hei"
  case "german":
    return "hallo"
  case "french":                    New line to check to
    return "bonjour"                see if your CI works
  default:
    return ""
  }

}
```

Don't forget to add the test! (See the following listing.)

Listing 4.5 `translator_test.go`

```go
func TestTranslate(t *testing.T) {
  // Arrange
  tt := []struct {
    Word        string
    Language    string
    Translation string
  }{
    ...
    {
      Word:        "hello",
      Language:    "french",
      Translation: "bonjour",
    },
  }
    ...
}
```

Commit and push your changes. Wait for the deployment to be done, and try making your call again, but this time with the language as French. This is a quick iteration with fast delivery and feedback to meet the needs of your customers. You are now continuously delivering a product at a minimum cost with the ability to learn and grow. At some point, you may find that your demand is growing, and you will need to scale to meet that demand. Or you may find that your product isn't meeting expectations and you need to pivot. Using a serverless pattern, you only pay for what you use, so the risk is minimized.

4.6 Platform as a Service

The benefits of FaaS are that they provide enough abstraction to make it fast and easy to develop and deploy an application. This abstraction comes at a cost of both financial expense and control. In general, you will find that the fewer abstractions you have, the cheaper it will be to run your applications, to a certain point. There is an expensive operating cost to trying to host your own servers and infrastructure for a product that hasn't been tested. Alternatively, you pay a premium for Amazon or Google to handle this for you. Eventually, you will need to shift if your product becomes popular. Now we will move from FaaS to PaaS.

PaaS allows you to hand over your source code, and then the platform will identify, build, and run your application for you. In 2007, Heroku become one of the first PaaS available, and it revolutionized the way people develop and deploy programs. Their platform provided an abstraction that was built on top of AWS cloud computing, which provided customers the benefit of developing an application without worrying about provisioning or paying for servers. This paved the way for other offerings from Amazon and Google to provide similar abstractions as offerings to their customers.

For many standalone services, it becomes important to check whether the application is running and healthy. Typically, this service can be used to great effect if there are dependencies involved, such as a database connection. Using a *health check* endpoint will tell the running platform that the service is working and ready. Otherwise, the platform may try restarting the application or mark the deployment as failed. Before we start moving our application to a PaaS, let's add a health check endpoint. We don't have any external dependencies, so we will use the code in the following listing to write a simple handler in the `handlers/health.go` file.

Listing 4.6 `health.go`

```
package handlers

import (
  "encoding/json"
  "net/http"
)

func HealthCheck(w http.ResponseWriter, r *http.Request) {
  enc := json.NewEncoder(w)
  w.Header().Set("Content-Type", "application/json; charset=utf-8")
  resp := map[string]string{"status": "up"}        ◁─┐  We just hardcode a response now
  if err := enc.Encode(resp); err != nil {              because we don't need to check the
    panic("unable to encode response")                  connection to any service. In the future,
  }                                                      we could add more details here about
}                                                        the status of specific dependencies.
```

Now that we have this endpoint, we need to make some slight modifications to our `main.go` file.

Listing 4.7 `main.go`

```
func main() {
  addr := fmt.Sprintf(":%s", os.Getenv("PORT"))
  if addr == ":" {
    addr = ":8080"
  }

  mux := http.NewServeMux()

  mux.HandleFunc("/translate/hello", rest.TranslateHandler)
  mux.HandleFunc("/health", handlers.HealthCheck)

  log.Printf("listening on %s\n", addr)

  log.Fatal(http.ListenAndServe(addr, mux))
}
```

> We add the health check to the /health endpoint to ensure we can call it.

Now that our application has a health check, let's deploy it to a PaaS.

Why didn't we add the health check to the FaaS? As a function, typically we don't expect it to have a long-running state. Instead, it is invoked and shut down. In some platforms, these functions stay running for a short period to reduce warm-up, which is the process of starting the application. Having a health check is typically something that is needed for a long-running service to know if it should be shut down or restarted.

It wasn't long after Heroku provided a PaaS that Google responded with Google App Engine. Originally focused on Java and Python applications, it now supports a wide variety of languages, including Go. App Engine will use your source code and run it in a *sandboxed* or isolated runtime to prevent your application from affecting other applications. This form of virtualization and abstraction ensures that your application will be safe and secure while providing an easy way of developing and deploying a scalable application. Google worries about whether the platform is running, as well as about upgrading servers and installing libraries, so you don't have to. This is the power of using a PaaS; it gives you control of a full application without worrying about the underlying runtime. Deploying to App Engine is as easy as deploying a Cloud function, with one addition: we need to provide an app.yaml in the root project folder file to describe the deployment. Let's create one at the root of our project using the code in the following listing.

Listing 4.8 `app.yaml`

```
runtime: go116
main: ./cmd
liveness_check:
  path: "/health"
  check_interval_sec: 30
  timeout_sec: 4
  failure_threshold: 2
  success_threshold: 2
readiness_check:
  path: "/health"
```

```
check_interval_sec: 5
timeout_sec: 4
failure_threshold: 2
success_threshold: 2
app_start_timeout_sec: 300
```

This is all Google needs to start our application and make sure things are running. To deploy this, we need to add a step to our pipeline. Instead of replacing the function, we deploy both. Below the function step, add the code in the following listing to our pipeline.

Listing 4.9 `pipeline.yml`

```yaml
name: CI Checks

on:
  push:
    branches:
      - main

jobs:
...
  deploy-paas:
    name: Deploy PaaS
    runs-on: ubuntu-latest
    needs: test
    steps:
    - name: Check out code into the Go module directory
      uses: actions/checkout@v2
      with:
        fetch-depth: 0
    - name: Deploy App
      id: deploy
      uses: google-github-actions/deploy-appengine@main
      with:
        credentials: ${{ secrets.gcp_credentials }}
    - id: test
      run: curl "${{ steps.deploy.outputs.url }}/translate/hello"
```

That's it! Now we can push our changes and call the endpoint that is output from the deployment. From here, we can grow and get feedback from our customers. This feedback will feed more growth and steer our application into something useful. The seamlessness we have between writing code and seeing it in production helps bolster the productivity and engagement of developers. No longer does it take hours or days to see the work; instead, it is there in a matter of minutes. Moving forward, we will enhance our pipeline to have better development practices, reduce bugs, and have more advanced deployments, but for now, we can reflect on how powerful and easy it is to build a pipeline.

You commit your changes and push them to your repository. At that moment you look up and see the PM walking toward you quickly. "Hey," they say, "are you ready for the demo?"

Summary

- Deliver the product with a description of what is changing to help customers adapt and use your product.
- Always deliver and deploy to receive customer feedback.
- A health check endpoint is an easy way of communicating the status of a deployed product.
- Each type of deployment has various levels of abstraction to help a developer quickly release products.
- FaaS helps create simple, easy-to-manage applications at a higher cost in the long run.
- PaaS helps give you a more complete server to run your application on, but with easy deployment options.

Part 2

Scaling

In part 1, we established a pipeline, testing procedure, and deployment, so in part 2, we can focus on hardening our process to reduce bugs and continue to deliver to our customer. We should get some feedback about how the product is being used and adopted and use this information to focus on adding more features and improving our performance.

At this point, your team will grow, and you will all need to get on the same page. Standardization and code quality checks will help avoid wasting developers' time by verifying that the code works before it is even run, and that is what we will work on in chapter 5. In chapter 6, we will see that testing becomes more important as we move toward a more modular system with our code and its organization. Finally, in chapter 7, we will make our application portable and accessible to other developers by packaging it in a universal way.

Code quality enforcement

This chapter covers

- Standardizing our code's format by using formatting tools and linters
- Reducing bugs and vulnerabilities in our code by introducing static code analysis tools
- Automating quality checks before pushing code to a repository
- Organizing our code and documenting it for clearer usage and reuse
- Creating a culture of learning through code reviews

"As you can see, we can structure our projects in a way that empowers our developers to deliver quickly, efficiently, and with quality, while lowering costs. We have written and deployed a new version of our translation application in a day with flexible deployment options along with automated quality checks."

Your project manager is smiling from ear to ear as they say this and sit back down. Your demo went really well. Without going into the nitty-gritty details, you were able to demonstrate your new application and even push a live change during

the demo to show the quick turnaround you can achieve. Your CTO looked intrigued but not convinced.

"What you have demonstrated looks promising, but I'm not convinced this will scale. We have a bunch of other developers, an entire QA team, and an operations team that all need work. I need to see a plan that shows me how we can spread this throughout the organization. I need to see how you can integrate with existing systems, teams, and developers before I consider doing this company wide. Can we meet on Friday to have these questions answered?"

You nod your head. It all makes sense to you since developers don't often work in a vacuum. Plus, this is an iterative process, and you just got a bunch of great feedback.

"Great!" says your project manager, "I'll get us something on the books. Please make sure you have a plan, documents, and another demo ready for Friday. You hit this one out of the park. Let's see if you can do it again."

5.1   *Reviewing code*

Thus far, you've worked in a vacuum—just you and your code. This isn't how software is usually made. Instead, most projects are a collaborative effort among several people. Over time this group of people becomes a team. As a team, they create sets of rules to operate by, learn from each other, and help improve each other. But how do we do this?

We have already introduced this tool: the repository. Not only does a repository store your code, but we can place it in a holding pattern until someone else allows it to be incorporated. Imagine again that our repository is a warehouse. When a shipment of goods comes in, someone needs to sign for it. If the boxes are damaged or missing, there is a trail back to the person who accepted the goods. There is a sense of accountability.

In the same way, we want to have our team sign off on whatever we are introducing to the code repository. To do this, we use a mechanism called a *pull request*, which is a review process of code against a repository. This will protect the source code and educate others about the changes you are making. Let's add this protection to our repository now.

To do this, we need to navigate to our repository. Click Settings → Branches. Here you will see a section called "Branch Protection Rules" where you will see a form on which you input the name of the branch you want to protect and the specific rules associated with it. Fill it in as in figure 5.1: add the branch you are protecting and what needs to be done to protect this branch. This will protect the main branch from direct commits (unless you are an admin) and will prevent merges until you have one review and checks have passed.

You should notice that we have also selected that checks should pass before merging. We already have some checks in place with our unit tests, and we will add these checks throughout the chapter (and book) to help aid our reviews and protect the developer's time. But for now, let us focus on the branch protection we just introduced. At this point, no one (other than an admin) will be able to commit directly to your main branch. Instead, they must submit a pull request for others to view. This

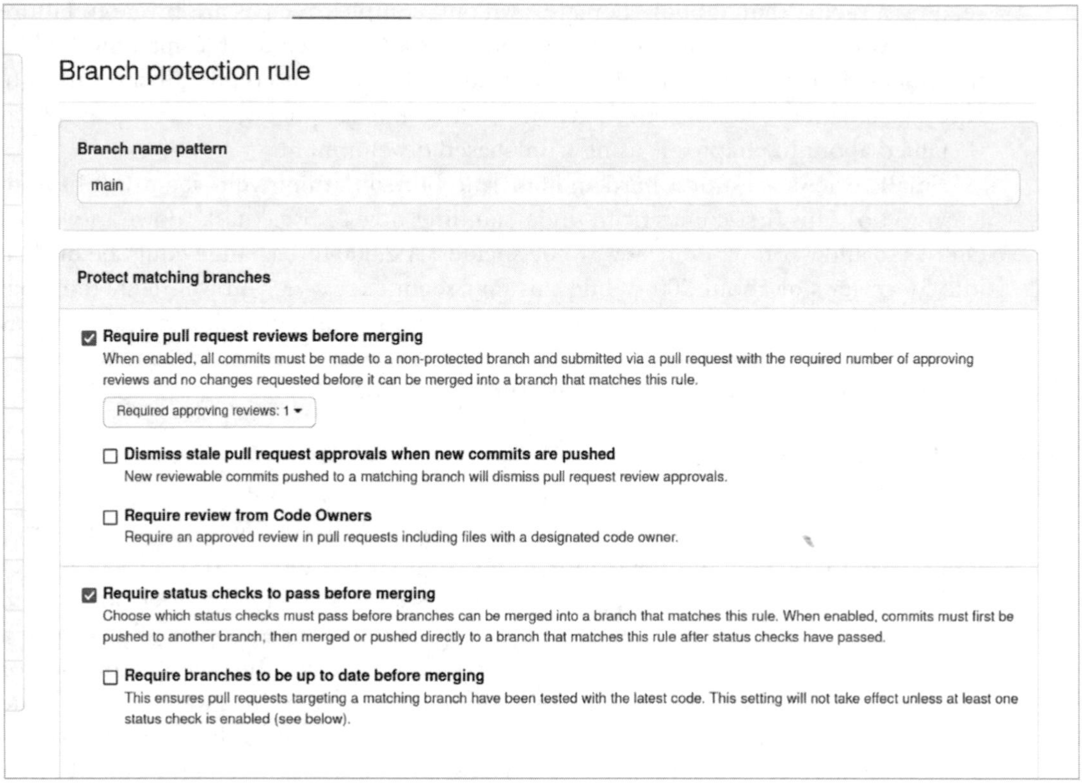

Branch protection rule

Branch name pattern

main

Protect matching branches

☑ **Require pull request reviews before merging**
When enabled, all commits must be made to a non-protected branch and submitted via a pull request with the required number of approving reviews and no changes requested before it can be merged into a branch that matches this rule.

Required approving reviews: 1 ▾

☐ **Dismiss stale pull request approvals when new commits are pushed**
New reviewable commits pushed to a matching branch will dismiss pull request review approvals.

☐ **Require review from Code Owners**
Require an approved review in pull requests including files with a designated code owner.

☑ **Require status checks to pass before merging**
Choose which status checks must pass before branches can be merged into a branch that matches this rule. When enabled, commits must first be pushed to another branch, then merged or pushed directly to a branch that matches this rule after status checks have passed.

☐ **Require branches to be up to date before merging**
This ensures pull requests targeting a matching branch have been tested with the latest code. This setting will not take effect unless at least one status check is enabled (see below).

Figure 5.1   Setting up branch protection in GitHub Repo

means that any changes require approval from one other person as a way of tracking accountability throughout the product. If a bug is introduced, it is no longer a single individual's mistake but that of the whole team since they didn't catch it in a review.

Code reviews seem to be a slow and cumbersome process when you are just trying to get work done. But I can assure you that they are not. They provide an excellent way of teaching others and informing your team about what you are changing. Even while working alone on a project, I find myself creating pull requests for *myself*. This helps me review what has changed and can help me identify bugs and problems. This is like reviewing a paper you've written and finding mistakes and glaring problems that you missed in the initial draft. What makes for an effective review, and what do you look for?

5.1.1   *Keep it small*

Limit reviews to 300 lines of code (including test code). Why? Because we as humans have a short attention span. Even if you can read a novel all day or a technical journal on a lunch break, you may not be able to handle a large review. A review is more like

reading a recipe than a book. Long, drawn-out, complex recipes are prone to failure because you may miss a step. Here, you may miss a line of code or a small bug. While this might be caught by some tools we'll introduce later, it could still slip through. Having a smaller review lets us focus on the task, merge quickly, and merge often, as we talked about in chapter 1, using trunk-based development.

Small reviews are not a hard-and-fast rule but something your team will have to learn to do. This first comes from understanding how to break tasks down into small chunks to allow your code reviews to be smaller. A 2,000-line change could be broken into 10 reviews of about 200. While this may seem excessive, you will likely find that your team can focus more on the small changes and point out problems. Also, it may not be just one person doing the development at one time, as demonstrated in chapter 1 with the task breakdown between API and UI work.

5.1.2   *Keep an open mind*

Code reviews are a team-building exercise and should be treated as such. They are not personal attacks or challenges to you as a developer. Nor are they a way to embarrass other developers. They are opportunities for you to learn and teach.

The author Stephen King says that the first step to becoming a good writer is to become an active reader. I believe that the same holds for developers. To become a better developer, you need to read more code. As a team, this allows more senior developers to show younger developers different techniques and ways to write code and solve problems. For younger developers, it becomes a way to show senior developers new techniques and solutions to problems. I personally love code reviews. I think it's a fantastic way to build and work with a team.

Treat code reviews as a philosophical discussion with friends rather than a political one. There are no hard-and-fast rules in development, but there are always areas in which to learn from others as in a philosophical discussion. Once it becomes personal, it becomes more difficult for others to learn, and often someone will start putting up their guard or being defensive and cease to learn instead of seeing the other side. To this day, I do not know how something as innocent as a code review can become such a sore spot for teams, but they often do. Here are some tips for how I think you can avoid this:

1 Treat others as you want to be treated.
2 Check your ego at the door.
3 Don't waste others' time with bad code.
4 Learn from feedback, and try not to repeat mistakes.
5 Take discussions offline instead of going back and forth in comments.
6 Keep an open mind as to what others are doing.
7 Make sure it works.

This list comes from experience with my past teams; 99% of the problems can be solved by communication, and the other 1% can be solved by process. Use code reviews as a way of connecting and building a team, not as a way of making yourself look better or others look bad.

5.1.3 Keep it moving

Reviews should be a priority because they are considered *work in progress* (WIP). As you've learned in earlier chapters, WIP is money stuck in the pipeline. Let's do some math. If a developer makes $100,000 a year, every hour of development amounts to about $50 worth of work. As that code sits in a review state, we do not receive any money from that work. I'm sure you are thinking, "If I'm reviewing code, I'm not writing code, and that is wasted time and money." If you spend time writing code while the code sits in the review, you increase the WIP and do not deliver the value. Soon a mass of reviews are in progress and nothing is completed.

It may also seem that switching tasks between writing code and reviewing code can be costly because you can forget where you are and what you were doing. The answer to this problem is learning to work reviews into your daily routine. Associate the task with something. When you find yourself with a fresh cup of coffee, do your reviews. I'd sit down every morning with my coffee, do my reviews, and then start my day. Once it was time for a second cup (or the ultimate conclusion of the beverage drinking occurred), I would do more reviews. We always find time for the things we want to do but rarely try to do things we don't want to do. We grow frustrated that no one reviews our code, but we don't take the time to review theirs.

> **NOTE** Build the time in and make sure others know that you are waiting on a review (politely).

Remind others that time stuck in review is time away from delivering to a customer.

5.1.4 Keep it interesting

Code review after code review can become dull, so it is important to keep things interesting. Talk with your team to see how things can change and improve in your review process. Go through your review, and ask questions or make comments. This is a great way of getting feedback from others. Have challenges to see who can eliminate the most code through a refactor or who can find a new way to write a unit test.

This seems dumb, but it helps with team morale. Like anything, it keeps people coming back for more. I once worked with a group that required a funny GIF as part of the pull request submission process, and reviewers not only needed to review the code but rate the GIF. Again, this helps build team morale, and while it seems like it is contrived or a waste of time, the cohesiveness of the team grows, and team members become more productive.

5.1.5 Keep it the same

While experimenting is fun and keeps people engaged, it is also important to establish some standards. GitHub allows for *pull request templates*, which allow you to create a standard format for a pull request, including a checklist. The checklist is a great way to remind others of what they need to do before submitting the request. To do this, open your source code, create a new directory called `.github`, and add a file called

PULL_REQUEST_TEMPLATE.md. The next listing shows an example template that can help with a pull request.

Listing 5.1   PULL_REQUEST_TEMPLATE.md

```
### Description
Please explain the changes you made here.

### Associated Task
Please list closed, fixed, or resolved issues here with a # and the number.

### Checklist
- [ ] Code compiles correctly
- [ ] Added tests that fail without the change (if possible)
- [ ] All tests passing
- [ ] Extended the documentation
```

Here, you have asked what was done and what sort of documentation you have for the work, as well as for a list of things that should be done before submitting.

When working as a team on the code review process, you should do regular check-ins about what is working and not working. In doing this, you can start to refine the process. There are still things you can do to automate the process and teach others. We'll see how to make it so the human doesn't have to bear all of the load of the review but work together with the machines to help guide and teach.

5.2   *Constraints on development*

There is an infamous scene from the famous show *I Love Lucy* where the main character Lucy and her friend Ethel work on an assembly line and it all goes wrong. Lucy and Ethel are working at a chocolate factory putting chocolates from the assembly line into wrappers. In the beginning, the two can keep pace with the flow of chocolates moving by them, but an unfortunate incident happens that causes them to fall behind. Panicking, the two go to comedic lengths to stem the flow of chocolates. To the public, this is an unfortunate and hilarious exposition of what can happen if workers fall behind on an assembly line. Industrial engineers watching this clip see only one thing: a constraint. A *constraint* is also known as a bottleneck. It is the location in an assembly line that determines the throughput of the factory.

In his novel *The Goal*, Eliyahu Goldratt outlines what is known as the "theory of constraints," in which he states that optimizations in any system that are not constraints are pointless. In our *I Love Lucy* example, enhancing the speed at which the chocolates are made is pointless if Lucy and Ethel cannot wrap them in time. This is demonstrated in figure 5.2. If A (Lucy) produces four items per minute and B (Ethel)

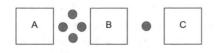

Figure 5.2   Step B can only process one item from step A. Work will eventually build up in front of B, and any enhancements to A or C will not help with the throughput.

can only process one item per minute, we will start overproducing items. Soon, excess inventory will begin to pile up, and the total throughput of our entire system will only equal one item per minute.

According to Goldratt, the focus of any company should be on trying to increase the throughput of the constraint and protecting its time from being wasted at that stage. This is known as *elevating the constraint*. There are several ways of elevating a constraint. In our *I Love Lucy* example, Lucy and Ethel may not have had a problem if additional workers helped them or if they had a machine that allowed them to wrap 10 times the number of chocolates. In another scenario, let's imagine Lucy and Ethel could keep a decent pace and were able to wrap 100 chocolates an hour, but 10% of them were defective for some reason. Their throughput would have gone down to 90 chocolates an hour. Once we've identified our constraint, we can find new ways of making it productive and protect it so that we have higher throughput.

Software development also has constraints. Almost the entire process is automated by a computer, which means that the slowest part of our pipeline is the developer. The actual thinking and development of features should be what determines the throughput of our pipeline. Code generation and reviews take time and are not automated tasks; therefore, time should be protected. A simple solution could be to add more workers. Adding more team members could mean more people writing code, but it gets complicated. As a team grows, a larger number of communication lines are required to maintain relationships and collaborate. Typically, most companies follow the *two-pizza rule*, in which a team should have no more people than can be fed by two pizzas. Any larger and you start seeing diminishing returns on team productivity.

> **NOTE** Fred Brooks famously said that adding more people to a project doesn't speed up delivery time, just as "nine women cannot make a baby in one month."

If adding more people isn't the solution, we need to make sure we protect their time. We can measure throughput for a company by measuring features and counting bugs as rework or work with defects. We can then focus on elevating our constraint by making it easy to develop code and catch bugs before they happen. This can be done by making our code easy to read, write, and fix and providing a mechanism for learning and teaching other developers about what we write. In this chapter, we check the quality of our code before we merge it and use this quality check as a way of learning and improving our system.

5.3 Standardizing our code through format and lint checks

It is common on assembly lines for the various stations to be standardized so that workers don't have to waste energy or time trying to determine which pieces go where. If we look back at Lucy and Ethel, we could only imagine how far behind they could have gotten if they needed to determine which wrapper color went on various pieces of chocolate. Instead, all of the wrappers and chocolates were standardized to help with the flow so that Lucy and Ethel could wrap them as quickly as they could.

Standardization then becomes an important element in helping with the flow through our development pipeline. As we outlined in chapter 2, standardizing the way we set up our environments and workstations is important to the overall developer experience, but that standardization needs to be extended. If we consider wrappers and chocolates as part of the materials flowing through Lucy's chocolate factory, we need to consider how we can standardize our materials through our pipeline. But how do you standardize code?

> **NOTE** It is important to distinguish here between industrial programming versus personal projects. *Industrial programming* means that others will be working with you on a product that others will consume. Here, standardization becomes important so that everyone is on the same page. *Personal projects* don't need this level of rigor if you are just experimenting with something. If a personal project becomes an industrial product, it is always best to consider rewriting it with these principles in place.

Each piece of code written must serve some special or individual purpose; otherwise, it wouldn't be written. You won't have the same unique chunks of code delivered by each of your developers. What can be standardized is the way the code looks and feels, its documentation, established patterns for pieces of code, and tests. Standardization then becomes a process of coming up with a general code style and deciding how to enforce that style so that when others look at your code, it is indistinguishable from that of code written by another teammate. This is typically done through a *style guide*, wherein the group establishes a set of rules about the format of their code. In general, this can be as simple (or controversial) as using tabs versus spaces, keeping brackets on the same line or the next line, spaces between functions, and many more. This will vary between languages and teams.

In addition to formatting rules, Go provides a guide for writing idiomatic Go code, which many linters will try to enforce. We will discuss linters later, but the following article also provides reasoning for the various format decisions that were made when writing the Go language: https://golang.org/doc/effective_go.

Go, however, has its own style, so this becomes a nonproblem. The running joke is "Nobody likes Go format, everyone loves Go format," meaning that there is most likely something that people don't like about some aspect of the Go formatting tool, but everyone likes the fact that a standard formatter exists and no one needs to worry about it. It is simple to use and built in. Go to your project directory, and type

```
go fmt ./...
```

You may see something change, or you may not. Go will move brackets to the same line as the function declaration, replace spaces with tabs, consolidate spaces between functions, and so much more. The point is that, as a developer, you should worry about things other than the format of your code. Additional tools are out there for other languages, such as JavaScript's `prettier` package and Python's `autopep8`. But it is one thing to have formatting standards and another to enforce their usage.

We need to do two things to help our developer: first, automate the process; second, enforce it. Let's start on the second portion so that we can see it in action and then automate it.

To enforce these rules, we should have already set some limitations on the main branch. We will set our pipeline to enforce checks before the merge button is allowed to be pushed.

Currently, our CI system only runs on changes to the main branch, so we will need to update the `pipeline.yml` file to run on pull requests. Open that file, and add the code in the following listing.

Listing 5.2 `pipeline.yml`

```
name: CI Checks

on:
  pull_request:          ◁─┐ Runs on pull
    branches:               requests to main
      - main
  push:
    branches:
      - main
...
  deploy-function:
    name: Deploy FaaS                          Only runs deployments on
    runs-on: ubuntu-latest                       pushes to the main
    needs: test                                branch, not pull requests
    if: ${{github.event_name=='push' && github.ref == 'refs/heads/main'}}  ◁─┘
    steps:
...
  deploy-paas:
    name: Deploy PaaS                          Only runs deployments on
    runs-on: ubuntu-latest                       pushes to the main
    needs: test                                branch, not pull requests
    if: ${{github.event_name=='push' && github.ref == 'refs/heads/main'}}  ◁─┘
    steps:
...
```

Additionally, we want to add a new check to see if formatting occurred before merging, so we will add a step to our pipeline. We will add this command to our Makefile (see the following listing).

Listing 5.3 Makefile

```
...
report:
  go tool cover -html=coverage.out -o cover.html
                                  This will check the results of running the
check-format:                     format command to see if there were any
  test -z $$(go fmt ./...)  ◁─┘   changes. If so, it returns a failing value.
```

Now we can update our pipeline to run this step, as in the following listing.

Listing 5.4   `pipeline.yml`

```
jobs:
  test:
    needs:
      - format-check
    name: Test Application
...
  format-check:
    name: Check formatting
    runs-on: ubuntu-latest
    steps:
    - name: Set up Go 1.x
      uses: actions/setup-go@v2
      with:
        go-version: ^1.18
    - name: Check out code into the Go module directory
      uses: actions/checkout@v2
    - name: Run Format Check
      run: make check-format
```

> Since formatting is less expensive than running tests, let's save time by checking the format first.

> Calls our check format command from the Makefile to see the results

Now create a branch called task/quality-check-enforcement-formatting, and commit your changes. Push the new branch, and create a pull request. Watch as the CI pipeline runs to make sure all of your changes work. Did it fail? If so, look into the failure. If it passes, feel free to try to make it fail by messing up the formatting and pushing again. Once everything is working, merge it. Congratulations! You have added a guard to your main branch. In fact, we've added two: formatting and testing now both need to pass in order to merge to main. This also relieves our team from needing to ask people to format. Next, we need to help our team by automatically finding bad code and security flaws that can't be found by linting but by another tool called static code analysis.

5.4   *Static code analysis*

Software is used to automate a formerly manual task. While humans are essential to reviews, they can make mistakes. Luckily, many bad coding practices and anti-patterns can be automatically recognized by software called *static code analysis* tools. These tools comb through your code looking for known patterns that are often related to bugs or security vulnerabilities. Some can be used to enforce good programming practices like documentation and spelling. Adding static code analysis tools to your pipeline can help reduce bugs and protect reviewers from wasting their time on "bad code."

To do this, we will use two tools. One is a tool built into Go, and the other is a community-supported tool that provides an extensive array of libraries to support additional checks. Let's first start with Go's internal command go vet, which is great for providing fast results about bugs in your code. Let's run it now to see if there are any problems. To do this, type

```
go vet ./...
```

The three dots, like in testing, tell the program to run the vet tool across all packages. Hopefully, you should see nothing as part of the results. Open `cmd/main.go`, and change one line (see the following code listing).

Listing 5.5 `main.go`

```
...
func main() {
  addr := fmt.Sprintf(":%s", os.Getenv("PORT"), "error")   ⬸── Adding an extra
  if addr == ":" {                                              variable can cause
    addr = ":8080"                                              this line to fail.
  }
  ...
}
```

Now run the `go vet` command, and you should see an error. The vet tool checks your source code and finds that you have a format command that has more variables than expected. This is great because it will catch a potential bug. We should add this to our pipeline so that we can do the checks. Once again, running this is much faster than running tests (or will be in the future), so we should add it before we test, but we can also run it after format checking. Let's update our pipeline to run these checks using the code in the following listing.

Listing 5.6 `pipeline.yml`

```
vet:
    name: Check formatting
    runs-on: ubuntu-latest
    steps:
    - name: Set up Go 1.x
      uses: actions/setup-go@v2
      with:
        go-version: ^1.18
    - name: Check out code into the Go module directory
      uses: actions/checkout@v2
    ...
    - name: Vet                    Runs built-in Go tool
      run: go vet ./...      ⬸──   for checking code
```

This will now run before we run our tests and after we check the formatting. This is great because it gives us a pipeline through which we can test the code quality and give specific feedback to our developers if something fails. We can think of this as various sieves through which we filter stones. Bigger holes allow larger rocks through, but as we progressively decrease the size, the smaller the stones become and the more easily you can see the individual stones. In the end, you are left with the different sizes of stones that you want.

In the same way, our code will move through, providing us with easy-to-digest errors and improvements to make until we are left with a product that is ready to review. The pipeline approach works well for targeting and pointing out the various problems but

can also result in longer lead time. *Lead time* refers to the time between the start and stop of a process from the moment an issue or feature is raised and gets delivered to the customer. The time between each of these steps is known as *cycle time*. If a cycle time is a subset of the overall lead time, we can focus on optimizing our cycle times to reduce the overall lead time to our customer. In figure 5.3, you can see that the overall lead time between a customer's request to delivery should be reduced to meet their needs. To do that, we can consider reducing the cycle times of each step in our pipeline.

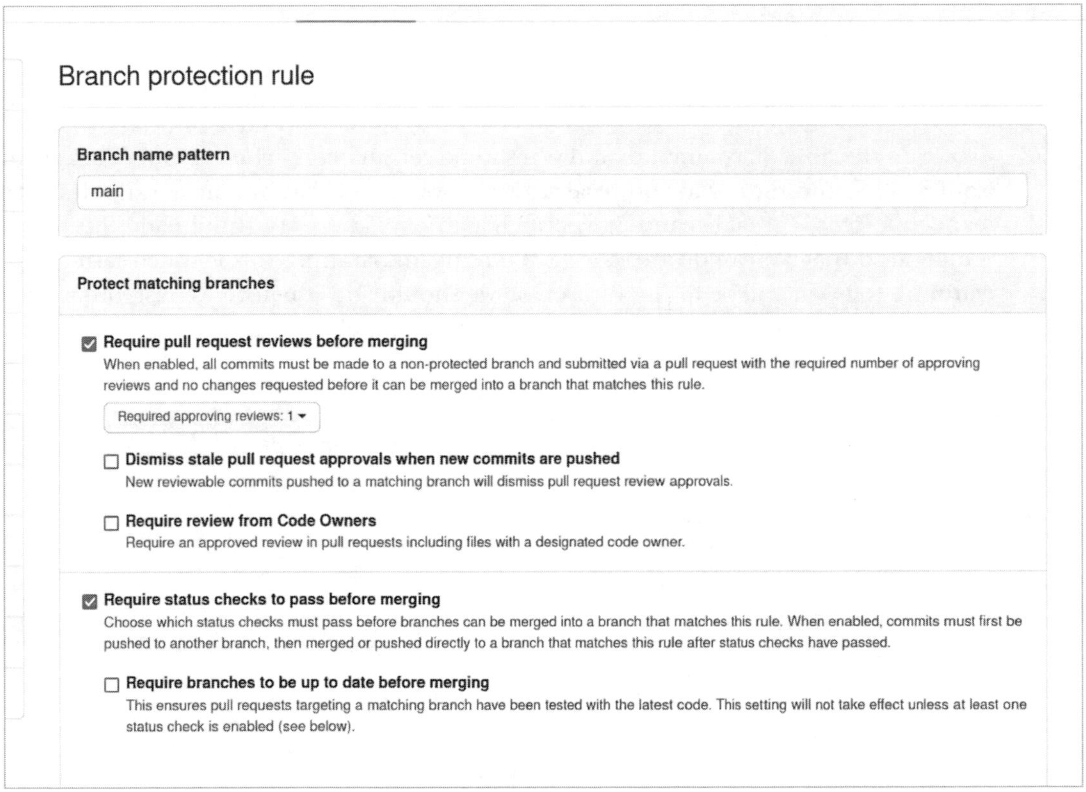

Branch protection rule

Branch name pattern

main

Protect matching branches

☑ **Require pull request reviews before merging**
When enabled, all commits must be made to a non-protected branch and submitted via a pull request with the required number of approving reviews and no changes requested before it can be merged into a branch that matches this rule.

Required approving reviews: 1 ▾

☐ **Dismiss stale pull request approvals when new commits are pushed**
New reviewable commits pushed to a matching branch will dismiss pull request review approvals.

☐ **Require review from Code Owners**
Require an approved review in pull requests including files with a designated code owner.

☑ **Require status checks to pass before merging**
Choose which status checks must pass before branches can be merged into a branch that matches this rule. When enabled, commits must first be pushed to another branch, then merged or pushed directly to a branch that matches this rule after status checks have passed.

☐ **Require branches to be up to date before merging**
This ensures pull requests targeting a matching branch have been tested with the latest code. This setting will not take effect unless at least one status check is enabled (see below).

Figure 5.3   Overall lead time is the time from the creation of the task to its delivery to a customer.

We can imagine that our pipeline could run multiple stages at the same time, such as linting, vetting, and testing. This becomes computationally expensive because you are running machines or processes in parallel, but you get your results faster and can see all problems that have occurred. This is another spot in which your team will need to determine how you want to run your pipeline. In this example, we will run a hybrid of parallel and sequential steps in our pipeline.

NOTE   GolangCI Lint is an aggregate linting tool that allows developers to select from a myriad of linters.

go vet is a great starting place for statically checking our code, but it doesn't need to stop there. A tool called golangci-lint can be installed on your machine and used as a pipeline step. GolangCI-Lint allows you to select from numerous linting and static-checking libraries to help extend your quality assessments. The full list is available on the libraries page, but we will use a few here to get started. By default, it will run several checks that will look for unused code, ineffective variable assignments, missing error checks, and much more. In addition, we will add a check for security. To do this, we need to create a new file called .golangci.yml. Create it in the root directory, and add the code in the following listing.

Listing 5.7 golangci.yml

```
linters:
  enable:
    - gosec        ←──┐ Adds linter
                        to the file
                                      Customizes the output
output:            ←───────────────── format of the linter
  format: colored-line-number

  # print lines of code with issue, default is true
  print-issued-lines: false

  # print linter name in the end of issue text, default is true
  print-linter-name: true
```

The linter we are using will automatically look for this configuration file when it runs within this project.

Code security is an often overlooked step in static code analysis, but a crucial one. Security checks can allow for things such as which randomization libraries and functions to use as well as what kind of hashing you may need. Your code may not use these things, but one day you may find (if you have your linter on) that you need to. Now that we have a broad understanding of what this tool can do, let's add it to our pipeline (see the following code listing).

Listing 5.8 pipeline.yml

```
jobs:
  test:
    needs:
      - format-check    ┐ Adds a lint check
      - lint          ←──┘ as a dependency
    name: Test Application
  lint:
    name: Lint
    runs-on: ubuntu-latest
    steps:
      - uses: actions/checkout@v2
      - name: Lint                                    ┐ Adds a lint action
        uses: golangci/golangci-lint-action@v2    ←──┘ to pipeline
```

Create a branch called task/add-static-check, commit your code, and create a pull request. What do you see? It should error! Why? Well, it looks like we are missing an error check on a function. If we had only seen this earlier, we could have saved ourselves some time. Let's remedy this by adding the installation and static check to our Makefile using the code in the following listing.

Listing 5.9 `pipeline.yml`

```
setup: install-go init-go install-lint
...
install-lint:                                      Grabs the content from
  sudo curl -sSfL \                                the linter locally
 https://raw.githubusercontent.com/golangci/golangci-lint/master/install.sh\
 | sh -s -- -b $$(go env GOPATH)/bin v1.41.1

static-check:
  golangci-lint run
```

Great, now we can run make `lint` locally and get the same errors. Fix the line by adding the code in the following listing.

Listing 5.10   Makefile

```
func TestTranslateAPI(t *testing.T) {
...

  for _, test := range tt {
    ...
    _ = json.Unmarshal(rr.Body.Bytes(), &resp)        This needs to capture the
  }                                                    error message even though
}                                                      we are not using it.
```

Commit your changes and push. Now everything should be green, and you can merge. This simple step will save you from several bugs and problems along the way. Situations like missing error checks can hide underlying problems that occurred while the system is running. Ineffective assignments are another common problem, wherein a variable is set but never used, which could lead to a bug. These tools add mild overhead but save you in the long run. Take the time as a team to evaluate and use them as you see fit, and let them evolve with your team.

5.5   *Code documentation*

Writing code should be like telling a story. You start with an idea and then define the structure. Most developers will not start writing code by first writing comments. They will most likely write a function just once and hopefully never need to come back to it. More frequently, someone will need to use the function or package for some reason or another, and it is the developer's job to tell the story of what the function does so that others don't need to dive into the code to figure it out. This comes down to making sure the title of the story is clear and the description is sound.

Because this is my first venture into writing, I can say that writing can be difficult. But I have found coming up with what to write on a function comment much more challenging. You need to first come up with a good name for the function that is helpful to people. This needs to be something that makes sense, like `Translate` and `TranslateFile` instead of `T` and `TFile`. Alternatively, you don't need to tell a story with a name like `TranslatesFileWithCaseInsensitiveAndUnixBasedHomeDir`. Instead, you would put in the comments how someone should expect the function to work. We've avoided package-level and function-level comments until now.

Go has built into it the capabilities of hosting a documentation server, wherein the library will parse your source code looking for comments above package declarations and above functions to create documentation. However, anything in the include directory will be skipped because it cannot be used in a dependency.

Since we don't have the documentation, we should remedy that. However, we also want to make sure that after we go through this exercise, no one follows us by not commenting on their code. This is known as a *scout philosophy*, in which you "leave it better than you found it." To do this, let's add a new *static code analysis* tool to check the comments. We will use a checker that requires comments on all exported functions and packages. Additionally, we will add a spell-check and ensure that all comments end in a period. Open `.golangci-lint.yml`, and add the code in the following listing.

Listing 5.11 `\golangci-lint.yml`

```
linters:
  enable:
    - gosec          Adds linters to check
    - godot     ◁─┘  comments and style
    - misspell
    - stylecheck     Settings for linter where
                     we want to capture
linters-settings:  ◁─┘ stylistic problems
  stylecheck:
    # Select the Go version to target. The default is '1.13'.
    go: "1.18"
    checks: ["all","ST1*"]

issues:
  exclude-use-default: false      ◁─┐ Some of these lint errors are
                                      hidden by GolangCI-Lint, so
output:                             │ we want to disable that.
  format: colored-line-number

  # print lines of code with issue, default is true
  print-issued-lines: false

  # print linter name in the end of issue text, default is true
  print-linter-name: true
```

Style checks will ensure that our comments are required and that we follow some other standards for comment writing. `godot` and `misspell` will make sure that our strings and comments are well punctuated and spelled correctly. Once you've added this file, run `make static-check` and see the results. Fix the code by adding comments that you feel are appropriate. Push your changes and merge. Remember, comments should explain what the function does, not how it does it. For example, the function `Translate` would have a comment such as "Translate will take a given word and language and will return the translation if available; otherwise, it will return an empty string."

5.6   Git hooks

We've protected our main branch, added quality checks, and then added various requirements on the main branch. We now need to focus on localizing the changes to our development environment. As a general rule, it is important to localize changes to your pipeline so that your developers can easily reproduce them locally. If you find that verifying changes locally becomes a problem, you should consider changing your pipeline. Localized functions allow developers to ensure their code should work before pushing it to a pull request. Imagine trying to guess if your code will pass before creating a pull request. This would create delays and problems along the way. For the most part, we have already automated a lot of the functions our pipeline has done, but we failed to ensure that developers are using them locally.

The policy will only get you so far. Often a developer will write some code in earnest, push it, create a pull request, and move on only to find in a few hours that the pull request failed for one reason or another. Similarly, when seeing a new pull request, developers will flock to review and approve it only to find that there are errors that prevent it from being merged. This wastes time for the developer, reviewer, and the CI pipeline. Moving these checks as close as possible to the source will help move the process along.

Git has a beautiful feature called *hooks* that ties into various functions supported by Git. A hook will run when a specific function is executed, either before or after. In our case, we want to create a *pre-commit hook* that will run before we commit our changes. This hook will verify that our code is properly formatted and that the static code analysis runs as expected. We need to ensure that these functions are installed for everyone, and they therefore should be part of our setup. First, we must create the script, which is just a simple shell script. Create a file called `scripts/hooks/pre-commit`, and add the code in the following listing.

Listing 5.12 `pre-commit`

```sh
#!/bin/sh

STAGED_GO_FILES=$(git diff --cached --name-only -- '*.go')
if [[ $STAGED_GO_FILES == "" ]]; then
    echo "no go files updated"
```

Grabs all Go files

If there aren't any, print the message.

```
else
    for file in $STAGED_GO_FILES; do
        go fmt $file          ◁───┐  Runs format on all files and
        git add $file              │  adds the file to the commit
    done
fi
                          ┌  Runs lint
golang-ci run    ◁────┘  check
```

Now we will create a script that adds this to our .git/hooks directory as part of initial-ization (see the following listing). Once there, it will run before any branch push, so be aware of error messages!

Listing 5.13 Makefile

```
setup: install-go init-go copy-hooks
...
copy-hooks:                        ┌  Creates a script
  chmod +x scripts/hooks/*   ◁──┘  and copies files
  cp -r scripts/hooks .git/.
```

Problems should now be caught in a local environment as a team tries to use these hooks to ensure that basic tasks are being completed, but be aware of the time cost of these functions. Notice that we did not add the test stage to the pre-push. This is because tests take a longer time to run as opposed to static checks. Try to find a happy medium. Make sure things don't take too long and interrupt the development flow. You and your team may find that these hooks are more obtrusive than helpful, in which case you should discuss their usage and function with your team.

5.7 Flow

A psychologist named Mihaly Csikszentmihalyi studied the way people work and how it relates to happiness and creativity. He believed that people enjoy what they do if they can establish a sense of *flow* or state of concentration and absorption in the task at hand. This is also known as "being in the zone." If you play sports or an instrument, I'm sure you've found yourself in a state of flow. You can see the next play, anticipate the next note, or become absorbed in what you are doing at the moment.

Csikszentmihalyi discovered that this pattern can be reflected in work as well, as long as it engages the worker in some way. Developers find this flow when writing code. Some of the most innovative and efficient code can come from an engaged development team. What can cause problems, though, is the interruption of flow, such as by these:

- Meeting overload
- Broken builds and tests
- Local development problems
- Heisenbugs, bugs that are inconsistently reproducible
- Coworkers popping in to talk or ask a question

Why does this matter? Because the flow of your team members is important. Making things easier will help to create a better flow for them. What we want to focus on is the flow that goes from an idea to implementation. The fewer disruptions we have at this stage, the better. This flow comes from the person doing the work, and anything that interrupts the flow interrupts their ability to be successful.

On the other hand, loose quality enforcement can lead to interruptions in the form of bugs and errors. There is no formula for what works best with teams. If you are a team of senior-level developers, you may require fewer guardrails. If you are a team of less experienced developers, you may find you need more. The key here is to communicate. Talk to each other regularly. Refine and enhance.

Overall, this chapter has been about helping your team work together. I realize that this is a challenging and unique area, as every team will be different, so you will notice that I have repeated a similar line time and again: do what works best for your team. We have built a pipeline, and we are adding to it. With each addition comes more complexity, but this complexity can often help teams as they grow and evolve. Most of these steps and protections will help your team in the long run. It may be by catching bugs or errors, but in some cases, it will keep people on their toes.

Parents often use timers as a way of communicating that it is time to leave rather than telling their kids it's time to go. This helps because the parent and the child have agreed that the timer is the thing that determines when it is time to go and not a seemingly arbitrary announcement from the parent. The timer is the communication tool. In the same way, team members will respond better to a program telling them to comment on their code rather than a team member because both have agreed on a single tool to keep them in check.

"Hey, do you have a minute?" Startled, you look up and see your project manager with someone you've never met before. "I want to introduce you to Yvonne, an intern who is going to help you meet the demo on Friday. She doesn't have a bunch of experience, but I'm sure you can help her get up to speed fairly quickly." Any help is welcome, especially now that you've standardized your work.

Summary

- Code quality checks can reduce bugs and standardize work.
- Formatting can standardize a workspace and make it easier for newcomers to onboard.
- Static code analysis will check your code for known anti-patterns and ask you to fix them.
- Moving quality checks to the front of the pipeline can reduce wait time and catch bugs before deployment.
- Constantly review and improve your development process to ensure the flow of the developer's work.

Testing frameworks, mocking, and dependencies

"So you want to sit with me and tell me what to code? Won't that be a waste of your time?" You've just given the intern permission to access the repository and sat down next to her at her desk. You explain that she should download the repository and follow the directions on the README, and you will sit there to answer any questions. After making some minor notes on where to expand the documentation, you move on to coding. The intern will add some new functionality to the system and write the code while you explain what to write.

This process of "pair programming" is a great technique to bring people on board and explain the code base. It also is a great team-building activity. One person can write the tests while the other implements the solution. In this case, you will write the test and explain what it does, and it will then be the intern's job to implement it with you there to guide her and provide pointers and input. Before you can do this, though, you need to define what you're going to build, so you pull up an editor and write the code in the following listing in your `translate.go` handler.

Listing 6.1 `translate.go`

```
type Translator interface {
    Translate(word string, language string) string    ◁┐  Extracting our method into an
}                                                       │  interface allows us flexibility
                                                        │  in the implementation.
```

"You want me to implement this interface in a new service? Why? Everything seems to work fine now. What will an interface do to help?" You smile; it's always fun to teach.

6.1 *Dependency inversion principle*

"Depend on abstractions, not concretions." This is the *dependency inversion principle*. This is a design principle that is found in software development. It is a fairly simple concept that helps developers create clean and focused code. Instead of using an implemented class or function directly, we depend on the abstraction.

The best way that I can explain this concept is to imagine a scenario where electrical plugs didn't exist. How hard would it be if you had to directly wire your lamp or TV to your home's electrical system? I'm sure you would think twice before you rearranged your furniture. Instead, we created plugs and outlets. We don't care about the wiring in our house, the circuit breaker (unless one is flipped), the line to the house, the transformer, or where the electricity comes from. It just simply works for us. If your lamp breaks tomorrow, it can be replaced, and you don't need to worry about putting in a new outlet. The plug should just fit.

This is what is known as an *interface*, an abstraction that allows someone to easily use something more complex behind the scenes. We talked about abstractions in chapter 4 and how they can be helpful in software development. It's no surprise that developers want to help abstract some of their code for others to use. Similarly, they want to be able to improve and change things without causing major refactors or problems. This is where interfaces come in. In software development, an interface defines the functions of a given struct or class. Once a struct has all of the request functions, it satisfies the interface and can be used in the place of another service that also satisfies the interface. Just like the lamps, we can change out pieces of code that help us grow and improve.

Some developers will forgo the creation of interfaces and instead create portions of code that are tightly coupled and intertwined. This makes it hard for us to test effectively and enhance our code in the future. We need to modularize our code so we can do a better job of testing it, which can be done through the use of interfaces.

6.2   *Defining an interface*

Interfaces are also called *protocols*, which help define boundaries between systems and provide a way to communicate between those boundaries. Protocols and interfaces create a definition of how to communicate through established structures or patterns. Just like different outlet faces on an electrical socket can

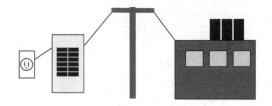

Figure 6.1   Various interfaces are designed to abstract the delivery of electricity.

tell us what sort of electricity is on the other side, an interface will tell our user how to use a service by defining method definitions (as seen in figure 6.1).

This allows our developers to write their code toward an interface definition rather than a concrete implementation, allowing us to make changes that don't affect the entire system. This is important as we develop because we may find that we need to slowly replace portions of our code while still supporting backward compatibility or testing features that are not ready for wide consumption. Later in this chapter, we will do this, but let's start with the simple example in the following listing.

Listing 6.2   `example.go`

```go
package main

import "fmt"

type Greeter interface {          ◁── The interface defines a
    Greet() string                      method that a struct needs to
}                                        have to satisfy the interface.

type spanishGreeter struct {}

func (g *spanishGreeter) Greet() string {    ◁── The spanishGreeter struct adds
    return "hola"                                  the method and therefore
}                                                   satisfies the interface.

type englishGreeter struct {}

func (g *englishGreeter) Greet() string {    ◁── In the same way, the
    return "hello"                                 englishGreeter also
}                                                   satisfies the interface.

func printGreeting(greeter Greeter) {    ◁── A generic method can
    fmt.Println(greeter.Greet())               then be written that uses
}                                               the interface as input.

func main() {
    printGreeting(&spanishGreeter{})
    printGreeting(&englishGreeter{})
}
```

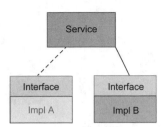

Figure 6.2   Interfaces allow us to swap between different services that satisfy the interface without changing our logic in the consuming service.

We created two structures that satisfy the same interface. This allows us to abstract the parameters of the function to take the interface and swap between the two structures. This can be seen in figure 6.2 where we have a service using an interface to hide the underlying implementation. Though this is a trivial example, we will see it be more powerful in the future as we customize our application. What we can see now is that we can implement any number of structs to satisfy this interface without changing the caller. Though I have never encountered this scenario, imagine using an interface for a backend datastore. With an interface, you could satisfy the interface using Postgres, RedisDB, MongoDB, or any number of technologies and not have to change your code. This rarely happens but prevents you from locking into a given implementation.

Why does this matter? By making use of interfaces, we can also simplify how we test our code. Let's look at our handler function as an example. Right now, it is dependent on the service struct for translations. If we were to change the underlying implementation of services, we would hope that this wouldn't affect our handler. But when we think about it, our handler should work independently of the underlying service. All the handler cares about is the output translation and nothing else, so we want to add an abstraction within the handler to make it easier to test (see the following code listing).

Listing 6.3   `translate.go`

```go
type Translator interface {
    Translate(word string, language string) string
}
```
◁───┐ **Extracting our method into an interface allows us flexibility in the implementation.**

You may wonder why we are defining this interface here and not somewhere else. The handler is the consumer of the interface and therefore defines the functionality it needs following the dependency inversion principle we discussed earlier. We define the interface we want and then create the implementation that satisfies this interface type. Go uses something called *duck typing* to help map an interface to its implementation. The term *duck typing* is a type system wherein the object needs to satisfy certain behaviors. It comes from a *duck test*: "If it walks like a duck and quacks like a duck, then it must be a duck." The handler can define what it expects from a structure through the use of an interface and ignore the underlying implementation. This means our implementation can come from anywhere, and a single implementation can satisfy many interfaces. As developers, we want to split our interfaces into small chunks known as *interface segregation* to help them be more composable and reusable. Go's standard library has a wonderful example of this (see the following listing).

Listing 6.4   `io.go`

```
type Reader interface {
    Read(p []byte) (n int, err error)        ◁    The reader interface only has
}                                                 one method to satisfy . . .

type Writer interface {
    Write(p []byte) (n int, err error)       ◁    . . . and so does the
}                                                 writer interface.

type ReadWriter interface {
    Reader                                   ◁    A composite interface can then be
    Writer                                        created from each of these interfaces.
}
```

A service may only want to implement `Reader` or `Writer` or both. You can treat interfaces like Legos that you assemble so that you can use what you need and nothing more. This is all well and good, but how do we use this composability? We create a structure that fulfills the interface and injects it into a consuming struct. This is known as *dependency injection*.

6.3   *Dependency injection*

I've always imagined dependency injection as putting a different engine in a different car. Many car bodies share the same engine, and many car bodies support different engines. For example, the 2022 Toyota Camry allows you the option to have a four-cylinder, six-cylinder, or four-cylinder hybrid engine all in the same type of car, in the same way that hybrid engines can also be used on other vehicles. This is a streamlined way for companies to reuse designs while giving their users the variety that they need.

> **NOTE**   We are going to wire these dependencies by hand, but there are tools out there that will do it for you. These include Wire, Fx, and Kit.

In the same way, we can build our code to use different services and elements while not affecting our current implementation. Code changes. Ideas change. Features get added. What is important is that these changes should not require an entire rearchitecting or rebuilding of our system. Instead, we should be able to define how the service should work in abstract terms and then satisfy them with concrete implementations so they are not *tightly coupled*, wherein a change in one service requires a change in another service. Instead, a change in a given service shouldn't affect the underlying functionality of another service. In the previous section, we talked about the merits of writing an interface. You can view your interface as a way of standardizing how a service will work. With this standard in place, you can then make changes as you need. You can attach the larger engine, the smaller engine, or the hybrid without doing a major overhaul. Let's see how this works. We've already written our interface for translation, and now we need to make the handler use it and the service satisfy it. Open your `translate.go` file, and add the code in the following listing.

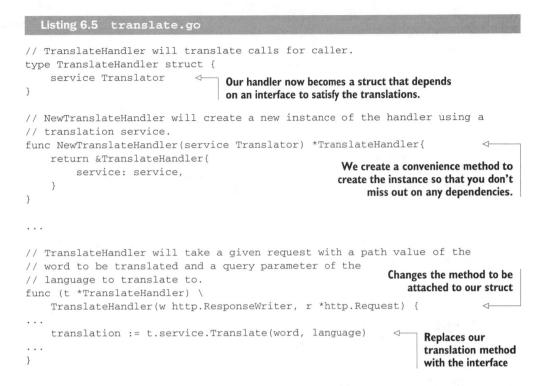

Listing 6.5 `translate.go`

```go
// TranslateHandler will translate calls for caller.
type TranslateHandler struct {
    service Translator
}
```
Our handler now becomes a struct that depends on an interface to satisfy the translations.

```go
// NewTranslateHandler will create a new instance of the handler using a
// translation service.
func NewTranslateHandler(service Translator) *TranslateHandler{
    return &TranslateHandler{
        service: service,
    }
}
```
We create a convenience method to create the instance so that you don't miss out on any dependencies.

```
...
```

```go
// TranslateHandler will take a given request with a path value of the
// word to be translated and a query parameter of the
// language to translate to.
func (t *TranslateHandler) \
    TranslateHandler(w http.ResponseWriter, r *http.Request) {
...
    translation := t.service.Translate(word, language)
...
}
```
Changes the method to be attached to our struct

Replaces our translation method with the interface

We've created a struct that holds our interface and allows us to call it in our handler function. Let's now update our service to satisfy the interface so we can still use it and get our system building again. Open `translator.go`, and add the code in the following listing.

Listing 6.6 `translate.go`

```go
// StaticService has data that does not change.
type StaticService struct{}
```
Creates a new struct to attach our existing function to

```go
// NewStaticService creates new instance of a service that uses static data.
func NewStaticService() *StaticService {
    return &StaticService{}
}
```
Creates a method to instantiate this struct

```go
// Translate a given word to a the passed in language.
func (s *StaticService) Translate(word string, language string) string {
...
}
```
Attaches the function to the struct and satisfies the interface needed by the handler

Now comes the dependency injection. As the name implies, we will inject the dependent services into the handler struct. Open `main.go`, and add the code in the following listing.

Listing 6.7 `main.go`

```
func main() {
...

    mux := http.NewServeMux()

    translationService := translation.NewStaticService()
    translateHandler := rest.NewTranslateHandler(translationService)
    mux.HandleFunc("/translate/hello", translateHandler.TranslateHandler)
...
}
```

Registers the function with the mux → `mux.HandleFunc(...)`

Creates the new static service → `translation.NewStaticService()`

Creates a new handler with the service as a dependency → `rest.NewTranslateHandler(translationService)`

As you can see, we create the service we need and pass it to our handler, which registers the translation function call. We now have control over what service the handler can use. We will take advantage of this later as we expand our services. Our FaaS will also fail now that we've made the change to the handler. See if you can fix it yourself.

What is interesting is that during this exercise you can witness how difficult it is to make small changes when your services become *tightly coupled*. We can see here that making our changes to our handler and service has broken several pieces of our code, including our tests. Right now, our code base isn't that big, so imagine what would have happened on a larger project!

Now we need to fix our tests. Let's do the minimum to fix this, and then we'll improve our tests to take advantage of the changes we've made. Open `translate_test.go`, and add the code in the following listing.

Listing 6.8 `translate_test.go`

```
func TestTranslateAPI(t *testing.T) {
...

    underTest := rest.NewTranslateHandler(translation.NewStaticService())
    handler := http.HandlerFunc(underTest.TranslateHandler)
...
}
```

Updates the tests to create the new handler → `rest.NewTranslateHandler(translation.NewStaticService())`

Registers the handler for the test → `http.HandlerFunc(underTest.TranslateHandler)`

Implement the changes to `translator_test.go` (see the following listing).

Listing 6.9 `translate_test.go`

```
func TestTranslate(t *testing.T) {
...

    underTest := translation.NewStaticService()
    for _, test := range tt {
        // Act
        res := underTest.Translate(test.Word, test.Language)
...
    }
}
```

Creates a new static service to test against → `translation.NewStaticService()`

Uses this for getting the results for the different test cases → `underTest.Translate(test.Word, test.Language)`

You'll notice that I used a variable called `underTest` in both of these files. This is a nice pattern to follow because it allows you to explicitly see what you are testing. Now we should be able to see all of our tests run without a problem. Commit your changes and push your branch.

Why did we go through all of the trouble of refactoring to not have anything change functionally?

The first reason is to underline the importance of creating interfaces early in development instead of doing it later. You can see the difficulty and pain of making these changes after the fact instead of planning them out before. I did this as a lesson. I remember as a junior developer being assigned the task of creating interfaces for all of the services in our system. It was tedious. It was painful. Worst of all, the interfaces were sloppy.

Sloppy interfaces are the ones that do too much and have too many parameters. They are too broad and difficult to reason about. They have *low cohesion* or *coincidental cohesion* because they are grouped arbitrarily and with little thought given to their function. Alternatively, if we were to think about our service at the onset, we could build something with *high cohesion* or *functional cohesion* and group them in a well-defined set of tasks. Functional programmers often tout the superiority of their languages because most functions will eventually fall into small, highly cohesive functions. But the same can be true of any language if you give it enough time and thought. See table 6.1.

Table 6.1 Cohesion is used to define how well a structure or class is defined.

High cohesion	Clearly defined purpose and method definitions
Low cohesion	Broad responsibilities that are often all in one class or struct

An easy example of this is a class named `Validation` versus a class named `UserRegistrationValidation`. In the first case, you have a class that houses too many functions for all types of validation within your system, whereas the second provides a more focused validation of a specific step in a business process. The second reason for putting you through all of this is so we can decouple our tests and make them more atomic, or independent, which in the long run, will give us stability and speed up our development. Let's take a look at what that will look like.

6.4   *Testing stubs*

With dependency injection, we give ourselves some control over a service that we didn't have before. In chapter 3, we introduced the concept of black box testing: we can't see inside the method or structure we are testing and must test it externally. As our applications become more complex, the service we are writing tests for may become more difficult to reason about. Dependency injection allows us to constrain and isolate various parts of the underlying code we are trying to test. This is known as *scientific control* within experiments to help minimize the effects of the *independent variable* or the thing

you are trying to test. In our current implementation of the handler, we cannot control how the underlying translation service will work, so we cannot control our tests.

Here is an example. Currently, in our handler tests, we expect `/translate/ hello?language=dutch` to return a 404 message. If we implement the Dutch translation in our underlying service, our test will break! This means that our handler tests are coupled with the underlying service, which is not what we want to test. Instead, we want to understand what will trigger the responses expected from the handler itself. If a result comes back as valid, we want to return a 200, which is the HTTP code for success, along with the corresponding value. If it is not found, a 404 error code will be returned.

But now that we can inject our own dependency, we can create our own service specifically for testing. This is known as a stub. Stubs are very simple implementations of any structure (service, repository, utility) that can be used in testing as well as in systems under development. A stub mostly lacks complicated logic and returns hard-coded values. This allows us to test the service with known expectations of the underlying stubbed service.

NOTE Stubs can be great placeholders while code is under development. In chapter 2, we talked about splitting up work among team members to get the smallest delivered code possible. This can be accomplished by looking at your code as layers and stubbing the underlying dependencies as you move forward. In this example, you would stub the service that feeds the code to the handler and solely focus on the handler. Once the handler is delivered, consuming applications can start the often painful integration process earlier while you continue to build out the business logic.

To see this in action, let's update our test code as in the following listing.

Listing 6.10 `translate_test.go`

```
type stubbedService struct{}     // Creates an empty struct to satisfy your interface

func (s *stubbedService) Translate(word string, language string) string {   // Satisfies the interface expected by the handler
    if word == "foo" {     // Creates a simple method within the interface to test against
        return "bar"
    }
    return ""
}

func TestTranslateAPI(t *testing.T) {

    tt := []struct {
        Endpoint            string
        StatusCode          int
        ExpectedLanguage    string
        ExpectedTranslation string
    }{
        {
```

```
                    Endpoint:            "/translate/foo",
                    StatusCode:          200,
                    ExpectedLanguage:    "english",
                    ExpectedTranslation: "bar",
            },
            {
                    Endpoint:            "/translate/foo?language=german",
                    StatusCode:          200,
                    ExpectedLanguage:    "german",
                    ExpectedTranslation: "bar",
            },
            {
                    Endpoint:            "/translate/baz",
                    StatusCode:          404,
                    ExpectedLanguage:    "",
                    ExpectedTranslation: "",
            },
    }

    h := rest.NewTranslateHandler(&stubbedService{})        Injects the stubbed
    handler := http.HandlerFunc(h.TranslateHandler)         service for testing

    ...

}
```

You'll notice that some things are different here. Mostly, we changed the test to focus on the results that come back from our service instead of trying to push the logic through to the service. What we want to test is this:

- That the default language is English if no language is passed
- That if a language is passed, the language is returned
- That if a word that is not translated, we expect a 404 and empty values

I personally like to make clear to the developer that they are test values, thus the use of foo, bar, and baz. This helps people realize that we are working with fake data instead of real data and focuses their attention on the actual logic. This will run well, but it lacks some fidelity. Specifically, we are missing the actual values passed to the service itself. Right now, we have a bug in our code that was left there intentionally. In our testing chapter, we talked about building services that are robust and that handle the standardization of input. While we built utilities to support this on the service, we failed to pay attention to this on the handler. We can make a call like in the following listing.

Listing 6.11 `translate_test.go`

```
func TestTranslateAPI(t *testing.T) {

    tt := []struct {
        Endpoint            string
        StatusCode          int
        ExpectedLanguage    string
```

```
        ExpectedTranslation string
    }{
        ...
        {
            Endpoint:            "/translate/foo?language=GerMan",
            StatusCode:          200,
            ExpectedLanguage:    "german",
            ExpectedTranslation: "bar",
        },
    }
}

    ....
}
```

Input here shows inconsistent capitalization from what we are expecting on the service.

The expectation is that the results should be lowercase.

Our test would fail. We want to make sure that the language is lowercase when we return the value. This way, the results are always standard and our consumers can develop against it properly. We want to not only verify that the returned value is lowercase but also make sure we are passing the lowercase version to our service. How do we do that?

We could add the logic to our stub to do the verification, but this becomes complicated. Instead, we can focus on using something that gives us more control around the testing logic by using a mock.

Before we get to mocking, let's circle back to what we are trying to achieve. We are not testing dependencies within our application; instead, we are testing how part of our application works *with* the dependencies. This distinction has to be clear because we want each piece to be independently testable and verifiable. Therefore, when you find that a portion of your code depends on an external library or service, you should consider how it will be incorporated into your testing strategy.

6.5 *Mocking*

In baseball, batters typically warm up with a pitching machine. This machine stands in for a person to help the batter practice their swing. In practice, the batter may face a live player who throws them the ball. This person isn't a pitcher but is someone who can give the batter just enough variation that makes it *higher fidelity* by making it more realistic. Finally, during the game, the hitter will encounter a real pitcher, and hopefully they are ready.

In testing we want to exercise our code in the same way. In the previous section we talked about stubs, which act as a placeholder for a service but with expected results. These stubs don't do very much, and you may find that you are adding strange logic code in your stub to make your tests work as expected. Before you go down that path you should consider mocking.

Mocking is like a stub but with more detail. With mocks you create a similar object, but you can attach methods that allow you to assert if certain methods were called and with what values. It can change functionality per test so that you can test error handling and strange values. Overall, it provides you with a deeper insight into how your function works and how you can test every edge case.

To help demonstrate this we will first add a feature to our system and then test it with a mock. If we cannot find the result in our database, we will call an external service using a client to fetch the result from the old system. To do this, we will first create an interface so that we can interchange them when we are ready to release the feature. Let's see what this service looks like:

```
touch translation/remote_translator.go
```

Next, add the code in the following listing.

Listing 6.12 remote_translator.go

```
package translation                              Verifies that the struct we are building
                                                 satisfies the interface. This will cause
var _ rest.Translator = &RemoteService{}    ◁──┘ a compile-time error if not satisfied.

// RemoteService will allow for external calls to existing service for
➥translations.
type RemoteService struct {
    client HelloClient      ◁──┐ Uses a new interface for
}                                making calls to external API

// HelloClient will call external service.
type HelloClient interface {
    Translate(word, language string) (string, error)   ◁──┐ Creates an interface for the
}                                                            client that calls and translates

// NewRemoteService creates a new implementation of RemoteService.
func NewRemoteService(client HelloClient) *RemoteService {
    return &RemoteService{client: client}
}

// Translate will take a given word and try to find the result using the client.
func (s *RemoteService) Translate(word string, language string) string {
    resp, _ := s.client.Translate(word, language)   ◁──┐ Uses the client to
    return resp                                            make external calls
}
```

Notice that we've added a new interface called `HelloClient`. Right now, all we have the service do is call the client and return the results. This will be the basis for our test. With mocking, you will find out that a lot of boilerplate occurs, so it is easier to organize our tests in `test suites` or groupings of tests that have a similar setup and tear down functionality. This means that we can establish our mock and test against it in various ways without conflicting setups or strange side effects.

6.5.1 Setting up our test suite

Luckily, there is a great testing tool kit called `testify` that will handle both suites and mocking. This library provides suites, assertion helpers, and mocks to help us with our testing. To use this, we will import our first external library:

```
go get -u github.com/stretchr/testify
```

NOTE GoMock is a popular alternative to Testify's mock tool. It has a mechanism for generating specific mocks for your interfaces.

Now let's create our test file and set up our suite:

```
touch translation/remote_translator_test.go
```

Next, add the code in the following listing.

Listing 6.13 `remote_translator_test.go`

```
package translation_test

import (
    "context"
    "errors"
    "testing"

    "github.com/stretchr/testify/mock"
    "github.com/stretchr/testify/suite"
    "github.com/holmes89/hello-api/translation"
)

func TestRemoteServiceTestSuite(t *testing.T) {
    suite.Run(t, new(RemoteServiceTestSuite))
}

type RemoteServiceTestSuite struct {
    suite.Suite
    client *MockHelloClient
    underTest *translation.RemoteService
}

func (suite *RemoteServiceTestSuite) SetupTest() {
    suite.client = new(MockHelloClient)
    suite.underTest = translation.NewRemoteService(suite.client)
}

type MockHelloClient struct {
    mock.Mock
}

func (m *MockHelloClient) Translate(word, language string) (string, error) {
    args := m.Called(word, language)
    return args.String(0), args.Error(1)
}
```

Go's testing framework expects tests to start with the word Test and have the (t *testing.T) method. This will be used to trigger our suite.

Builds a suite that houses whatever dependencies we need to run our tests

Extends the Suite struct to use default methods

SetupTest will run before each test. Here, we initialize the mocked client and the service to test.

Creates a Mock struct to satisfy the interface

Extends Mock to use methods to track calls

Asserts that the values were called with the expected values

Satisfies the interface for the Mock

Returns the values from the mock

We have wrapped our traditional testing mechanism from the testing library in a struct that extends a `Suite` struct. With this structure, `testify` can use the `SetupTest` function to run before we run any tests. We then use the `Mock` structure to extend the functionality we will need to verify and manipulate the test so that we can try various edge cases. Testify allows you to use various setup and teardown commands to help reduce duplication of code, and in the case of mocks, reset their values.

We will explore some additional setup and teardowns in the next section, but for now, you can see how we are organizing our suite so that we can focus on the actual tests.

6.5.2   *Using our mocks in test*

We have written a service that calls a remote endpoint for a value and returns it to the user. This obviously isn't what we want long term, but we'll let the tests drive the writing of this service. First, let's get our tests written (see the following listing), and then we will work on enhancing our service.

Listing 6.14   `remote_translator_test.go`

```
package translation_test

...

func (suite *RemoteServiceTestSuite) TestTranslate() {
    // Arrange
    suite.client.On("Translate", "foo", "bar").Return("baz", nil)

    // Act
    res := suite.underTest.Translate("foo", "bar")

    // Assert
    suite.Equal(res, "baz")
    suite.client.AssertExpectations(suite.T())
}
```

Tells the mock what to expect as input and what to return

Suites have assertion libraries that act as convenience methods in testing. Here, we check if the values are equal.

Asserts the calls were made on the mock

Now run your tests, and see if they pass. This gives us more control over the dependency to verify that the service was called along with asserting the values by which the service was called. This is powerful because all too often, bugs can happen because a service may expect values to come in a certain format that the calling service may have forgotten or missed. Mocks provide a way for us to verify the values as part of the setup (see the following listing).

Listing 6.15   `remote_translator_test.go`

```
package translation_test

...

func (suite *RemoteServiceTestSuite) TestTranslate_CaseSensitive() {
    // Arrange
    suite.client.On("Translate", "foo", "bar").Return("baz", nil)

    // Act
    res := suite.underTest.Translate("Foo", "bar")

    // Assert
    suite.Equal(res, "baz")
    suite.client.AssertExpectations(suite.T())
}
```

This is the same expectation we had before from our mock. We will try to see if our method passes the expected input to the service it's calling.

Here, we change the input so that the test will fail.

Run this, and you should see a failure. It says it expected the input to be foo, not Foo. Here, the mock verifies the expectations we set earlier. Now we need to change our function to reflect this requirement (see the following listing).

Listing 6.16 `remote_translator.go`

```go
package translation

import (
    "strings"
)
...
// Translate will take a given word and try to find the result using the client.
func (s *RemoteService) Translate(word string, language string) string {
    word = strings.ToLower(word)
    language = strings.ToLower(language)          // Lowercases the input
    resp, _ := s.client.Translate(word, language) // so that your tests pass
    return resp
}
```

Now your tests should pass. Not only can we use a mock to verify the input, but it allows us to control the output. Here, we can add a simple test with minimal changes to see what happens if we get an error (see the following listing)

Listing 6.17 `remote_translator_test.go`

```go
package translation_test
...

func (suite *RemoteServiceTestSuite) TestTranslate_Error() {
    // Arrange
    suite.client.On("Translate", "foo", "bar").Return("baz",
    ➥ errors.New("failure"))                    // Now we return an error
                                                 // to see how we handle it.
    // Act
    res := suite.underTest.Translate("foo", "bar")

    // Assert
    suite.Equal(res, "")                          // We should not get
    suite.client.AssertExpectations(suite.T())    // an answer back.
}
```

Ah, we aren't handling the error in our service! Let's fix that using the code in the following listing.

Listing 6.18 `remote_translator.go`

```go
package translation

import (
    "strings"
    "log"
```

```
)
...
// Translate will take a given word and try to find the result using the client.
func (s *RemoteService) Translate(word string, language string) string {
    word = strings.ToLower(word)
    language = strings.ToLower(language)
    resp, err := s.client.Translate(word, language)
    if err != nil {              ◁─────┐ Handles
        log.Println(err)               │ the error
        return ""                }
    }
    return resp
}
```

Now we can verify how we handle this error. See how we could easily extend the test without changing how our mock is created? Stubs don't provide this level of control by default and need to have special programming to handle these types of cases. Instead, our mock provides us with the ability to inject errors and verify inputs without needing to change the underlying implementation.

> **NOTE**   Why even test the error? It may seem pointless in this example, but it can be helpful in most cases. Errors happen constantly in code, and business rules need to be associated with each type of error. Here, we just log the error and return an empty string. Our test verifies that no matter what, we should return an empty string in the case of a failed translation.

The final feature we want to add to our service is a cache. Most times, when calling an external or remote service, it is important to save the values to reduce the number of calls. This makes your service faster because it doesn't require waiting on a response from a server; it also makes it dependable, and in some cases, it saves you money. We want to verify that if we make the call with the same value, it only happens once. Our mock can keep track of this for us (see the following listing).

Listing 6.19   `remote_translator_test.go`

```
package translation_test
...
                                                         Asserts that this
                                                         command was
func (suite *RemoteServiceTestSuite) TestTranslate_Cache() {    only run once
    // Arrange
    suite.client.On("Translate", "foo", "bar").Return("baz", nil).Times(1)  ◁─┘

    // Act
    res1 := suite.underTest.Translate("foo", "bar")
    res2 := suite.underTest.Translate("Foo", "bar")        ◁─────┐
                                                  Makes the call twice to test the
    // Assert                                     cache. Notice that we are using
    suite.Equal(res1, "baz")                    capitalization so we know that our
    suite.Equal(res2, "baz")                  business logic should lowercase the
    suite.client.AssertExpectations(suite.T())     value before looking in the cache.
}
```

You should see a failure when you run your test. Let's fix this by using an in-memory map in the next listing.

Listing 6.20 `remote_translator.go`

```go
package translation

import (
    "fmt"
    "log"
    "strings"

    "github.com/holmes89/hello-api/handlers/rest"
)

// RemoteService will allow for external calls to existing service
⮕ for translations.
type RemoteService struct {
    client HelloClient
    cache map[string]string          ⟵  Uses an in-memory
}                                         map for a cache

...
// NewRemoteService creates a new implementation of RemoteService.
func NewRemoteService(client HelloClient) *RemoteService {
    return &RemoteService{
        client: client,
        cache: make(map[string]string),   ⟵  Creates the map as
    }                                         part of initialization
}

// Translate will take a given word and try to find the result using the client.
func (s *RemoteService) Translate(word string, language string) string {
    word = strings.ToLower(word)
    language = strings.ToLower(language)
                                                    Creates a key for your map
                                                    to store the translation
    key := fmt.Sprintf("%s:%s", word, language)  ⟵

    tr, ok := s.cache[key]        ⟵   Checks the cache
    if ok {            ⟵              for the key
        return tr         If the value was
    }                     found, returns it
                                                    Makes the
                                                    translation call
    resp, err := s.client.Translate(word, language) ⟵
    if err != nil {
        log.Println(err)
        return ""
    }
    s.cache[key] = resp      ⟵   Stores the value
    return resp                   in the cache
}
```

Perfect! Now run your tests and see that they all pass. Mocks can be a powerful tool for testing, but be warned that they can become complicated and your tests can become

hard to follow. This is where as a team you will need to focus on the *compatibility* or easy assembly of services and functions and the relationship between them. If a test becomes burdened with a bunch of mocks, the service may need to be broken up. If a mock needs to be changed constantly because of a changing interface, you may need to rethink your abstraction. Mocks aren't the silver bullet for testing; they're just one tool to help you test your code in isolation and enhance your unit testing.

6.6   *Fake*

Finally, we will add one more set of unit tests for a client that calls an external API. Here, we come up against a different type of interface testing, this time with an API that we don't control. Like our other interfaces tests, we can establish a *contract* or definition of what this API should look like and use a fake to simulate it.

> **WARNING**   We don't have control over the other API, just our own, and if something were to change on the other API, we could end up with failures. This fake is simulating an *external dependency*, or a system outside our control, and therefore should be monitored and heavily logged in case failures such as outages occur. Advanced system patterns such as Circuit Breakers should be used, but they are outside the context of this book. I suggest *Cloud Native Patterns* (Manning, 2019) by Cornelia Davis.

A *fake* is an object, struct, or service with limited capabilities. So far, we have described stubs and mocks in the context of testing. We will use the term *fake* as a definition of an object that stands in for an external service. Fakes provide this last category of tools to help us verify the base units of our code before we start moving toward integrating with external integration.

Go provides the ability to create a test server to call against, which makes our testing easier. We will use a fake HTTP server to build our fake to test a client we create. Let's set up our suite before we get into the details of the implementation. First, create the files using

```
touch translation/client.go
touch translation/client_test.go
```

and then add the code in the following listing.

Listing 6.21   `client_test.go`

```
package translation_test

import (
    "encoding/json"
    "io"
    "io/ioutil"
    "net/http"
    "net/http/httptest"
    "testing"
```

```
        "github.com/stretchr/testify/mock"
        "github.com/stretchr/testify/suite"
)

func TestHelloClientSuite(t *testing.T) {
        suite.Run(t, new(HelloClientSuite))
}

type HelloClientSuite struct {
        suite.Suite
        mockServerService *MockService
        server            *httptest.Server
        underTest         translation.HelloClient
}

type MockService struct {
        mock.Mock
}

func (m *MockService) Translate(word, language string) (string, error) {
        args := m.Called(word, language)
        return args.String(0), args.Error(1)
}
```

Use a test server to run against ←

We are going to be testing the interface defined here. ←

Similar mock to the ones we've seen before to help us inject values into the handler ←

To set up our client test, we will need to create a handler that captures the message to test what the client passes (see the following listing).

Listing 6.22 `client_test.go`

```
func (suite *HelloClientSuite) SetupSuite() {
        suite.mockServerService = new(MockService)
        handler := func(w http.ResponseWriter, r *http.Request) {
                b, _ := ioutil.ReadAll(r.Body)
                defer r.Body.Close()

                var m map[string]interface{}
                _ = json.Unmarshal(b, &m)

                word := m["word"].(string)
                language := m["language"].(string)

                resp, err := suite.mockServerService.Translate(word, language)
                if err != nil {
                        http.Error(w, "error", 500)
                }
                if resp == "" {
                        http.Error(w, "missing", 404)
                }
                w.Header().Set("Content-Type", "application/json")
                _, _ = io.WriteString(w, resp)
        }
        mux := http.NewServeMux()
        mux.HandleFunc("/", handler)
        suite.server = httptest.NewServer(mux)
}
```

SetupSuite is used because we don't want to create a new server for each test, just this group of tests.

Use the mock to get information and then handle the response using the correct error codes. ←

Start the test server. ←

```go
func (suite *HelloClientSuite) TearDownSuite() {
    suite.server.Close()        ◁─┐  Shut down the server
}                                 │  at the end of the suite.
```

> **NOTE**   We are setting up a database within the context of our test. Alternatively, you can use tools such as WireMock, which is language agnostic.

We are setting up a fake server with an HTTP handler that uses a mock so that we can test how the client handles various message types. Specifically, we want to see what happens when an error occurs, the result cannot be found, or a good result is found. The actual test cases will need to be written out once we've built the client, but you can see here how the setup of our suite will drive that design from the start. Let's use the code in the following listing to write our client and then write our tests.

Listing 6.23   `client.go`

```go
package translation

import(
    "errors"
    "log"
    "encoding/json"
    "io/ioutil"
    "net/http"
)
                                           ┌─ Types check to make sure
                                           │  it fulfills the interface
var _ HelloClient = &APIClient{}    ◁──────┘

type APIClient struct {
    endpoint string     ◁─┐  Stores the passed-in
}                         │  endpoint to call

// NewHelloClient creates instance of client with a given endpoint
func NewHelloClient(endpoint string) *APIClient {
    return &APIClient{
        endpoint: endpoint,
    }
}

// Translate will call external client for translation.
func (c *APIClient) Translate(word, language string) (string, error) {
req := map[string]interface{}{
        "word":     word,
        "language": language,
    }
    b, err := json.Marshal(req)
    if err != nil {
        return "", errors.New("unable to encode msg")
    }

    resp, err := http.Post(c.endpoint, "application/json",   ┆ Makes the external
    ⮑ bytes.NewBuffer(b))                                ◁───┘ call to the server
```

```
    if err != nil {
        log.Println(err)
        return "", errors.New("call to api failed")
    }
    if resp.StatusCode == http.StatusNotFound {          ◁──┐  Checks the status codes to
        return "", nil                                        properly handle the response
    }
    if resp.StatusCode == http.StatusInternalServerError {
        return "", errors.New("error in api")
    }
    b, _ = ioutil.ReadAll(resp.Body)
    defer resp.Body.Close()                    ┌─  Uses a generic struct to
    var m map[string]interface{}           ◁──┘   get values from the JSON
    if err := json.Unmarshal(b, &m); err != nil {
        return "", errors.New("unable to decode message")
    }
    return m["translation"].(string), nil
}
```

Now the client will make the call to a server based on the provided endpoint and handle the results, giving the calling service the translated text. As you can see, we have plenty of paths to go down for tests, and most of them are failure cases. We will go through a few cases, but I'll let you finish up the others. Since we have almost everything already set up, the last thing we need to do before writing our tests is add our new client to the test suite (see the following listing).

Listing 6.24 `client_test.go`

```
func (suite *HelloClientSuite) SetupSuite() {            Creates the client in the suite and
    ...                                                  passes the unique server URL to it
    suite.underTest = translation.NewHelloClient(suite.server.URL)    ◁──┘
}
```

Now we can start writing some tests. We can use the mock the same way we did in our other tests to manipulate the output of our fake server. First, we will take the happy path rather than two failure cases (see the following listing).

Listing 6.25 `client_test.go`

```
func (suite *HelloClientSuite) TestCall() {
    // Arrange
    suite.mockServerService.On("Translate", "foo", "bar").Return(`{
    ➥ "translation":"baz"}`, nil)            ◁──┐  Makes the system
                                                  return valid JSON
    // Act
    resp, err := suite.underTest.Translate("foo", "bar")

    // Assert
    suite.NoError(err)          ◁──┐  Checks to see that
    suite.Equal(resp, "baz")        there wasn't an error
}
```

```
func (suite *HelloClientSuite) TestCall_APIError() {
    // Arrange
    suite.mockServerService.On("Translate", "foo", "bar").Return("",
    errors.New("this is a test"))

    // Act
    resp, err := suite.underTest.Translate("foo", "bar")

    // Assert
    suite.EqualError(err, "error in api")
    suite.Equal(resp, "")
}
```
➡ Returns an error to test the error status (annotation pointing to `errors.New("this is a test"))`)

Checks the returned error value to make sure the right error was passed (annotation pointing to `suite.EqualError(err, "error in api")` / `suite.Equal(resp, "")`)

```
func (suite *HelloClientSuite) TestCall_InvalidJSON() {
    // Arrange
    suite.mockServerService.On("Translate", "foo", "bar").Return(`invalid
    json`, nil)

    // Act
    resp, err := suite.underTest.Translate("foo", "bar")

    // Assert
    suite.EqualError(err, "unable to decode message")
    suite.Equal(resp, "")
}
```
➡ Makes the system fail by sending the wrong content (annotation pointing to `json`, nil)`)

Can you add tests for bad input and not found responses?

6.7 *Just the base of the pyramid*

In chapter 3, we talked about how unit tests provide us with the base we need for the rest of our tests. In that chapter, our tests were fairly simple, but as you can see, once other functions and systems get involved, they become more complicated. This dependency can be avoided by creating abstractions, but those abstractions need to be tested in a realistic way. It is up to you to find this out and explore ways of keeping your services as simple as possible. If your test code becomes complicated, it might cause you to pause and look at your code to see if it can be simplified and refactored. See table 6.2.

Table 6.2   Comparing stubs, mocks, and fakes

Type	Pros	Cons
Stub	Easy to create and manipulate	Verification can become complicated.
Mock	Records interactions for later verification	More complex setup and teardown.
Fake	Higher-fidelity interactions with a simulated system	Complicated to write and maintain.

Our introduction to stubs, mocks, and fakes gives you tools to help you write better tests. Be aware that these tools should not preempt good design. When writing code,

you will sometimes find that you have a ton of mocks floating around or that your fake becomes too complicated. These are canaries in your coal mine, and these should raise some flags about your implementation. Maybe your code needs to be broken up. Maybe you need to rethink your design. In any case, you need to watch and think about how you are testing and writing your code. Tests provide an excellent mirror to what you are doing. Complicated structs are hard to write tests for and therefore are more prone to errors. Cracks in the foundation of your testing pyramid, as seen in figure 6.3, will lead to a decrease in confidence about your code, so take your time to think about what you are writing and how you are structuring your tests and your code.

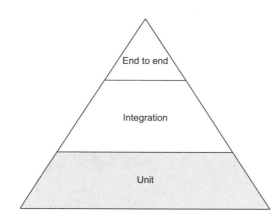

Figure 6.3   We have now covered the base of our pyramid using these techniques.

We find ourselves slowly crawling up the pyramid and still have the middle and top layers to add to our system to help us establish some confidence in what we are building. But these tests are going to become even more complicated to manage and less dependable, and therefore will require a different part of our pipeline. The theme I'm trying to establish in this book is this notion of starting from a place of simplicity and moving toward the complex. Complexity should be avoided if at all possible but is sometimes unavoidable as a trade-off. You alone will be able to determine when it is time to move toward complexity based either on features or the size of your team. Working together, you and your team will figure out the best way to build, test, and run your application.

"Wow, that was neat. I didn't realize I would be contributing something so important on my first day." You smile. It is really nice to see someone learn something new and help them understand how your system works. A few more pair programming sessions like this and the intern will be ready to teach the next person who comes on board. So far, she's been able to contribute both test code and feature code. Now it's time to teach her the infrastructure.

Summary

- Interfaces can be used to define the communication between services and act as an abstraction to isolate your code.
- Services that satisfy an interface can then be passed into a service as a dependency allowing you to inject the code you want to support the service.
- Suites allow you to set up and tear down tests and groups of tests in a uniform way.
- Stubs are lightweight structures that can help you test a service without external dependencies in a simple way.
- Mocks add more dimensions to your tests by allowing you to verify calls and their content.
- Fakes can be used in conjunction with mocks and stubs to stand in completely for another service.

Containerized deployment

"Listen, I understand that this project is now gaining some traction, but we need to be able to integrate with it as soon as we can. The old service is at the center of everything we do, so you will need to give us documentation on how to run what you already have," says Carol. You are just sitting down with your lunch when she sits down at the same table. Carol has been the team lead over at the mobile application team for several years now. She runs a tight ship and doesn't like surprises—like to one your PM put you in charge of developing. You smile and say you'll get her team something by the end of the day. Something simple that they won't have to do anything crazy to use.

"It would be nice if it's the exact system you are using in production and can be used locally." This is important. Having a system work the same on your machine as it does in production is huge. Of course, you could point her team to the binary you publish on your repository, but your binaries are compiled for Linux, not for macOS or Windows, which the mobile app team uses. You need something more universal.

What can you do? How can you deliver a product in a way that runs uniformly in any environment? How can you ensure that it runs efficiently and is secure? The answer is containers.

If you look at some trucks driving down the highway, you will see a large metal cargo container on the back. These are the same containers you see at shipping docks in harbors and on the backs of trains. They are all the same ISO containers that adhere to ISO standard 668:2020 and have the dimensions of 8 feet wide, 20 or 40 feet long, and 8 feet 6 inches high. This standardization allows items to be transported easily by all of these different vehicles, as demonstrated in figure 7.1.

Prior to the invention of these containers, ships, trucks, and trains had *break bulk cargo* or essentially loosely bound, nonstandard containers such as barrels and boxes. Trying to find space for such items became a complicated puzzle and required extra manual labor to move items from one vehicle to another. The transition to containers made it so that shipping products were standardized in a way that made the transportation of goods easy and efficient.

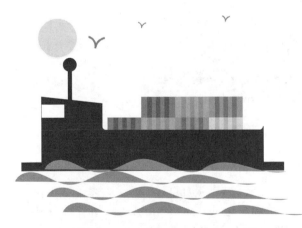

Figure 7.1   Container vessels have a flat surface that allows for many containers to be moved at once.

Shipping software today can often feel like break bulk cargo if you consider the state of the operating systems and computer architectures. Suppose we want to write code that supports Linux, macOS, and Windows but also runs on 32-bit or 64-bit Intel or ARM architectures. How many binaries would we need to ship? If we take three operating systems and four architectures, we would have 12 different binaries that would need to be built and run for that specific machine. This becomes the same problem of irregular barrels and boxes that the shipping industry had and often falls victim to the

meme "it works on my machine." As mentioned before, we want uniformity in the items we build and the products we ship.

How can we solve this problem? The same way the shipping industry did: containers.

7.1 *What is a container?*

To better understand how a container works, we need a brief overview of how an operating system works. An operating system's job is to manage various resources within the physical machine. This includes storing information in memory or on a hard disk or deciding which programs to execute. A *container* is a self-contained operating system that is *virtualized*, meaning it runs on a machine that doesn't use a physical machine directly. This *virtual machine* works with the underlying operating system to run various applications. Container runtimes are virtual machines that work with the host operating system to share the same *kernel*, or the service that chooses which applications run. These abstraction layers give us the ability to hide the underlying implementation layers, as seen in figure 7.2.

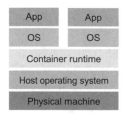

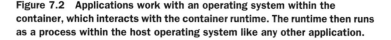

Figure 7.2 Applications work with an operating system within the container, which interacts with the container runtime. The runtime then runs as a process within the host operating system like any other application.

> **NOTE** In this book, we use one of the more popular container tools: Docker. Alternatively, you can use Podman, which is gaining popularity.

What does this mean for you? When we create a container, we create a standardized format to run on a given runtime. Containers are built from *images* or snapshots of what our system should look like. You can think of this as being sort of like a template or a saved file that gets loaded and runs on the system. A single image can be used to create many containers. These images are defined and built for a given runtime, much like our application binaries, but the runtime allows our container to run anywhere that implements this specification. Currently, the most common runtime for most developers is Docker, so much so that Docker and containers are often used interchangeably (like calling a tissue a Kleenex), but there are many different implementations of the container specification.

You may be thinking, "What does this mean for you?" Well, as you can imagine, as your company grows, you may not all be using Go. Python or JavaScript may be introduced. Or you may have dependencies like databases and queuing systems. All of these pieces require configuration and setup. If you are working in Go, you may not want to have to go through the hassle of installing Python to integrate with another team's product. You don't want your developers taking precious time trying to install

or update to the latest version of Postgres. Instead, you can rely on Docker to help manage, maintain, and run all of these dependencies. This frees you up to focus on your development.

Because Docker is a common runtime for containers, many developers will have it installed on their machines to help them run their applications and application dependencies uniformly. But as you move away from your host machine and want to ship your container to a hosted environment, you may find that there are other ways of optimizing and building your containers to have them run more efficiently in that environment. There is a joke that the "cloud" is just someone else's machine. This joke, though, is true. It is all just some other machine somewhere else, and with many different cloud providers building and implementing their hardware and custom runtimes, it can sometimes be better to build images optimized for their runtimes. This can be done by using their base images or allowing them to help build the images for you, which is known as *Buildpacks*.

7.2 *What is a Buildpack?*

In chapter 4, we deployed our application using a PaaS framework in Google Cloud. In both of those deployments, we did not need to focus on how those applications were being run or where they were running; they were abstracted. We can imagine, though, how all of this works. At the very base of everything are physical machines running the code, but there are layers of virtualization and abstraction. You, as the developer, do not need to worry about things like security patches and kernel upgrades; just focus on your code. There is some hidden magic that determines what code you are running and how to deploy it, and suddenly it works.

The cloud is just someone else's computer.

Buildpacks work in a very similar way and are inextricably linked with how many PaaS work under the hood. In fact, this technology was first developed by Heroku in 2011 and has been used by various other companies such as Pivotal and Google to help run their PaaS. The concepts are simple: you provide the code, and they'll build the image. Under the hood, PaaS are building their custom images based on the libraries and dependencies that their platforms need to make the code run as efficiently as possible and deploy them as containers in their hosting environment. This gives you resilience and substantial uptime, and they can get the most out of their hardware by running isolated, secure, and maintainable applications.

If you are building an application, Buildpacks will give you a lot of features that will make your application more robust, such as advanced caching, multiprocessing, language detection, and much more. The recent Buildpacks game-changer is the notion of *Cloud Native Buildpacks* which allows you, as the developer, to take advantage of the PaaS-like ecosystem of building an application with the portability of using containers.

What goes on inside of a Buildpack? When triggering a Buildpack, it goes through two stages: detection and builds. When triggering a build, the Buildpack analyzes your source code to first determine if it can recognize the source code and build the container; this is known as the detection stage. In our case, it will look for Go files or a

.mod file. If we were building a Javascript application, it would look for a `package` `.json` file, or if a Java application, it would look for a `pom.xml` file.

When entering the building stage, the Buildpack will determine what the runtime should be, how the library should be built, the installation of dependencies, and the compilation and running of the application itself. It does this through the use of a *builder*, which is an image specifically used for creating the application based on the detection done in the previous step. The building and running of an image are done through a *stack*, which combines the build and run environments.

Docker is just one container runtime. There are many other container runtimes out there that aren't as popular.

All of this can allow different groups to create a process for identifying and building applications specific to their runtimes and environments. This means that Google, Amazon, Heroku, and Microsoft can build their own container runtimes that are optimized for their hardware, and you can tap into that performance by using their Buildpack. Let's try it with Google.

7.3 Let's build a container

To start, we will use a Buildpack to build and run our container locally. Then we will use the same process to deploy the container to production. Following that, we will work on building our own container using our own definition and deploy that as well. This way, you will know how to build and maintain your own containerized deployment and local development. First, we must install our container runtime, in this case, Docker.

Docker has three different installation types depending on your operating system, so it will be best if you follow the directions for the one that best suits you. Directions can be found at https://docs.docker.com/get-docker/. This will give us our container runtime. Now we need to create a container. To do this, we will use a Buildpack and install `pack`, which is a tool built and maintained by Cloud Native Buildpacks. It can be installed by following the directions at https://buildpacks.io/docs/tools/pack/.

`pack` will help us choose and build our application into a container using a defined Buildpack. To demonstrate this, let's see what `pack` suggests we use to build our application. Type `pack builder suggest` and see what options come up:

```
Google:             gcr.io/buildpacks/builder:v1    Ubuntu 18 base image
    with buildpacks for .NET, Go, Java, Node.js, and Python
Heroku:             heroku/buildpacks:18            Base builder for
    Heroku-18 stack, based on ubuntu:18.04 base image
Heroku:             heroku/buildpacks:20            Base builder for
    Heroku-20 stack, based on ubuntu:20.04 base image
Paketo Buildpacks:  paketobuildpacks/builder:base   Ubuntu bionic base image
    with buildpacks for Java, .NET Core, NodeJS, Go, Python, Ruby, NGINX and
    Procfile
Paketo Buildpacks:  paketobuildpacks/builder:full   Ubuntu bionic base image
    with buildpacks for Java, .NET Core, NodeJS, Go, Python, PHP, Ruby,
    Apache HTTPD, NGINX and Procfile
Paketo Buildpacks:  paketobuildpacks/builder:tiny   Tiny base image (bionic
    build image, distroless-like run image) with buildpacks for Java Native
    Image and Go
```

Notice that these packs are not focused on a specific language but rather provide a broad foundation for multiple languages. You may also notice that these languages are those that are supported for FaaS and PaaS offerings on Google. This is because underneath, our FaaS and PaaS are running within a container using a Buildpack. Now let's build our application by typing the following:

```
pack build hello-api --builder gcr.io/buildpacks/builder:v1
```

Let's look at what it did. The builder identifies that our application is a Go project from our module file and looks for a `main` package to run. Some configurations can be done if you have more than one main function. Each Buildpack will have its own configuration. To see how our container runs, type

```
docker run hello-api
```

You should see your server run. Call your translation endpoint and see that your application is running in a nice, neat, portable package. Now that you can build a container, let's publish it so that others can use it.

7.4   Adding a container build to your pipeline

Now we want to make this an artifact available through our releases, just like we did with our binary. Why do we want a container if we already have the binary? Remember what containers are: a universal runtime for your application independent of the underlying operating system. Since our other development teams want to use our application, we can simply share a container with them so that they don't need to worry about dependencies, libraries, or runtimes. This way, they don't need to have any underlying knowledge of Go or even of how to start our application and instead can run the container like they would any other application. They don't even need to build our container; we can provide it for them in a *registry*.

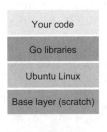

A *container registry* is just a storage area for images that are created for a container. The default registry on Docker is `hub .docker.com`, in which you can find all sorts of images to use. Each item in the registry can be pulled to run or be used as a *base* image for other images to be built from. Like Legos, images can be stacked on top of each other to build products. The image from which a container starts is known as the *base*. Figure 7.3 shows how this could work.

Figure 7.3 Layers of containers

At the bottom, you have an image such as an operating system. This layer can then be the base for another layer, such as a language. Then you can use that layer for building your application. These layers can add up over time and become complex, but they all get stored in this registry. When you run a container, more often than not, you want to pull it from a registry rather than build it on your own. Registries can act as private places for you and others to store and run your containers. In this chapter, we will publish our application to two repositories: one for public consumption and one for us to run in

Google Cloud. Since we can now build our container using a Buildpack, we can publish the container to a registry.

To publish our container, we want to add it to our pipeline so that it is continuously delivered. Open your `pipeline.yml`, and add a container build section using the code in the following listing.

Listing 7.1 `pipeline.yml`

```
containerize-buildpack:
  name: Build Container buildpack          Only builds our container
  runs-on: ubuntu-latest                   after the source code has
  needs: test                       <───┘  passed unit tests
  steps:
  - name: Check out code into the Go module directory
    uses: actions/checkout@v2                      Installs Pack through
  - name: Install Pack                             curl for our build stage
    run: (curl -sSL "https://github.com/buildpacks/pack/releases/download/
    v0.21.1/pack-v0.21.1-linux.tgz" | sudo tar -C /usr/local/bin/
    --no-same-owner -xzv pack)                                      <───┘
  - name: Build
    run: pack build gcr.io/${{ secrets.GCP_PROJECT_ID }}/hello-api:latest
    --builder gcr.io/buildpacks/builder:v1          <──┐ Uses the pack command
  - name: Set up Cloud SDK                               to build our container
    uses: google-github-actions/setup-gcloud@master     targeted for GCP
    with:
      project_id: ${{ secrets.GCP_PROJECT_ID }}
      service_account_key: ${{ secrets.gcp_credentials }}
      export_default_credentials: true
  - name: Configure Docker                         Configures Docker to use GCP
    run: gcloud auth configure-docker --quiet  <──┘ for the container registry
  - name: Push Docker image to GCP
    run: docker push gcr.io/${{ secrets.GCP_PROJECT_ID }}/hello-api:latest <──
  - name: Log in to the GHCR
    uses: docker/login-action@master  <──┐                Pushes the container
    with:                                 Logs into GitHub    to GCP registry
      registry: ${{ env.REGISTRY }}       Container Registry
      username: ${{ github.actor }}
      password: ${{ secrets.GITHUB_TOKEN }}   Retags the image
  - name: Tag for Github                      for GitHub
    run: docker image tag gcr.io/${{ secrets.GCP_PROJECT_ID }}/hello-api
    :latest ${{ env.REGISTRY }}/${{ env.IMAGE_NAME }}:latest
  - name: Push Docker image to GHCR                           <──
    run: docker push ${{ env.REGISTRY }}/${{ env.IMAGE_NAME }}:latest
                                                 Pushes the new tag to
                                                 GitHub Container Registry
```

If you commit and push your changes, you should see a container now listed on your artifacts page. To test this, we can simply do the following:

```
docker run ghcr.io/holmes89/hello-api:latest
```

Now that you've automatically built and pushed your containers, we need to run them. To do this, we will use a container runtime.

7.5 *Deploying to a container runtime*

We've created a container using a Buildpack. We've published the container to the Google Container Registry. Now let's deploy our container. What advantage does using a container runtime provide? Why did we go through all of this?

For the first time in this book, we have a point of inflection between how an application is run in the cloud and how it runs on our machine. Our container now runs in a universal runtime. This is the closest we can get to an abstraction that we can run locally the same way it's run in the cloud. This is a powerful tool because it solves the problem of "it runs on my machine" and "I'm struggling with this framework." This is why containers are such a popular solution in today's development process.

A famous (or infamous) container orchestration tool is Kubernetes, which gives developers tools to deploy applications built on containers within a resilient, clustered environment. It's a big, complicated, and powerful tool. Kubernetes is beyond the scope of this book, but I mention it here because it is the foundation of some other container runtimes that we will use. These containers are underneath the hood of products such as Google Cloud Run and FaaS; you can't see the container, but it's there. Google runs your container for you using Kubernetes in an isolated process, but you don't need to worry about maintaining the cluster, writing deployments, and setting up incoming requests. Instead, you follow a pattern and deploy the container, and Google takes care of the rest.

In figure 7.4. we can see that we continue to move toward less abstraction and more control over our deployment process. We can now define the container and have it run in a universal runtime. We will use Google Cloud Run, but we could just as easily ship this product onto AWS ECS or a Kubernetes cluster.

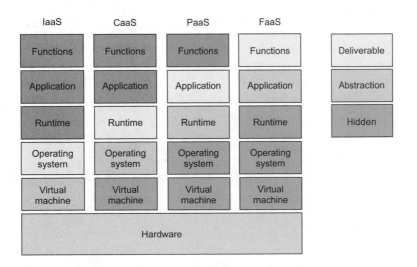

Figure 7.4   We are now using our container as our shippable product.

Now we can set up a container deployment just as easily as all of the other deployments we've completed thus far. We just need to open our `pipeline.yml` and add the code in the following listing.

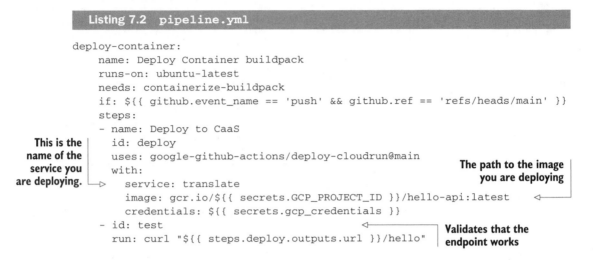

Listing 7.2 `pipeline.yml`

```
deploy-container:
    name: Deploy Container buildpack
    runs-on: ubuntu-latest
    needs: containerize-buildpack
    if: ${{ github.event_name == 'push' && github.ref == 'refs/heads/main' }}
    steps:
    - name: Deploy to CaaS
      id: deploy
      uses: google-github-actions/deploy-cloudrun@main
      with:
        service: translate
        image: gcr.io/${{ secrets.GCP_PROJECT_ID }}/hello-api:latest
        credentials: ${{ secrets.gcp_credentials }}
    - id: test
      run: curl "${{ steps.deploy.outputs.url }}/hello"
```

This is the name of the service you are deploying.

The path to the image you are deploying

Validates that the endpoint works

7.6 *Writing your own image*

What if you don't want all of the extra stuff that's in the Buildpack container? Remember, the Buildpack is structured to run well in the containerized environment with underlying libraries, configurations, and services to all help your products run well in their runtime. But with these libraries comes some additional overhead, in this case, space. For a deployed environment, this may not be a big deal, but what if we wanted to make it smaller or debug information?

Why smaller? For a development team, it may make sense to have smaller images floating around or a special development image for debugging purposes. In either case, we can't rely on the Buildpack abstraction to do this for us, so we will need to define our Dockerfile to build them.

The beautiful thing about Go is that it compiles into a binary and in most cases does not rely on external libraries to run. This means that you can make a binary and put it on the smallest base image possible. A *base image* is the starting place from which our container is built. If you look through different container definitions, you will find images for Ubuntu, Debian, Windows, and so forth. These images are built and maintained by teams that install security patches, upgrades, libraries, and in some cases applications. This way, you can run something like Postgres without installing it on your machine, or use a base image for Go so that you don't need to install Go. Let's see how this works by creating a Dockerfile. Type `touch Dockerfile` in the root of your directory. The following listing shows the result.

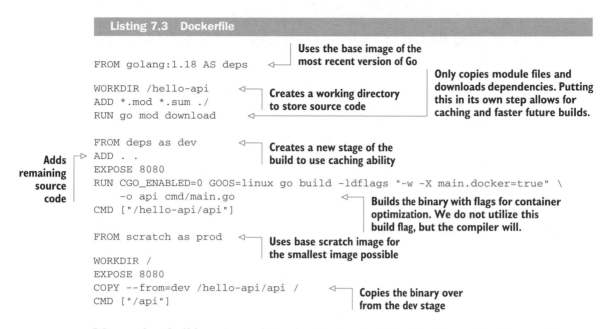

Listing 7.3   Dockerfile

```
FROM golang:1.18 AS deps

WORKDIR /hello-api
ADD *.mod *.sum ./
RUN go mod download

FROM deps as dev
ADD . .
EXPOSE 8080
RUN CGO_ENABLED=0 GOOS=linux go build -ldflags "-w -X main.docker=true" \
    -o api cmd/main.go
CMD ["/hello-api/api"]

FROM scratch as prod
WORKDIR /
EXPOSE 8080
COPY --from=dev /hello-api/api /
CMD ["/api"]
```

Uses the base image of the most recent version of Go

Creates a working directory to store source code

Only copies module files and downloads dependencies. Putting this in its own step allows for caching and faster future builds.

Creates a new stage of the build to use caching ability

Adds remaining source code

Builds the binary with flags for container optimization. We do not utilize this build flag, but the compiler will.

Uses base scratch image for the smallest image possible

Copies the binary over from the dev stage

We can then build our image by typing `docker build -t hello-api:min .` and for our dev image `docker build -t hello-api:dev --target dev .`. Now that both images are built, let's compare how large they are! We can simply type `docker images`, and you'll see your three image definitions, their tags, their size, and when they were built:

```
hello-api          dev          78b80879b282      4 minutes ago      962MB
hello-api          min          64d767be4d62      4 minutes ago      4.74MB
hello-api          latest       a6052d265459      41 years ago       129MB
```

Wow! Our dev image is obviously the largest, but our min image is 3% the size of the Buildpack image! Why is that? Earlier we talked about how containers work. Each image is based on another image. Each time a new container is built, a layer gets added to your image. You can see this when you pull images as part of this build. Beneath all of those layers is the very base image that all images come from, as you can see in figure 7.5. It is called `scratch` and is completely empty, so your application needs to be self-contained—just like our Go binary! That means we can copy our binary over to the `scratch` image, and it will interact with the runtime to run, just like any other container but without the bloat. This way, you don't have to worry about outdated libraries

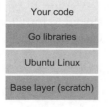

Figure 7.5   Containers use layers to help construct the image. The more layers you have, the larger your image becomes, and the more security vulnerabilities arise.

or security patches. However, you can't debug because there isn't a command line. It's a trade-off, but it can be extremely useful to ship around to other users.

Now let's add these containers to our pipeline and publish them to our registry using the code in the following listing.

Listing 7.4 `pipeline.yml`

```
containerize:
    name: Build Containers
    runs-on: ubuntu-latest
    needs: test
    steps:
    - name: Check out code into the Go module directory
      uses: actions/checkout@v2
    - name: Build Min
      run: docker build -t ${{ env.REGISTRY }}/${{ env.IMAGE_NAME }}:min .      ◁   Builds the min image and tags it
    - name: Build Dev
      run: docker build -t ${{ env.REGISTRY }}/${{ env.IMAGE_NAME }}:dev
      ➥ --target=dev .      ◁   Builds the dev image using dev as the target for the build
    - name: Log in to the GHCR
      uses: docker/login-action@master      ◁   Logs in to GitHub Container Registry
      with:
        registry: ${{ env.REGISTRY }}
        username: ${{ github.actor }}
        password: ${{ secrets.GITHUB_TOKEN }}      ◁   Pushes the min image to the registry
    - name: Push Docker min image to GHCR
      run: docker push ${{ env.REGISTRY }}/${{ env.IMAGE_NAME }}:min
    - name: Push Docker dev image to GHCR      ◁   Pushes the dev image to the registry
      run: docker push ${{ env.REGISTRY }}/${{ env.IMAGE_NAME }}:dev
```

When your code is pushed, you should now see that you have three different containers. This can become extremely helpful when we start tagging our product for stable releases. These can be considered our latest builds for the time being and are used to test new features that may not be stable. Now that we are shipping our containers, we can integrate them into our development process, and others can as well.

7.7　*Local environment organization*

You have a containerized service. You are shipping it for other developers to use. But your development is becoming dependent on other services as well. Is there something containers can do to help you in your development and shipping?

As you start down the path of using containers in your development environment, you will find that things such as environmental variables, port numbers, and runtime args can get a little clunky. You will find that you are going back to restarting a container and forgetting how it was configured. Or you may find that running a full integration of your application requires more than one container. This is where tools like `docker-compose` can help. `docker-compose` is a tool for running and organizing multiple containers. By writing a simple YAML file, you will be able to build and run containers in a simple, universal environment. As has been emphasized throughout this book, it is

important to have simple-to-use tools to help developers. The compose file will even integrate into our CI pipeline by organizing our build parameters.

To begin, let's install Docker Compose. If you are using Mac or Windows, you are in luck! It is already installed as part of your Docker Desktop installation. If you are on Linux, you will need to follow the simple install here: https://docs.docker.com/compose/install/

Once you have it installed, you will find a list of commands to use by typing `docker-compose`. Here, you will see options to build, create, and run services or commands. Compose requires the presence of a `docker-compose.yml` file to work. It will progressively look into parent directories until a suitable file is found. This YAML file is specially structured to give every service a unique name to reference, along with the image name, parameters, and many other options to help developers configure their containers to start. The names used in the file can also act as DNS entries for an internally run network that `docker-compose` builds, allowing services to reference each other if need be. We will explore this in upcoming chapters. For now, we will make a basic file to create our containers. Create and open `docker-compose.yml` in the root directory of your project, and add the code in the following listing.

Listing 7.5 `docker-compose.yml`

```
version: "3.8"
services:
  api-min:                    Specifies the name of the        Labels the service as part of
                              service for internal use         the prod group for targeted
    profiles: ['prod']                                         deployments and builds
    image: ghcr.io/holmes89/hello-api:min
    port: 8080:8080                                            The image you wish
    build: .            Separates the dev service target       to use for this service
  api-dev:                for debugging purposes
    profiles: ['dev']                                          Labels the service as part of the dev
    image: ghcr.io/holmes89/hello-api:dev                      group for additional testing features
    port: 8080:8080
    build:              The image you wish
      context: .        to use for this service
      target: dev       Specifies the target if you are using
                        this for building your Docker image
```

We can see that we have defined both of our builds in `docker-compose`, which allows us to simply type `docker-compose build api-min` to build our min file. Try it out! Additionally, we have added the concept of profiles, which will help as our application grows. Try `docker-compose --profile prod up` to see the min file start. Try this with your `dev` profile too.

This will become important once we add dependencies and advanced testing, but for now, we will use this for shipping. We can now update our pipeline to reference our compose file rather than bake our configuration into the build command directly. This will save us time and energy as we move along in our development.

Now that we have successfully deployed a tool to help us build our application and run it, we are poised to expand our capabilities. We can slowly and efficiently start

building our application with its dependencies for easy local development. We can ensure that our services work the same on our machine as they do in our deployed environment because we are using the same artifact. Our compose file can act as a loose definition of our infrastructure that we can eventually evolve to suit our needs and act just like our production environment. This loose coupling of services allows us to focus on our code instead of trying to focus on the infrastructure.

7.8 Containers, containers everywhere

Containers are popular, and I'm sure you can see why. Portability and simplicity were game changers in the development world. Now entire operating systems can be shipped with products inside of them with minimal setup on the user end. Entire infrastructures and systems are built using containers. They run as cloud applications, build systems, and even robots. This is the peak of software development, right?

Not really. The gains we have with containers are certainly helpful for developers and with the developer experience but are sometimes unnecessary. As we saw in previous chapters, sometimes software can be written to be a simple function that does everything you need. Or you can have a simple application that is hosted on a shared platform. Containers may lie underneath the surface of many of these technologies, but developers may not need to use them. Building and maintaining containers means that you are responsible for things like upgrades, security patches, and how to best build your application. This can create complexity in its own right.

There is no silver bullet in technology, so always be wary of people who preach otherwise. Consider the technical cost of running and building containers before adopting them. The portability of the product is the most important aspect. If you find that you are struggling with a container, you may be using it wrong. Remember that there are trade-offs to everything. You need to consider them before adopting a technology. In this case, a container may not be the best solution for instances of high-performing applications because you are running a virtual machine. Containers can be great for running tests in a clean environment, but the tests shouldn't be reliant on the container to run tests locally.

But, as we will see in the upcoming chapters, containers have their place in the development cycle and can help us be more productive. As always, work with your team, and find what works best for you.

Summary

- Containers provide an abstraction with the local operating system to help create a universal runtime for applications.
- Buildpacks focus on creating containers that run efficiently on managed platforms.
- Use container runtimes to use your container locally as well as in a production environment.

Part 3

Going public

If you've made it this far, you may find that your team and customer base have grown to a point that you are swamped with feature requests and a more complicated product. This is a good problem to have! It means that not only are you are writing new features for customers, but you have a large enough team to explore how to configure your system to experiment with your customers' experience.

To do this, in chapter 8, we will look at configuring our application to change without changing its code. We will use this configuration to help us focus on writing tests based on feature requests running against an entire system instead of the modular pieces of code in chapter 9. Then we'll move our application to a larger production ecosystem in chapter 10 using containers. Chapter 11 is a summary of all you have learned.

Configuration management and stable releases

8

This chapter covers

- Creating configuration management to change application functions
- Exploring different options for configuration management
- Hiding new or incomplete features with configuration feature flags
- Communicating software changes through release notes and versioning

"I just can't see how we can safely roll this out while we are still testing or how we can easily cut over to the new system once we are comfortable," the QA lead says during a kickoff meeting. "I mean, we've been happy with the automated testing, and it has caught a few bugs already, but we can't sign off on releasing this into the wild yet."

"We can't just have this sitting around, though. We need to be able to show that this rewrite is worth it. We have shown that we can make changes quickly and release often, but we need some real traffic to see how this is going to hold up, and the only way we can do that is if we start letting our customers use it." Your project

133

manager is beyond exasperated at this point. You've just gone through an entire roll-out plan meeting, and once again, it feels like QA is stopping any sort of progress.

But as you sit there, you have to feel that QA has a point. We aren't sure how this will operate under different loads, and we aren't sure how this will work in our entire ecosystem. You mention this, but when you get a sideways glare from your project manager, you start to propose a solution rather than point out a problem.

You mention that the new system relies on the old system for translations we don't currently have in the database. You also mention that the current storage device for your system is just an in-memory key-value store—definitely something you need to change if you want this to be in production.

"Exactly my point: there are just too many changes that need to happen before we can even start testing it and sign off on it in production," someone from QA interjects.

You patiently correct them. "No, we will continue to release but will slowly cut people over once we are sure things are working as expected. Similarly, you will only ship one binary, but it will be able to change based on various settings."

"We need to list what we want to start integrating with in order to go live." Your project manager stands up, grabs a marker, and writes the following:

- Change API port.
- Add ability to change client endpoint for legacy systems.
- Turn off client calls.
- Add a database for long-term storage.

"Do you think you can get this done in a week? We need to get this rolling soon," your project manager says. You nod; using configuration management, you can build a system that you can use to turn various features on and off.

8.1   Configuration

All programs deal with two things: input and output. Programs take in data and emit data. Some will simply print "Hello World!" (that's the output). Some will only read log messages and store them in a database (that's input). But you can imagine providing input to an application to make it change its functionality.

Take, for instance, an application that is a counter. It may look something like the code in the following listing.

Listing 8.1 `main.go`

```go
package main

import (
    "bufio"
    "fmt"
    "os"
)
```

```go
func main() {
    fmt.Println("Welcome to advanced counter. Press Enter to increment value.")
    reader := bufio.NewReader(os.Stdin)
    count := 0
    for {
        fmt.Printf("Count is: %d\n", count)
        _, _ = reader.ReadString('\n')
        count++
    }
}
```

This is simple enough, but instead of having the counter increment by one, maybe we want it to increment by two, so we change the line count++ to count = count + 2. Great! But now you want to increment by 100. I hope you can see where we are going here. This is not scalable or transferable to other use cases. What if we could use just one piece of code to do this and not need to recompile it each time? We would provide input to the application when it started, which would affect its output. This input to change the functionality is known as a *configuration*. To configure this application, we will use what is known as an *environmental variable*: a variable stored in your terminal session. We will explore other configuration techniques in the following sections.

To allow configuration, we would use something like the code in the following listing.

Listing 8.2 `main.go`

```go
package main

import (
    "bufio"
    "fmt"
    "os"
    "strconv"
)

func main() {
    fmt.Println("Welcome to advanced counter. Press Enter to increment value.")
    reader := bufio.NewReader(os.Stdin)
    count := 0
    inc, err := strconv.Atoi(os.Getenv("INC"))
    if err != nil {
        fmt.Println("invalid incrementor, defaulting to 1")
        inc = 1
    }

    for {
        fmt.Printf("Count is: %d\n", count)
        _, _ = reader.ReadString('\n')
        count += inc
    }
}
```

If you run this code, you will see the warning message, but if you were to run something like `INC=2 go run counter.go`, you would see the values increment by two. This seems simple but is extremely valuable, especially for things like

- Database connection information
- Password salts
- Client endpoints
- Log levels

> **NOTE**   We will build our tools for configuration management. However, you can use the popular Viper library to manage configuration that way.

How can we add configuration to our API? Can we manage the configuration in different ways?

8.2   *Advanced configuration*

For our application, we will look at adjusting our application functionality by loading various configurations. First, let's identify the features we want to be modified:

- Custom port number
- Storage type (database, in memory)
- Storage connection information (if a database)
- External client endpoint (if none, do not call)

Let's define this as a struct we can pass around in our application. Create a new package called `config`, and in it, create a file called `core.go`. In that, we will define a struct as in the following listing.

Listing 8.3 `core.go`

Stores the port as a string, but we will validate that it is in the proper format later.

This is the endpoint for our client to call and can be injected if it is not an empty string.

Actively passes in the database type for future enhancements

This is similar to the legacy endpoint in that if it is empty, we will use the in-memory database.

```go
type Configuration struct {
    Port            string `json:"port"`
    DefaultLanguage string `json:"default_language"`
    LegacyEndpoint  string `json:"legacy_endpoint"`
    DatabaseType    string `json:"database_type"`
    DatabaseURL     string `json:"database_url"`
}
```

Notice we put JSON text decorators on the struct. This is because we are going to load our configuration in three different ways:

- With environmental variables
- With files
- With flags

Typically, these are the three most common ways to configure an application. There are other ways as well, but we'll focus mainly on these. By defining a core structure around our configuration, we can create a common function that will allow us to go through these steps to configure our system. First, we load whatever variables we can through the environment, then override them from a JSON file, and finally rely on flags to load information into our application.

Let's write out our load function to work in this way. To start, we can come up with a set of values to start with, which we will call `defaultConfiguration`. Our default configuration can look like the following listing.

Listing 8.4 `core.go`

```
var defaultConfiguration = Configuration{
    Port:            ":8080",          ◁─┐ Creates a basic structure with
    DefaultLanguage: "english",          │ just the port number as default
}
```

Given this default state, we can add various ways of changing the configuration.

8.2.1 *Environmental variables*

Environmental variables are stored in a user session in the system. These values can be hardcoded or passed into an application by prepending the command with the variable. This is an easy way to inject values into a system before it starts and can be used dynamically if your system calls the environmental variable repeatedly. We will add a method to the `configuration` struct to load the variables from the environment and then return them to the calling method using the code in the following listing.

Listing 8.5 `core.go`

```
package config

import "os"
...

// LoadFromEnv will load configuration solely from the environment
func (c *Configuration) LoadFromEnv() {
    if lang := os.Getenv("DEFAULT_LANGUAGE"); lang != "" {     ◁─┐
        c.DefaultLanguage = lang                                 │ Inline checks if the language
    }                                                            │ is set in the ENV and then
    if port := os.Getenv("PORT"); port != "" {                   │ updates the structs variable.
        c.Port = port                                          ──┘
    }
}
```

We are checking for two variables, `DEFAULT_LANGUAGE` and `PORT`. If they are set, we override the configuration settings; otherwise, we use the defaults. We also introduce a helper method because people often want to forgo the colon in the port definition,

so we will create a method to make sure it's there and is a valid number (see the following listing).

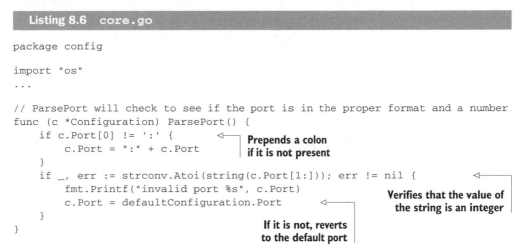

Listing 8.6 core.go

```go
package config

import "os"

...

// ParsePort will check to see if the port is in the proper format and a number
func (c *Configuration) ParsePort() {
    if c.Port[0] != ':' {
        c.Port = ":" + c.Port
    }
    if _, err := strconv.Atoi(string(c.Port[1:])); err != nil {
        fmt.Printf("invalid port %s", c.Port)
        c.Port = defaultConfiguration.Port
    }
}
```

Prepends a colon if it is not present

Verifies that the value of the string is an integer

If it is not, reverts to the default port

8.2.2   File

While environmental variables provide an easy way of loading configurations, there is still a more portable way: by using a file. JSON or YAML files are common ways of storing and loading configuration within a system and allow for portability between environments. The common configuration file can be modified for your local environment and your production environment without changing the underlying code. We add a new flag to allow us to pass in a configuration file explicitly and create a new function to parse the file and load variables. Let's first create a new function to load a configuration file through JSON using the code in the following listing.

Listing 8.7 core.go

```go
import (
    "encoding/json"
    "errors"
    "io/ioutil"
    "log"
    "os"
    "strconv"
)

...

// LoadFromJSON will read a JSON file and update the configuration based
// on the file.
func (c *Configuration) LoadFromJSON(path string) error {
    log.Printf("loading configuration from file: %s\n", path)
    b, err := ioutil.ReadFile(path)
    if err != nil {
        log.Printf("unable to load file: %s\n", err.Error())
```

Reads the contents of the file from the path

```
        return errors.New("unable to load configuration")
    }
    if err := json.Unmarshal(b, c); err != nil {        ⟵┐  Parses the content
        log.Printf("unable to parse file: %s\n", err.Error())   into the struct
        return errors.New("unable to load configuration")
    }
    // Verify required fields
    if c.Port == "" {                                   ⟵
        log.Printf("empty port, reverting to default")
        c.Port = defaultConfiguration.Port
    }
    if c.DefaultLanguage == "" {
        log.Printf("empty language, reverting to default")
        c.DefaultLanguage = defaultConfiguration.DefaultLanguage
    }
    return nil
}
```

Unmarshalling the JSON will not overwrite existing values if they are not present, but we want to validate for invalid settings.

8.2.3 Flag

There are times when a user may want to inject variables more explicitly. This is useful when you switch environments, because environmental variables can be stored in a session using export DEFAULT_LANGUAGE=Finnish and will not need to prepend the command with the variable setting. Using flags is a common way of passing in variables to servers at runtime. More often than not, you've used flags in other areas when starting an application. Any time you've done ./foo -h, you've passed an h flag to the service, indicating you want help with that application. We will add a flag to set the port, which is a common feature most servers provide.

To do this, we will create a LoadConfiguration function that will tie all of our configuration pieces together (see the following listing). We will layer our configuration, so pay attention to which variables may be overwritten. In our configuration function, we will have the following order of operations:

1 Use the default configuration.
2 Load a file if provided.
3 Use environmental variables.
4 Use flags.

Listing 8.8 `core.go`

```
import (
    "encoding/json"
    "errors"
    "flag"
    "io/ioutil"
    "log"
    "os"
    "strconv"
)
...
```

```
//LoadConfiguration will provide cycle through flags, files, and finally
➥ env variables to load configuration.
func LoadConfiguration() Configuration {
    cfgfileFlag := flag.String("config_file", "", "load configurations from
    a file")                                                        ◁──┐  Adds flag and
    portFlag := flag.String("port", "", "set port")                    │  description of flag

    flag.Parse()              ◁──┤  Processes flags
    cfg := defaultConfiguration
                                                          ┌───  Checks to see if
    if cfgfileFlag != nil && *cfgfileFlag != "" {    ◁──┘   a file is passed in
        if err := cfg.LoadFromJSON(*cfgfileFlag); err != nil {
            log.Printf("unable to load configuration from json: %s, using
            default values", *cfgfileFlag)
        }
    }
                                           ┌──  Loads environmental
                                           │    variables
    cfg.LoadFromEnv()     ◁──┘

    if portFlag != nil && *portFlag != "" {    ◁──┐  Checks to see if the port
        cfg.Port = *portFlag                       │  value is set and not empty
    }

    cfg.ParsePort()      ◁──┐  Parses our port to
    return cfg                │  make sure it's valid
}
```

We have built a system that allows you to change the functionality without changing the code itself. You can imagine larger files with more configurations available to hide features that are under development or change functionality without needing to rebuild. This is a powerful tool that can be used by your team to help build a robust product.

8.3   *Hiding features*

Next time you are in your car, look at the steering wheel and the dashboard. Do you notice any pieces of plastic that look as though a button could go there? These are known as *blanks* and are for different types of car packages. This means that the same steering wheel or console can be made for all types of cars, but only specific cars will have buttons for those features, as shown in figure 8.1. An example is a button for managing heated seats. If you bought a basic car, this would be blank, but if you bought the luxury package, it would be there.

This is a form of feature flagging, wherein you can build something the same way but adapt to which features are available to customers. This practice can be used to hide features from users who haven't paid for them (free versus paid tier), features that are still under development, or features you want to roll out to only a few customers for testing.

Now that you've built the ability to change your configuration, let's update our code to use it. Here, we will explore modifying our application as well as modifying

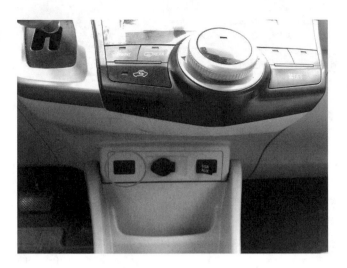

Figure 8.1   **Plastic fills expansion slots in various vehicle models.**

our service. In it, you will also find how this will relate to and be used with our dependency injection. To start, we will adjust our port number, and then we'll move on to updating our client and storage code.

8.3.1   *Updating the port*

Since we have built our configuration struct, we now need to load it in our main method. To do this, we will simply call our `LoadConfiguration` method. Once we have the configuration, we can start using it in constructing our main function in our main binary, and not our function for simplicity. That being said, all of the configuration changes we explore can also be attached to our function or whatever application we are writing. Let's see what updating our port number in our `cmd/main.go` file looks like in the following listing.

Listing 8.9   `core.go`

```go
import (
    "log"
    "net/http"

    "github.com/holmes89/hello-api/config"
    "github.com/holmes89/hello-api/handlers"
    "github.com/holmes89/hello-api/handlers/rest"
    "github.com/holmes89/hello-api/translation"
)

func main() {

    cfg := config.LoadConfiguration()      ⟵  Loads our
    addr := cfg.Port                            configuration
                              ⟵  Replaces the hardcoded string
....                             with the configuration port
    log.Printf("listening on %s\n", addr)
```

```
        log.Fatal(http.ListenAndServe(addr, mux))
}
```

Now let's test these different configuration changes. First, create a configuration JSON file called `config.json`. It should look like this:

```
{
    "port": 8079
}
```

Notice that we are missing some fields. This is okay since we handle the default values as part of the loading of the file. Let's run through some different tests to see our configuration in action:

```
go run cmd/main.go --config_file config.json
2022/03/31 14:19:44 loading configuration from file: config.json
2022/03/31 14:19:44 listening on :8079
```

Great! Now let's test our ENV var, which can be set in several ways on Unix-like systems. One way is to use the `export` variable, which is then stored in the session. The alternative way is to set the variable before the command. Here is an example:

```
PORT=8081 go run cmd/main.go --config_file config.json
2022/03/31 14:21:59 loading configuration from file: config.json
2022/03/31 14:21:59 listening on :8081
```

Notice how the ENV variable is now taking precedence over the config file. Finally, we can test the port flag:

```
PORT=8081 go run cmd/main.go --config_file config.json --port 8082
2022/03/31 14:23:36 loading configuration from file: config.json
2022/03/31 14:23:36 listening on :8082
```

All three ways of configuring our system are working. At this point, we can move on to using our configuration to change our connections to external services.

8.3.2   External client

In chapter 6, we explored dependency injection and interfaces. In that chapter, we built a static client and remote client. Here, we will decide which client to load based on whether the client URL is set in our configuration. To do this, let's again open our `cmd/main.go` file and add the code in the following listing.

Listing 8.10   `main.go`

```
func main() {

    cfg := config.LoadConfiguration()

...

    var translationService rest.Translator   ⬅──  Creates a variable that is of
                                                   the type of the interface to
                                                   pass into the handler
```

If the legacy
endpoint is
set, creates a
new client

```
translationService = translation.NewStaticService()        ◀─┐  By default, creates
if cfg.LegacyEndpoint != "" {                                 │  the static service
    log.Printf("creating external translation
    ⮕ client: %s", cfg.LegacyEndpoint)
    client := translation.NewHelloClient(cfg.LegacyEndpoint)
    translationService = translation.NewRemoteService(client)  ◀─┐
}                                                                 │
                                           Inserts that client into the
                                           creation of a remote service

translateHandler := rest.NewTranslateHandler(translationService)  ◀─┐
}                                                                   │
                                                     Injects the service
                                                       into the handler
```

You should see that we are using our interface to help load the client we want and pass it into our handler. Again, we can change the environmental variables to affect the client endpoint. Setting it will allow you to call an external service. In this case, if we pass in the URL http://hello-api.joelholmes.dev and call the endpoint, we should hopefully see it respond with a valid response.

We still have some different features to build out, such as a persistent storage backend (e.g., a database), but we'll handle them in the next chapter. We also did not incorporate the default language into our handler. I'm going to leave that up to the reader to handle.

Now we have something we can pass off to our QA folks to test while we move forward with our development. We can continuously deploy our application with minor bug fixes and changes without affecting the overall system. Testing can now occur in parallel with development, and only after we feel that everything is working as planned can we release it. But now we are facing a new potential problem. With bugs being fixed and features being developed, how can we know what version of our software we are testing or releasing? How can we communicate this to our users and team members?

8.4 Semantic versioning

To communicate with others what software version they are using, we will use two tools: versioning and a change log. Every time you update the software, you should notice that a special indicator is given about the software version being installed. The most common way of doing this is called *semantic versioning*. Figure 8.2 shows an example.

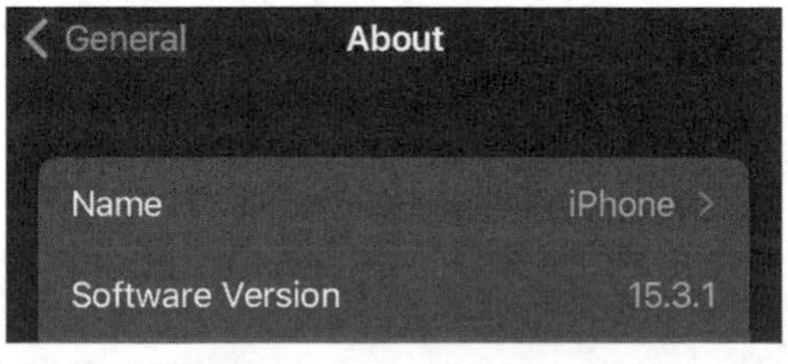

Figure 8.2   iPhone software version

Now that we are releasing a product, it is important to indicate to users which version they should be using. Often, developers like to be on the bleeding edge of releases because some new features and problems have been fixed. However, this means you are on the bleeding edge of bugs as well. Software versioning solves this problem.

These releases often look like v1.2.3, 1.2.3-e5ad2, or 1.2.3-alpha. This is to indicate some information about the stability of the software along with the compatibility of the changes. Releases with a partial hash (e5ad2 above) or a Greek letter (alpha, beta, etc.) are often known as *developer builds*, which indicate they are not quite ready for everyone to use. A released software version typically has a structure like the one shown in figure 8.3.

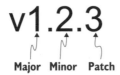

Figure 8.3 **Semantic versioning helps distinguish between large, possibly breaking, changes and minor fixes. The usage of this is up to the discretion of the team and should be communicated to consumers of products, as they may be dependent on certain features.**

As you can see, things such as "major" and "minor" changes are very subjective. The most important thing to focus on is breaking functionality. If an endpoint is removed or a method call is redefined, that is most likely a change in the major version, while a bug fix or feature may be a minor or patch fix.

Git tags are a great way of communicating these kinds of changes and a way for us to integrate them into our release strategy. We want to constantly integrate but may not be ready to always release to the public, so we add special rules to our build process if a tag is pushed versus when we push small changes. In later chapters, we will construct a deployment process that supports the latest development build and a release to our production system.

Some APIs provide what is known as an /info endpoint to help communicate the product version to the developers and the users. An /info endpoint is extremely helpful when someone is trying to see if a release was successful or where a bug may have been introduced. Let's add one to our application. In the handlers directory, create an info.go file (see the following listing).

Listing 8.11 `info.go`

```
package handlers

import (
    "encoding/json"
    "net/http"
)

var (
    tag  string
    hash string
    date string
)

func Info(w http.ResponseWriter, r *http.Request) {
    enc := json.NewEncoder(w)
    w.Header().Set("Content-Type", "application/json; charset=utf-8")
```

These are variables that will be set through the compilation process. We want these values to be linked to the binary instead of read through an environment variable because it should be associated with the binary itself.

```
    resp := map[string]string{                     ←——   Maps the values
        "tag":  tag,                                       to the response
        "hash": hash,
        "date": date,
    }
    if err := enc.Encode(resp); err != nil {
        panic("unable to encode response")
    }
}
```

Let's add this handler to the `main.go` file (see the following listing).

Listing 8.12 `main.go`

```
func main() {

    ...

    mux.HandleFunc("/health", handlers.HealthCheck)
    mux.HandleFunc("/info", handlers.Info)        ←——   Just like the health check, we need
                                                          to add this handler to our service,
    log.Printf("listening on %s\n", addr)                 but this time at the info endpoint.

    log.Fatal(http.ListenAndServe(addr, mux))
}
```

Now we need to pass values to these variables through our build command. The information we are passing is the most recent tag information, the hash, and the build date. This can help us determine the exact change that occurred based on the hash and the general time since it has been released based on the build date. To populate these fields, we need to update our build process. Open your Makefile, and edit the `build` command to add some additional flags (see the following listing).

Listing 8.13 Makefile

We use the git command to get the most recent tag version from our repo and store it as a variable.

We use the git command to get the most recent hash from our repo and store it as a variable.

```
GO_VERSION := 1.18.5
TAG := $(shell git describe --abbrev=0 --tags --always)   ←——
HASH := $(shell git rev-parse HEAD)                       ←——
```

We use the shell to grab the current timestamp of the build to help us determine how long it's been since a deployment.

```
DATE := $(shell date +%Y-%m-%d.%H:%M:%S)    ←——
LDFLAGS := -w -X github.com/holmes89/hello-api/handlers.hash=$(HASH) -
    X github.com/holmes89/hello-api/handlers.tag=$(TAG) -X github.com/
        holmes89/hello-api/handlers.date=$(DATE)    ←——
....
```

We combine all of these values into build flags that target variables in the handler package we defined so that they are embedded in the binary.

```
build:
    go build -ldflags "$(LDFLAGS)" -o api main.go    ←——
```

Adding the ldflags adds the build flags we want to the go build command.

Type make build, run your application using ./api, and call the /info endpoint by using the following:

```
curl localhost:8080/info
```

You should see the results come back with the information populated. Since we made the change to the build command in the Makefile, we don't need to make any changes to our pipeline to support this feature. What we do want to do is create a release only if our repository is tagged. Open your pipeline file again, and add a special rule to only do a release when we push a tag, as in the following listing.

Listing 8.14 pipeline.yml

```
name: CI Checks

on:
  push:
    branches:          We want to run our build
      - main           on tags as well as pushes
    tags:        <──┘  to the main branch.
      - v*
jobs:
  ...
  deliver:
    name: Release
    needs: build                                          Only run this step if
    runs-on: ubuntu-latest                                it is being tagged.
    if: github.event_name == 'push' && contains(github.ref, 'refs/tags/')  <──┘
    steps:
```

8.5   Change log

Now that we are capturing various versions, we should have a better description of the changes between the release. We can automate this process by using a tool that will look at the commit messages we make and add them to the body of the release. This is great because it forces us to remember that the messages we write will be read by others. We will enhance this in future chapters, but let's get the basics in place now. We need to edit the deliver section of our pipeline (see the following listing).

Listing 8.15 pipeline.yml

```
name: CI Checks

on:
  push:
    branches:
      - main
    tags:
      - v*

jobs:
  ...
```

```
deliver:
  name: Release
  needs: build
  runs-on: ubuntu-latest
  if: github.event_name == 'push' && contains(github.ref, 'refs/tags/')
  steps:
    - name: Checkout code
      uses: actions/checkout@v2
    - name: Download binary
      uses: actions/download-artifact@v2
      with:
        name: api
    - name: Changelog
      uses: scottbrenner/generate-changelog-action@master
      id: Changelog
    - name: Create Release
      id: create_release
      uses: actions/create-release@v1
      env:
        GITHUB_TOKEN: ${{ secrets.GITHUB_TOKEN }}
      with:
        tag_name: ${{ github.ref }}
        release_name: Release ${{ github.ref }}
        body: |
          ${{ steps.Changelog.outputs.changelog }}
        draft: false
        prerelease: false
    - name: Upload Release Binary
      uses: actions/upload-release-asset@v1
      env:
        GITHUB_TOKEN: ${{ secrets.GITHUB_TOKEN }}
      with:
        upload_url: ${{ steps.create_release.outputs.upload_url }}
        asset_path: api
        asset_name: api
        asset_content_type: application/octet-stream
```

Uses this library to automatically create a Changelog to append to the release

Adds the output of the library to the body of the release

Makes these releases official by resetting the draft to false and release to false

Commit your changes and push them. Then we will tag our release with the v0.0.1 release:

```
git add .
git commit -m "created info endpoint"
git push
git tag "v0.0.1"
git push origin v0.0.1
```

Check your releases now, and you can see v0.0.1 has been released! Download the file, and test to see if your info endpoint works. Now go to your deployment, and call the info endpoint. What do you see? Hopefully, you can see the version as well as some other information required to identify the build.

When you look at the release, there should be a description that reflects the commit messages you've been writing. This becomes another location for accountability on the part of you and your teammates. Just as comments such as "updated text"

aren't very helpful to developers, they also will not be helpful to your customers. Instead, you should consider putting a process in place of having effective comments that outline the changes you've done. A good example of this is "Corrected the spelling error on the About Page" or "Created new stub API endpoint for Issue #43" where Issue #43 refers to some internal ticketing system.

By automating this process, you help build accountability and thoughtfulness into your work. The main goal of a team is to find a way to work together and communicate effectively. Through this process, your team will gain a level of resilience and independence to help them feel empowered to solve existing problems and handle new ones that arise. This does not happen overnight but is a culture you need to help create.

8.6 *Accountability and handling failure*

Mistakes are going to happen. They happen to every person and every team. Companies will often see a mistake as a failure in process or people and will add additional constraints and extend deployment timelines to be sure there aren't any bugs or problems. Teams will be created to ensure the quality of a product before it is shipped, often leading to longer and longer lead times (deployment timelines).

But let's consider the alternative. What if we accepted a failure-tolerant culture, that mistakes are going to happen no matter what we do? How does our culture change? Who finds the problems, and who solves them? How quickly can we fix them, and how can we learn from our mistakes?

This mindset is what Kent Beck often refers to as "bravery" in his various programming books. He describes putting processes in places such as automated testing, code standardization, pair programming, and many more to allow for fast development practices that rely on "brave" developers to be able to confront problems that may arise. Toyota has a similar process where anyone on an assembly line has the opportunity to stop all production by pulling what is called the "andon cord." This simple process halts the line and triggers a light to indicate where the problem is located. Then everyone will swarm to that spot to see what the problem is, solve the problem, and learn.

This process of learning from a problem allows the organization as a whole to think about mitigating problems in the future and participating in the feedback cycle established within its culture. This is known as a *generative culture*, where the organization prioritizes improvement in capacity, quality, and innovation. How does this compare to the risk-averse culture described before? Surely everyone means well in extending timelines and adding special teams to ensure quality. If we compare the generative culture to a *bureaucratic culture*, we see small differences. Where generative organizations investigate failure, bureaucratic organizations look for who caused the problem. Generative cultures provide freedom to their employees to make and improve the company and its processes, while bureaucratic cultures restrict responsibilities and silo groups from helping each other improve.

Ron Westrum studied various organizations and created this typology model. His findings were that generative cultures can mitigate risks and increase organizational safety. In the development world, this means fewer bugs and major outages happening

in production. If a problem occurs, the organization will learn from it and find ways to make sure it doesn't happen again without restricting others' abilities to contribute. In table 10.1, you can see a breakdown of the two distinct types of company cultures.

Table 8.1   Types of company cultures

Bureaucratic	Generative
Information may be ignored.	Information is actively sought.
Messengers are tolerated.	Messengers are trained.
Responsibilities are compartmentalized.	Responsibilities are shared.
Bridging between teams is allowed but discouraged.	Bridging between teams is rewarded.
Organization is just and merciful.	Failure causes inquiry.
New ideas create problems.	New ideas are encouraged.

What does this mean for our development team?

As an organization, you need to create a generative culture for your developers that gives them the ability to move fast but learn from mistakes. Give a voice to everyone in the organization to express concerns, and try to solve problems as they arise. Do "blameless postmortem" meetings to help find the root cause and invest in improving your process. Everyone should have a voice about technical problems as well as team dynamics and improvements.

Since we are building tools and pipelines to move our code from implementation to running in production, we can use our pipeline to add more checks, guards, and analysis to our code before it goes to production. We can focus on making deployments so seamless that we can patch bugs quickly and efficiently as they happen or provide the ability to roll back our changes by reverting our code and redeploying a previous version.

The final and most important step is the visibility of problems as they occur. When a build or deployment fails, it becomes the responsibility of everyone on the team to not point fingers. This should be done through some alert system (email, Slack message, throwing a rubber chicken). The team should be able to solve the problem and resolve the build and deployment process before any additional work is done. Once the problem is resolved, work can continue. What is important is that just like at Toyota, everyone learns from the experience and thinks of ways to improve the system.

If you have the capacity on your team, having someone monitor and gather metrics about your process and system can create a great feedback mechanism for finding areas to improve. Situations like flaky tests, long build times, frequent build failures, and dependency timeouts can be the result of poorly written tests, a slow build server, a bad development environment, and the need for artifact caching. But you will not know that these problems are there or how they should be prioritized if you aren't gathering metrics and talking to your team.

As you type away in your editor, you hear the ding of your email. You stop, open it, and read the following from the QA team, "I saw you just released an update of the software that integrates with our existing API. The document says I can test this locally, and I assume it's not running in production. This is pretty great! Any chance you can start implementing something similar with a database? It would be great to start moving in that direction with the product. Thanks!"

You smile. It looks like you've convinced them you can develop hidden features without affecting your system. Time to start planning the database.

Summary

- Configuration allows you to modify an application's function without changing its code.
- Configuration combined with dependency injection can allow you to hide incomplete or untested features.
- Semantic versioning communicates the scale of changes to a system.
- Change logs provide a synopsis of the work that has been completed.
- Generative cultures allow for growth and change within an organization.

Integration testing 9

This chapter covers

- Converting user requirements to descriptive tests
- Writing tests that follow a behavior-driven design pattern
- Integrating external dependencies into tests using containers

You are sitting in the conference room with your project manager, a QA lead, an Ops lead, and the CEO. The project manager stands at the front of the room and starts the presentation.

"It's called a strangler application. The name 'strangler application' comes from the strangler fig tree, which builds itself around a host tree until the host tree dies. As sad as it sounds, we want to eventually sunset our old application. We feel our application has been tested enough to start rolling it out to a select group of customers. The new service will start out depending on the old service like it does today, but over time, we can gradually phase the old one out once we are satisfied that we haven't missed anything."

You look around the room and notice everyone nodding their heads.

"This seems to mitigate some of our risks because we can always switch back to the old service if we have any problems," the QA lead adds.

"Exactly. We have built a system for writing flexible software that can be responsive to our needs. What are the final pieces we are missing?" your project manager adds, looking around the room.

The Ops lead chimes in, "A database with all of the translations will be needed if we want to shut down the old system."

Someone from QA adds, "Additional testing around that would be helpful. Can we automate that?"

A few weeks ago, you would have never expected that, but now you have established some credibility around automated testing. Your team is buying into this new development process, and it's showing.

You walk up to the board and write

- Convert client calls to database calls.
- Migrate old data.
- Establish integration tests that meet feature requirements.

"Looks like we have a plan. Great work, everyone," the CTO says as they stand up and walk out of the room. That is your cue to get started.

9.1   *Phasing out the old*

Strangler applications are great at converting old code into new code a little bit at a time. We already started the process of creating a link between the old system and the new system when we created the external client back in chapter 6. If you remember, we call the external system if we do not have the value in a cache. Our interface looks like this:

```
type Translator interface {
    Translate(word string, language string) string
}
```

Up to this point, we've built a framework of flexibility. This allows us to slowly phase out the old application by using our configuration management along with dependency injection to change how the new system interacts with the old system. First, we need to choose a database to store our data. Once we are convinced everything is working as expected, we will remove the external client and hopefully shut the old system down.

To manage this, we will overload our configuration to have a database connection. If we see this connection, we will override the external client. We will need to add some values to our configuration (see the following listing).

Listing 9.1   `core.go`

```
type Configuration struct {
    Port            string `json:"port"`
    DefaultLanguage string `json:"default_language"`
    LegacyEndpoint  string `json:"legacy_endpoint"`
```

```
    DatabaseURL      string `json:"database_url"`
    DatabasePort     string `json:"database_port"`
}
```

Adds Database URL for connection

Adds port in case the standard port is not in use

To create all of this, we should consider how to verify that our changes are working, so we will write some integration tests that test the system as a whole. Thus far, we've mostly focused on basic unit tests and have simulated external integrations. Instead of simulating these integrations, we should also create a set of tests to verify these interactions. The most common integration point is often between an application and a database. Now we want to move our system over to connect to a database instead of calling the external client, but we want to have the flexibility to turn the client call on and off.

First, we will focus on creating a new connection that matches our existing interface. Then, based on our configuration, we will make an external service call, a database call, or a hybrid that makes an external call only if the value is not present in the database. Before we do anything, we should write some tests to validate the existing functionality, and then integrate the database and verify that it works. These tests will validate the user's experience rather than the overall functionality of a module of code, so we will take a slightly different approach than what we did before.

9.2 Behavior-driven design

In chapter 3, we talked about test-driven development (TDD), which helped us focus on how a unit of code was intended to function. This meant that we could focus on providing the proper inputs to get the expected outputs. We spent time verifying that portions of the system were called by mocking them, and it required a little bit of our technical knowledge to understand how everything should work. We can take this same format and abstract it a bit more. Imagine that your project manager, CEO, or even your customers wrote the tests and that you wrote the implementation. This is exactly what *behavior-driven design* is supposed to do. We start looking at things at a macroscopic level and then look at a larger picture of how the product or feature will be used. Instead of focusing on Arranging our tests, Acting on our function, and Asserting our values (remember the three As from chapter 3), we instead focus on a Given, When, Then structure that can be written in clearer text and tested against. The following listing provides an example that we can use for our application.

Listing 9.2 `app.feature`

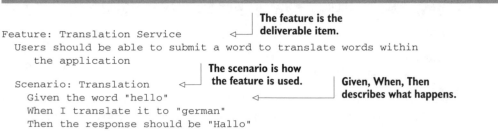

The feature is the deliverable item.

```
Feature: Translation Service
  Users should be able to submit a word to translate words within
    the application

  Scenario: Translation
    Given the word "hello"
    When I translate it to "german"
    Then the response should be "Hallo"
```

The scenario is how the feature is used.

Given, When, Then describes what happens.

This domain-specific language (DSL) is known as Gherkin and is used to allow non-technical people to write requirements that can be converted automatically into tests. Once in your testing framework, these requirements become your validation criteria or assertions in our Arrange, Act, Assert pattern. What's great about this is that you are validating against requirements that someone else wrote or that can be referred to as part of your development process. No longer can a project manager say you didn't meet the requirements if they wrote the descriptions and all of the tests passed!

> **NOTE**   We are focused on running our BDD tests using a Go runner; however, you can write more comprehensive integration suites using Selenium or Cypress.

What is special about the Gherkin language is that multiple libraries can use it. Each one of these features can be tied to specific unit tests or used to test user interfaces. The point is that our project managers can start writing code for us in this special language, and we can then use it to verify that a feature is complete through multiple means. For example, let's assume we are creating a UI with our API. We can use this same feature file to write our Go backend tests, JavaScript UI tests, and automated QA end-to-end tests. As long as the feature is there but the tests are not implemented, our build will fail. This is intentional because the requirements of our system have changed.

Taking this feature request, we can plug it into our testing pipeline; however, we will not test individual packages but instead test the `main` package, which runs the whole application. At a high level, we can verify that we meet the expectations of our users. We will use this feature definition to drive our tests. To do this, we will use a library called Godog, which falls under the Cucumber project, the top open-source project for BDD. Cucumber has written other libraries for other languages that support Gherkin as well.

9.3   *Writing BDD tests in Go*

To start, we will set up our BDD testing by writing our feature definitions and tests. We will set up our tests and write them, but the expectation is that they will fail. Once they are written, we will work on fixing them by attaching our database. By the end of the chapter, we will be able to verify that our services work entirely as expected.

The first thing we need to do is install a new tool called Godog. To do this, let's first add an entry to our Makefile (see the following listing).

> **Listing 9.3   Makefile**

```
setup: install-go init-go install-lint install-godog
...
install-godog:
    go install github.com/cucumber/godog/cmd/godog@latest    ⟵── Installs the
                                                                  Godog binary
```

Next, run the installation to verify that it works. We should be able to copy our feature to a directory to test. Godog has many different ways to run tests, but for now, we will

rely on the default behavior, which is to look for feature files in a local directory called features. Since we will test the API binary, we will create that directory in the cmd directory.

Once you've created the cmd/features directory and copied over our app .feature, we can navigate to the cmd directory and type godog run. You should see a snippet of generated code like in the following listing.

Listing 9.4 `console`

```
func iTranslateItTo(arg1 string) error {          ◁─┐ Our text is converted into
        return godog.ErrPending                        functions with similar names
}                                                       capturing particular input.

func theResponseShouldBe(arg1 string) error {
        return godog.ErrPending                   ◁─┐ Until implemented, we can
}                                                      use this special error type.

func theWord(arg1 string) error {
        return godog.ErrPending
}
                                                      ┌ Tests enter here to set up
func InitializeScenario(ctx *godog.ScenarioContext) {  ◁─┘ and run each scenario step.
        ctx.Step(`^I translate it to "([^"]*)"$`, iTranslateItTo)      ◁─┐
        ctx.Step(`^the response should be "([^"]*)"$`, theResponseShouldBe)  │
        ctx.Step(`^the word "([^"]*)"$`, theWord)                         │
}                                                      Each step has a special capture
                                                       group that provides input to
                                                       the appropriate function.
```

Obviously, this code is incomplete but gives us a basis to start. Copy the text, and create a new file called main_test.go in that directory. We will also create a struct to help capture some of the input we need for our tests. The code will look like the following listing.

Listing 9.5 `main_test.go`

```
package main        ◁─┐ We use the main package so that
                         we can reference the methods
import (                 inside to start the application.   ┌ Use the Godog library
    "github.com/cucumber/godog"               ◁─┘           to help set up the tests.
)
                                 ┌ This struct will help store
type apiFeature struct {}   ◁─┘ information throughout the tests.

func (api *apiFeature) iTranslateItTo(arg1 string) error {
    return godog.ErrPending
}

func (api *apiFeature) theResponseShouldBe(arg1 string) error {
    return godog.ErrPending
}
```

```go
func (api *apiFeature) theWord(arg1 string) error {
    return godog.ErrPending
}

func InitializeScenario(ctx *godog.ScenarioContext) {
    api := &apiFeature{}

    ctx.Step(`^I translate it to "([^"]*)"$`, api.iTranslateItTo)
    ctx.Step(`^the response should be "([^"]*)"$`, api.theResponseShouldBe)
    ctx.Step(`^the word "([^"]*)"$`, api.theWord)
}
```

> Functions are now within the context of our feature struct.

Our test is set up, but we are unable to access and run our main function, so we want to create the ability to start a server the same way main() does. This is typically done by creating a function that houses the logic of the application creation and having the main function call it. We will refactor our main.go file to match this pattern (see the following listing).

Listing 9.6 main.go

```go
package main

import (
    "log"
    "net/http"

    "github.com/holmes89/hello-api/config"
    "github.com/holmes89/hello-api/handlers"
    "github.com/holmes89/hello-api/handlers/rest"
    "github.com/holmes89/hello-api/translation"
)

func main() {

    cfg := config.LoadConfiguration()
    addr := cfg.Port

    mux := API(cfg)

    log.Printf("listening on %s\n", addr)

    log.Fatal(http.ListenAndServe(addr, mux))
}

func API(cfg config.Configuration) *http.ServeMux {

    mux := http.NewServeMux()

    var translationService rest.Translator
    translationService = translation.NewStaticService()
    if cfg.LegacyEndpoint != "" {
        log.Printf("creating external translation client: %s",
    cfg.LegacyEndpoint)
```

> The main function just runs the server now instead of configuring the service's HTTP and service endpoints.

> This function will assemble the service and HTTP endpoints to be passed to the server.

```
        client := translation.NewHelloClient(cfg.LegacyEndpoint)
        translationService = translation.NewRemoteService(client)
    }

    translateHandler := rest.NewTranslateHandler(translationService)

    mux.HandleFunc("/translate/hello", translateHandler.TranslateHandler)
    mux.HandleFunc("/health", handlers.HealthCheck)

    return mux
}
```
← **The mux router is returned to be attached to an HTTP server.**

You should be able to start your application and have it still work. Now we can wire our Godog tests. To verify our results, we will call our API and parse the results. While Go has the capability of calling HTTP endpoints, we'll use a library to help us make the code a little easier to read. To do this, install `go get github.com/go-resty/resty/v2`. Resty helps make writing API calls a little clearer. For example, if we wanted to call our API using Resty, it would look something like the following listing.

Listing 9.7 Resty example

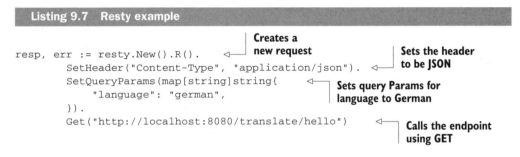

```
resp, err := resty.New().R().
        SetHeader("Content-Type", "application/json").
        SetQueryParams(map[string]string{
            "language": "german",
        }).
        Get("http://localhost:8080/translate/hello")
```

Creates a new request
Sets the header to be JSON
Sets query Params for language to German
Calls the endpoint using GET

We need the input for this call in order to verify our tests. Remember earlier when we looked at the methods Godog generated for us? They have string inputs that we can set in a feature test structure. Let's add the code in the following listing to our struct.

Listing 9.8 main_test.go

```
type apiFeature struct {
    client   *resty.Client
    server   *httptest.Server
    word     string
    language string
}
```

Shared client for tests
Creates a test server to avoid port conflicts
The word being used
The language being translated to

Now we can store the values in the various steps (see the following listing).

Listing 9.9 main_test.go

```
func (api *apiFeature) iTranslateItTo(arg1 string) error {
    api.language = arg1
    return nil
}
```

Saves the values to the struct

```
func (api *apiFeature) theWord(arg1 string) error {
    api.word = arg1
    return nil
}
```

Let's initialize our feature struct using the code in the following listing to have a server start up and shut down for each scenario.

Listing 9.10   `main_test.go`

```
func InitializeScenario(ctx *godog.ScenarioContext) {

    client := resty.New()          Creates a shared client
    api := &apiFeature{            Creates a new feature
        client: client,            struct for sharing
    }

    ctx.Before(func(ctx context.Context, sc *godog.Scenario)
      (context.Context, error) {          Uses before and after hooks
        cfg := config.Configuration{}     to manage the server
        cfg.LoadFromEnv()

        mux := API(cfg)                            Creates the same mux
        server := httptest.NewServer(mux)          as the main function

        api.server = server
        return ctx, nil
    })

    ctx.After(func(ctx context.Context, sc *godog.Scenario, err error)
      (context.Context, error) {
        api.server.Close()          Closes the server
        return ctx, nil             after the scenario
    })

    ctx.Step(`^I translate it to "([^"]*)"$`, api.iTranslateItTo)
    ctx.Step(`^the response should be "([^"]*)"$`, api.theResponseShouldBe)
    ctx.Step(`^the word "([^"]*)"$`, api.theWord)
}
```

Loads the config from Env (could also use default) — points to `cfg.LoadFromEnv()`

Creates the test server — points to `mux := API(cfg)` and `server := httptest.NewServer(mux)`

Finally, we can test the call. We will do this in the `theResponseShouldBe` function. In it, we assemble the API call and verify the results as in the following listing.

Listing 9.11   `main_test.go`

```
func (api *apiFeature) theResponseShouldBe(arg1 string) error {
    url := fmt.Sprintf("%s/translate/%s", api.server.URL, api.word)

    resp, err := api.client.R().                         Creates the URL to call
        SetHeader("Content-Type", "application/json").   based on the word
        SetQueryParams(map[string]string{
            "language": api.language,          Sets the language
        }).                                    to translate
```

```
        SetResult(&rest.Resp{}).    ◁──┐  Captures the result
        Get(url)                        │  in a known struct

    if err != nil {
        return err
    }

    res := resp.Result().(*rest.Resp)       ┌─  Verifies
    if res.Translation != arg1 {         ◁──┘   the word
        return fmt.Errorf("translation should be set to %s", arg1)
    }

    return nil
}
```

And there we have it! Type godog run again, and see what the results are. Now create another scenario for another language if you want! Does it work? Next, let's add our requirements for the database.

9.4 Adding a database

To start, we'll add a new requirement that requires us to move outside of our static data set and instead uses an external database. This same set of tests could have been used for connecting to our external service. Imagine for a minute that the QA team is writing all of these requirements against the old system originally. Then you move them to the new project as you start your strangler application. You will know when you've reached a level of parity when all of the tests pass. Once we've flipped a configuration to use the database, we can once again verify that everything is ready to be deployed (see the following listing).

Listing 9.12 `app.feature`

```
Feature: Translation Service
  Users should be able to submit a word to translate words within the applica
      tion

  Scenario: Translation
    Given the word "hello"
    When I translate it to "german"
    Then the response should be "Hallo"

  Scenario: Translation
    Given the word "hello"
    When I translate it to "bulgarian"
    Then the response should be "?????????"
```

If we run our tests now, we should see a failure. Think back to chapter 3 and remember our fail, pass, fail pattern. This means our project manager or someone else can monitor our progress on a feature as we develop it. Reports can be generated to show the coverage and progress toward completing all scenarios within a given feature and can be dubbed *feature complete*.

It's also extremely important to note that this set of app features can be tested on both a backend API and a frontend screen. The completeness of a feature can be verified by a series of integration tests, not just a single one!

As for our feature, we can imagine a larger collection of translations that we need to verify. Our current solution of keeping all our translations in a switch statement in code is not scalable, nor does it allow us to add or remove languages without restarting the service, so we will add a database to our system. Databases are specialized data storage applications that do a much better job of managing and handling our various pieces of data. We will then test the integration between our service and the external dependency, which in this case is a database.

There are many database options, but we will use the extremely simple (yet powerful) key-value store called Redis, which is very lightweight and will work very similarly to the caching mechanism we implemented earlier. We'll break down this work into development and then testing. We need to have a way to establish a connection before we can set up our tests. Remember, all we need is a service that implements our `Translator` interface, and we can drop it right into our existing handler.

First, let's add Redis to our infrastructure. Remember in chapter 7 when we introduced `docker-compose` to help us build our containers? We will use the same technology to manage our dependencies. Let's add Redis as a dependency to our `docker-compose.yml` file, as in the following listing.

Listing 9.13   `docker-compose.yml`

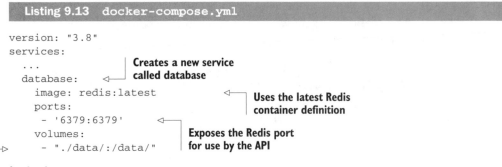

```
version: "3.8"
services:
  ...
  database:          Creates a new service
    image: redis:latest          called database
    ports:                       Uses the latest Redis
      - '6379:6379'              container definition
    volumes:
      - "./data/:/data/"         Exposes the Redis port
                                 for use by the API
```
Mounts the database
backup for testing use

If you run `docker-compose up -d database` and then type `docker exec -it database redis-cli`, you should see a prompt appear. If you type `ping`, you should get a `pong` response. Congratulations! You've just started a database!

Let's create a connection. We already updated our configuration to handle the connection string to the database. Now we'll create a new file in the `translation` package. We'll call it `database.go`. The first thing we do is create a function that returns a connection struct. We'll use this struct to implement the `Translator` interface. We'll create just enough code to be able to start writing our tests. Let's write the code in the following listing.

Listing 9.14   database.go

```go
package translation

import (
    "context"
    "fmt"

    "github.com/go-redis/redis/v9"
    "github.com/holmes89/hello-api/config"
    "github.com/holmes89/hello-api/handlers/rest"
)

var _ rest.Translator = &Database{}

type Database struct {
    conn *redis.Client
}

func NewDatabaseService(cfg config.Configuration) *Database {
    rdb := redis.NewClient(&redis.Options{
        Addr:     fmt.Sprintf("%s:%s", cfg.DatabaseURL, cfg.DatabasePort),
        Password: "", // no password set
        DB:       0,  // use default DB
    })
    return &Database{
        conn: rdb,
    }
}

func (s *Database) Close() error {
    return s.conn.Close()
}

func (s *Database) Translate(word string, language string) string {
    return ""
}
```

This is a type verification so that we know our service satisfies the interface.

Returns a new connection struct using database configuration

A close function is needed to clean up a connection.

Just do the minimal amount of work to get started.

Now we can create our integration tests. Thanks to our operations team, we were able to get a backup of the production database, so as part of our tests, we will load the backed-up database into a Docker container and run our service against it. This will simulate, as closely as possible, a production environment to test. Let's create the setup for our suite (see the following listing).

Listing 9.15   main_test.go

```go
var (
    pool     *dockertest.Pool
    database *dockertest.Resource
)

func InitializeTestSuite(sc *godog.TestSuiteContext) {

    var err error
```

This will run before each suite, which differs from the setup that runs on each scenario.

```
                sc.BeforeSuite(func() {
  Creates a   ┌─▷  pool, err = dockertest.NewPool("")
  new docker  │    if err != nil {
  connection  │        panic(fmt.Sprintf("unable to create connection pool %s", err))
  pool        │    }

                     wd, err := os.Getwd()
                     if err != nil {
                         panic(fmt.Sprintf("unable to get working directory %s", err))
  Mounts the  │    }
  database    │
  backup      └─▷  mount := fmt.Sprintf("%s/data/:/data/", filepath.Dir(wd))

                     redis, err := pool.RunWithOptions(&dockertest.RunOptions{     ◁─────────┐
                         Repository: "redis",                                                │
                         Mounts:        []string{mount},                      Runs the docker
                     })                                                          container    │
                     if err != nil {
                         panic(fmt.Sprintf("unable to create container: %s", err))
                     }
                     if err := redis.Expire(600); err != nil {
                         panic("unable to set expiration on container")
                     } //Destroy container if it takes too long
                     database = redis
                })

                sc.AfterSuite(func() {         ┌ Shuts down the
                     database.Close()          │ container when finished
                })                        ◁────┘
           }
```

Now we need to update our scenario setup as well (see the following listing).

Listing 9.16   main_test.go

```
func InitializeScenario(ctx *godog.ScenarioContext) {

...
     ctx.Before(func(ctx context.Context, sc *godog.Scenario)
       (context.Context, error) {
           cfg := config.Configuration{}
           cfg.LoadFromEnv()
 The Docker library │                                        ┌ Sets the database to connect
 randomly creates a │      cfg.DatabaseURL = "localhost"   ◁─┘ to Docker on your machine
 port to connect to.└─▷    cfg.DatabasePort = database.Port("6379")

           mux := API(cfg)
           server := httptest.NewServer(mux)

           api.server = server
           return ctx, nil
     })
...
}
```

Finally, we edit our main file to use the new URL from the database we just started (see the following code listing).

Listing 9.17 main.go

```go
if cfg.DatabaseURL != "" {
        db := translation.NewDatabaseService(cfg)     ◁─┐  If the database is set, we use
        translationService = db                          │  this as our service through
    }                                                     │  dependency injection.
```

Now we can run our tests and see them fail. Great! Let's update our implementation code to retrieve files. According to the documentation, the translated values are stored in a format of language:word, where all word variables are in English, so our logic becomes fairly simple, as in the following listing.

Listing 9.18 database.go

```go
func (s *Database) Translate(word string, language string) string {
    out := s.conn.Get(context.Background(), fmt.Sprintf("%s:%s",
    word, language))
    return out.Val()   ◁─┐ Returns the        ◁─┐ Queries the database by
}                         │ string value          │ constructing the key from
                                                   │ the word and language
```

Run our tests again, and you should see them pass!

> **NOTE** Hopefully, some of you were wondering why we didn't create tests specifically to test the database instead of relying on the integration tests. This is because it was out of the scope for this chapter, but it is a great exercise. You can use the same database setup as earlier or look into some other in-memory database testing solutions.

Can you think of other tests that could be added? Or other features that we perhaps didn't cover?

9.5 Releasing

Let's look at our testing pyramid (figure 9.1).

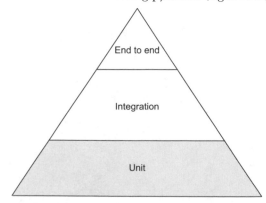

Figure 9.1 End-to-end tests are smaller at the top because they are more expensive and not as dependable. They should be supported by larger suites of integration and unit tests. Each layer should run on its own, starting with unit tests and progressing up the pyramid in different phases.

We have covered all tiers of the pyramid, starting with our unit tests from chapter 3, our acceptance tests from chapter 6, and now our integration tests from this chapter. Does this mean we're done? No, not even close. This is when you and your team need to start monitoring how much coverage you have and how long these tests take. Ideally, you don't want your test suites to run more than 5–10 minutes for them to be effective. Integration tests can be separated into various groups for speed. For example, a subset of tests can run against the core features, while a longer suite could be used for all regressions (old problems). This group of tests is often referred to as *functional testing*, or tests that verify the specifications of the application. Table 9.1 gives a brief overview of these different types.

Table 9.1   Types of functional tests

Type	Description	Answers the question
Smoke test	Preliminary test to check for basic functionality	Does it turn on?
Sanity test	Validates high-level calculations such as aggregations or mathematical calculations	Is the count of items correct?
Regression test	Verifies that previously reported bugs have been addressed	Did this used to work?
Usability test	Evaluates customer interactions with the product	How do people use this feature?

When would it be appropriate to run these tests in our chain? In the previous chapter, we discussed releases: we want to release only when our code is stable, so we want to use these tests as a way of knowing that everything is stable to release. In theory, all of our unit tests and acceptance tests should support our integration tests, so there shouldn't be any surprises when we tag or release. Yet we want one final guard against releasing broken code, so we will add an integration testing phase in our build (see the following code listing) that will happen only after a release has been made but before it is pushed to production.

Listing 9.19   `ci.yaml`

```
smoke-test:
      name: Smoke Test Application
      needs:
      - test
      runs-on: ubuntu-latest
      steps:
      - name: Set up Go 1.x
      uses: actions/setup-go@v2
      with:
          go-version: ^1.18
      - name: Check out code into the Go module directory
```

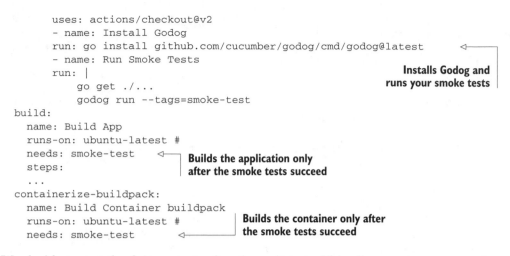

```
      uses: actions/checkout@v2
      - name: Install Godog
      run: go install github.com/cucumber/godog/cmd/godog@latest
      - name: Run Smoke Tests
      run: |
          go get ./...
          godog run --tags=smoke-test
build:
  name: Build App
  runs-on: ubuntu-latest #
  needs: smoke-test
  steps:
  ...
containerize-buildpack:
  name: Build Container buildpack
  runs-on: ubuntu-latest #
  needs: smoke-test
```

Installs Godog and runs your smoke tests

Builds the application only after the smoke tests succeed

Builds the container only after the smoke tests succeed

We decide to put the feature tests after the unit tests. This allows us to move up the testing tree before we start to build. The way we constructed our integration tests means we can get insight if our system works when it starts up. In the days of hand-soldered circuit boards, this was known as a *smoke test* because if it smoked when it was plugged in, there was a problem. Today's smoke tests verify that a system starts and has basic functionality. Therefore, our integration tests can be our smoke tests as well.

Often, labels are given to certain tests to denote if they are part of a smoke test or a larger *regression test* suite. These can correspond to the functional testing types. We can possibly run additional checks after our smoke tests run. A smoke test failure will stop the pipeline, but a regression suite may be a flag for someone to verify that something has changed. This becomes an automated QA system that can allow QA members to spend most of their time exploring the system to find additional bugs. In the next listing, let's adjust our scenarios to use labels and update one last flag to our CI for smoke tests.

Listing 9.20 `api.feature`

```
Feature: Translate API
  Users should be able to submit a word to translate

  @smoke-test
  Scenario: Translation
    Given the word "hello"
    When I translate it to "german"
    Then the response should be "Hallo"
  @smoke-test
  Scenario: Translation unknown
    Given the word "goodbye"
    When I translate it to "german"
    Then the response should be ""
  @smoke-test
  Scenario: Translation Bulgarian
    Given the word "hello"
    When I translate it to "bulgarian"
    Then the response should be "?????????"
```

```
@regression-test
Scenario: Translation Czech
  Given the word "hello"
  When I translate it to "Czech"
  Then the response should be "Ahoj"
```

A separate test type to be run

Edit our CI to run only the smoke tests first and then a second step to test regressions (see the following listing).

Listing 9.21 ci.yaml

```
smoke-test:
...
    run: |
        go get ./...
        godog run --tags=smoke-test
regression-test:
    name: Regression Test Application
    needs:
    - test
    runs-on: ubuntu-latest
    steps:
    - name: Set up Go 1.x
    uses: actions/setup-go@v2
    with:
        go-version: ^1.18
    - name: Check out code into the Go module directory
    uses: actions/checkout@v2
    - name: Install Godog
    run: go install github.com/cucumber/godog/cmd/godog@latest
    - name: Run Smoke Tests
    run: |
        go get ./...
        godog run --tags=regression-test
```

Establishes a longer or more comprehensive test suite to run periodically

Specifies the regression suite

As you see your pipeline turn green, the QA manager walks by. Now is a great time to show them what you've been able to accomplish. You show the different feature tests and explain how we can take all of the requirements they want and put them in the various test suites. Upon seeing the green scenarios, they smile, the first time you've seen them do so.

Summary

- Using behavior-driven development helps the whole team establish requirements.
- Gherkin provides a universal language to write behavior-driven tests that can be implemented by different teams.
- External dependencies for integration tests can be provided by using containers to replicate real-world services.
- Tags can be used to help focus test suites and shorten the overall runtime of tests.

Advanced deployment 10

This chapter covers

- Creating a Kubernetes cluster
- Deploying an API in Kubernetes
- Deploying a database using Helm
- Configuring your API to use the database

"If you look at these charts, you can see that our new service has actually helped drive more traffic to our services. Our mobile application team was able to whip together a quick application using some of the same techniques adopted for the translation service. This application has had wide adoption and is trending in all app stores. However, since the translation service is still running as an on-demand service, we find that it is more expensive than running dedicated servers, so we are left with two options: use a dedicated container orchestrator like Kubernetes or build dedicated virtual machines to run the service."

Everyone looks at the graphs the DevOps lead is showing. There are some nods of an agreement, but the CTO finally speaks up.

"I thought the whole point was to move away from dedicated services and toward a 'serverless' approach. Won't this reduce our delivery to market? Are there alternatives?"

The DevOps lead advances the slide and says, "We have a longer-term goal of moving toward a container orchestration framework like Kubernetes. This is because we may not get 100% utilization out of a dedicated virtual machine to handle more applications on the same level or resources. We are working with various teams to start implementing container creation for their products so that we can host all of them on a Kubernetes, or K8S, cluster. However, none of us have worked with Kubernetes before, so there could be a bit of a learning curve. The alternative is to create custom images and deploy them to virtual machines. We call this the *classic deployment* process. It is error-prone right now because we have little process around it. However, we've learned from this process that having as much as possible in the repository helps with productivity overall, so we will adopt 'infrastructure as code' on some of our older services to help us maintain our infrastructure more clearly. Unfortunately, we don't have anyone with experience in this area and are swamped, so we may rely a bit on the development team to get things started. Would that be okay?"

You smile and nod. The fact that these initiatives and ideologies are now starting to spread to other teams shows tremendous improvement overall by the company. Working on a more robust deployment process for the entire company can seem a little daunting, but it will be well worth the value.

"In an attempt to not seem too trendy, I think it's worthwhile to do a research spike on both. Do you think you can get me some estimates of the level of work for the Kubernetes cluster first? If we can move the entire company in that direction, I think it will make sense for us financially, but we need to make sure it won't monopolize developer time. We can then experiment with the infrastructure as code at a later date."

10.1   *Not quite IaaS*

We have come to a crossroads in our deployment progression. Remember that we are treating various abstractions with our deployments and using them as a service. In previous infrastructure chapters, we explored using a function as a service (FaaS), wherein a small, lightweight, on-demand application runs only when requested. We then moved to a platform as a service (PaaS), wherein we simply hand over our binary, and a server is magically created around it. Our last deployment used containers as a service (CaaS), wherein a container is built and run, giving us exposure to an underlying virtualized environment for more system-level integrations.

At this point, if you find that we need fewer abstractions and even more control, we can go one of two different ways. One is to go on a full Infrastructure as a Service (IaaS) route by building and running our physical infrastructure using virtual machines and load balancers to direct traffic to our application. The other way is to set up, run, and manage a container orchestration tool such as Kubernetes. In this chapter, we choose the latter because it is trendy due to its varied development toolset and developer-friendly interfaces. Appendix D briefly outlines the alternative for those who may want to take the true IaaS route. Instead, we are going to be in the middle of the IaaS and CaaS stacks shown in figure 10.1.

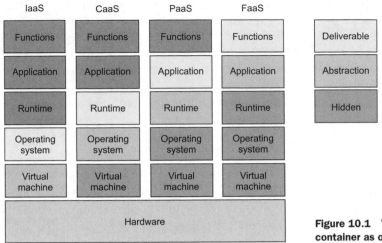

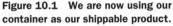

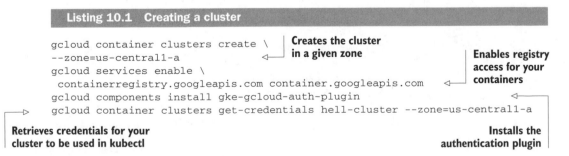

Figure 10.1   **We are now using our container as our shippable product.**

Kubernetes is not quite IaaS. It lives somewhere between the CaaS and IaaS realms. This is because Kubernetes handles much of the underlying infrastructure through abstractions. Features like node scaling and load balancing are all created and maintained by the Kubernetes cluster. As the developer, you are only concerned with defining the types of resources you want and submitting them to the cluster to then run. This building of resources in an abstract way is the core of IaaS. Tools like Terraform are used to maintain and build actual infrastructure, just like Kubernetes.

Instead of servers and load balancers, Kubernetes works with deployments and services. These abstractions allow Kubernetes to shift workloads across different server instances based on the load on the server. Kubernetes reduces a lot of the maintenance and management around your applications because it handles tasks such as load balancing, service restarts, and so on. Because of this, Kubernetes has become a very popular option for many teams that have scaled from on-demand to dedicated services for optimal uptime.

10.2   *Your first cluster*

We need to first create a cluster (see the following listing). Instead of installing Kubernetes locally, we will rely on GCP to create one for us. To do this, we will use the GCP tool.

> **NOTE**   If you don't want to go through the hassle of setting up a cluster in the cloud, there are plenty of local tools, such as Minikube and KinD.

And you should have access to your nodes. That's it. Google makes it very simple for you. If you wish to use another cloud provider, there may be additional steps. Now you are ready to deploy.

For a full list of regions and zones that are closer to where you live, visit http://mng.bz/91Ro.

10.3   *Building blocks*

You can find countless books, talks, and blog posts about Kubernetes and all of its building blocks, so I will not go into it here. We need to worry about two things: deployments and services. *Deployments* run a container or group of containers (*pods*) that scale (replica sets), which is exactly what GCP's Cloud Run did for us in chapter 7. A *service* creates an endpoint that directs calls to our deployment. This essentially acts as a load balancer that can distribute calls equally among multiple server instances.

Let me explain each of these two core elements in more detail. A deployment can be thought of as a wrapper around two lower entity definitions for Kubernetes. Pods are groups of containers (a play on the Docker Whale; a group of whales is a pod). If you want more than one copy of your pod to run, wrap it in a *replica set*, which runs multiple instances of your pod. Finally, a deployment wraps the scaling in health checks and definitions to call the pod.

A service acts like a router to your application. It can be as simple as a forwarding port to your underlying application, similar to a DNS lookup that a browser does when loading a website or as complicated as a load balancer with specific rules for how to route calls for A/B testing or feature testing.

Both of these definitions lack a lot of detail, which should suffice for what we are trying to accomplish. However, I encourage you to look at Marko Luksa's *Kubernetes in Action* (Manning, 2017) for more details.

Let's start by creating our deployment. First, we need to create a new directory called k8s in your root directory and a directory beneath it for the service called hello-api. Here, we will create a new file called deployment.yml. In it, we need to write our deployment definition. The key is to have one instance of our container running. Luckily, we have a container image uploaded that we can use. The code in the following listing shows the deployment definition, which will be /k8s/hello-api/deployment.yml.

Listing 10.2   `deployment.yml`

```
apiVersion: apps/v1            The type of Kubernetes
kind: Deployment         ◁──   object we are creating
metadata:
  name: hello-api         ◁──────────────   The name of the
spec:                                        deployment
```

```
    replicas:         ◁──  The number of
    selector:               pods to run
      matchLabels:
          app: hello-api
    template:
      metadata:
        labels:
          app: hello-api
      spec:
        containers:
        - name: hello-api
          imagePullPolicy: Always
          image: gcr.io/PROJECT_NAME/hello-api:latest
          ports:
          - containerPort: 8080    ◁──  This port matches what the
            name: hello-api-svc          container is listening on.
```

How to reach this application ⟶ (points to `name: hello-api-svc`)

Now we apply our deployment using `kubectl`. If it is not installed, you can do so by following the instructions on https://kubernetes.io/docs/tasks/tools/. Once installed, you simply need to run `kubectl apply -f k8s`, and all files in that directory will be applied. If we type `kubectl get pods`, we should now see our running API pod.

Now let's set up the service in `/k8s/hello-api/service.yml`. Our service is very simple, as it just needs to open a port to point to our deployment, as shown in the following listing.

Listing 10.3 `service.yml`

```
apiVersion: v1
kind: Service
metadata:              ◁──  The Service type will route incoming
  name: hello-api            requests to deployments.
spec:
  selector:
    app: hello-api           The Load Balancer will utilize
  type: LoadBalancer    ◁──  underlying cloud infrastructure to
  ports:                     route messages to your deployment.
  - port: 80
    protocol: TCP            Maps to the port the
    targetPort: 8080    ◁──  deployment depends on
```

Now we can call `apply` and see our service show up. We can test it by calling the endpoint provided at `kubectl describe service hello-api`.

10.4 Scaling and health status

A service critical to any system should have some sort of redundancy. In software, you want your customers to avoid any downtime and be able to meet the demands that people are asking on your system. This is known as *scaling*: the system can grow to meet the demands put upon it by distributing the requests among several running services. In doing so, you reduce the chances of a system running out of memory or having long responses. There are two types of scaling: vertical and horizontal. *Vertical*

scaling allows you to add more power to a machine to handle the increased load. *Horizontal scaling* allows you to create additional instances of servers to handle the load. In this section, we will focus on scaling horizontally for our deployments.

We haven't had to worry too much about scaling up to this point because the system we are deploying the application on has handled all of our scaling. If you were to make 1 million requests against our FaaS, PaaS, or CaaS services we put up, you would see that they have multiple running instances to handle the load. Meanwhile, our Kubernetes deployment would not be able to scale at this point because we haven't given it the proper settings to do so. We will only focus on manual scaling and health checks here, but books like *Kubernetes in Action* can show you other methods.

Again, we do not want outage time, so we need to allow Kubernetes to know when a deployment is ready so that it can shut down the old deployment. This is known as a *rolling deployment*. To do this, we tap into the health check endpoints we added in chapter 4. Here, we will add liveness (Is the service running?) and readiness (Is it ready to receive requests?) checks. Both will let Kubernetes know that our pod is ready. To do this, we need to modify our deployment file by adding the code in the following listing.

Listing 10.4   deployment.yml

```yaml
apiVersion: apps/v1
kind: Deployment
metadata:
  name: hello-api
spec:
  replicas: 1
  selector:
    matchLabels:
        app: hello-api
  template:
    metadata:
      labels:
        app: hello-api
    spec:
      containers:
      - name: hello-api
        imagePullPolicy: Always
        image: gcr.io/PROJECT_NAME/hello-api:latest
        ports:
        - containerPort: 8080
          name: hello-api-svc
        livenessProbe:
          httpGet:
            path: /health          ⟵  This call will check every
            port: 8080                  3 seconds to see if it is
          initialDelaySeconds: 3        returning a 200 response.
          periodSeconds: 3
        readinessProbe:
          httpGet:
            path: /health
            port: 8080
```

```
        initialDelaySeconds: 3
        periodSeconds: 3
```

The liveness probe will check to see if the container is up and running, while the readiness probe will start directing traffic to the pod. In this instance, we will use the health endpoint. Here, we determine if the system is ready by checking if the HTTP server responds. If not, the pod will be shut down and a new one will start in its place.

In this instance, our liveness probe and readiness probe are the same. This, however, is not always the case. Let's say, for example, that you had two processes running in your pod, an API and a cache. Caches can sometimes be *warmed* or preloaded with data. In this case, the liveness probe would be healthy, but the pod would only be ready to accept messages after the cache was warmed. Think of it as starting your car versus putting it into gear. If either of the checks takes longer than expected, the pod will be deleted and a new one created to start the process over.

With the liveness and readiness probes in place, we can now scale the service by adding replicas. To do this, we just need to edit one line, as shown in the following listing.

Listing 10.5   `deployment.yml`

```
apiVersion: apps/v1
kind: Deployment
metadata:
  name: hello-api
spec:
  replicas: 3          ⬅──┐  Increases the number
  selector:               │  of instances to 3
    matchLabels:
        app: hello-api
  template:
    metadata:
      labels:
        app: hello-api
    spec:
      containers:
      - name: hello-api
        imagePullPolicy: Always
        image: gcr.io/PROJECT_NAME/hello-api:latest
        ports:
...
```

This will create three separate pods for this service. Commit these changes. We will be able to see how all this works after we create automatic deployments. But at the moment, Kubernetes gives us the control to add and remove advanced deployment practices with a few lines of code. In the past, this configuration would have been difficult to maintain and monitor because you would have been dealing with physical machines, load balancers, and monitoring tools. Instead, Kubernetes provides all of this for you so that you can get started on deploying. Because it is all code, it becomes much easier for us to update our deployments.

10.5 *Automatically deploying*

In the past, we deployed our code when we merged to main. This gave our customers the bleeding edge of our development each time we merged our pull requests. However, in chapter 8, we introduced the concept of tags, which allow us to mark a deployment as stable. With this stability, we can easily track what code has been deployed and what fixes and features we can target for future releases. Once this cadence is established, we can easily estimate the time it takes to deliver new releases to our customers.

All of this is to say is that tagging your products and codebases is extremely important. It also meshes well with our containerized releases because containers also use release tags. Our deployment code has a reference to a `latest` tag, which loosely translates to "I don't care what version it is; I want the newest." We feel like we have moved past this point (maybe this would be a good setup for a development environment!) and now want to tag, so we should create a container build process that pushes a new tagged version of our container when our code is tagged. We will use the same tagging strategy we discussed in chapter 8, but this will also be based on what your team decides. Let's modify our code to do that, as in the following listing.

Listing 10.6 `pipeline`

```
containerize-buildpack:
    name: Build Container buildpack
    runs-on: ubuntu-latest #
    needs: smoke-test
    if: github.event_name == 'push' && contains(github.ref, 'refs/tags/')
    steps:
  ...
```

Let's try it out:

```
git tag v0.0.1
git push origin v0.0.1
```

You should see a new container tagged and pushed to GCP. Now that we can tag our containers, we need to have a process of updating our deployment. There are two rules of thought with managing these types of deployments: automated or retroactive. In the automated world, you create a process that runs `apply` whenever a file is changed in the K8s directory. This means that you change the code, and the pipeline keeps track of the cluster credentials and state. This is a great place to get to, but until those processes are clearly defined and working efficiently, many will update their repo with the applied changes retroactively. This is typically done by putting a PR up with the changes and waiting for approval. Once it's approved, you apply the code and then merge.

We now have a CD process in place using Kubernetes. We aren't running our production-level system. To do that, we need our database and configuration.

10.6   Deploying Redis using Helm

Many platforms like Kubernetes that use infrastructure as code allow additional tools and abstractions to extend it or be built on top of it. In this case, Kubernetes works well with a tool called Helm. Helm is like a package manager but for your Kubernetes cluster. It will use a similar deployment mechanism known as a Helm Chart to deploy applications. Helm charts are used mostly for out-of-the-box functionality in production but can be tweaked to suit your needs.

In this instance, we will use Helm to deploy Redis for our cluster, but first we need to install Helm. To do so, follow the instructions at https://helm.sh/docs/intro/install/.

I'm hoping that you have been wondering where our Makefile was for this section. We need it now to help us manage our deployments. First, we will create the Helm deployment and then the steps to deploy our app. Helm allows us to configure our deployments by passing specific settings as we apply the chart. These settings are often things like scaling or security values. In our case, we want our Redis database to be secure by using a password. To do that, we edit our Makefile so that we can have a deployment command with some configurations (see the following listing).

Listing 10.7   Makefile

Uses a specialized Kubernetes
deployment of Redis

```
install-redis:
  helm repo add bitnami https://charts.bitnami.com/bitnami
  helm install redis-cluster bitnami/redis --set password=$$(       ◄──
  ➥ tr -dc A-Za-z0-9 </dev/urandom | head -c 13 ; echo '')    ◄──  Generates
                                                                    a random
deploy:                                                             password to use
  kubectl apply -f k8s
```

Run `make install-k8s-redis`, and we should be able to watch the new pods come online. The database is now running, so we can configure our system to run against it. For that, we need to create a configuration map.

10.7   Updating deployment configuration

In chapter 8, we went through the work of making our application change its functionality through configuration. Now we can use this same mechanism using Kubernetes. Since Kubernetes clusters do not consist of a single machine, we can't simply set environmental variables on each system, nor can we add a configuration file to the individual server.

Instead, Kubernetes treats this as a resource, just like a deployment or service. We can create and reference a *configuration map*, which defines a set of similarly used configuration values that decouple our environmental variables from the consuming container. This means we will have a configuration map for our service to consume. Since

we are now in production, we should also consider updating our Redis server by using a special configuration type called a *secret*. First, let's make our map.

Configuration maps are just like any other Kubernetes resource in that we can create them using a file. Let's create a new `config.yml` file under the `k8s/hello-api` directory. In it, we will add the code in the following listing.

Listing 10.8   `config.yml`

```
apiVersion: v1
kind: ConfigMap
metadata:
  name: hello-api
data:                                    Sets ENV vars in
  database_url: "redis-cluster"   ◁──┘   the config map
```

Apply it by typing `kubectl apply -f k8s/hello-api/config.yml`, and you should see a notification that a new resource was created.

Before we attach the configuration to our service, we should also create a secret for our Redis server. Secrets are a little different than configuration maps in that you don't want to store them as files on our system because of a security risk, nor do you want to make them easily visible within our cluster.

> **NOTE** While Kubernetes has a special field called a secret, it does not mean this is encrypted or secure, only that it is obfuscated from the end user. A robust production system should consider a secret manager like Vault.

Secrets are mostly used for things like usernames and passwords. They don't need to be like your email or bank login that you need to remember. Instead, as we saw earlier, we can provide a random string to be the password, and Kubernetes will manage it for us. When we created our Redis deployment, a password was provided. We don't need it; we can just reference it in the same way as a configuration map. To put these values in our deployment, we need to set some environmental variables. Let's open that and add the code in the following listing.

Listing 10.9   `deployment.yml`

```
apiVersion: apps/v1
kind: Deployment
metadata:
  name: hello-api
spec:
  replicas: 1
  selector:
    matchLabels:
        app: hello-api
  template:
    metadata:
      name: hello-api
```

```
  labels:
    app: hello-api
spec:
  containers:
  - name: hello-api
    imagePullPolicy: Never
    image: holmes89/hello-api:v0.3
    ports:
    - containerPort: 8080
      name: hello-api-svc
    env:
    - name: DATABASE_URL        ◁─┐  Sets DB URL from the
      valueFrom:                   │  configuration map
        configMapKeyRef:
          name: hello-api
          key: database_url
    - name: DATABASE_PASSWORD   ◁─┐  Sets Password from
      valueFrom:                   │  the Helm secret
        secretKeyRef:
          name: redis-cluster
          key: redis-password
          optional: false
```

These values should match the values we had in our application configuration when we run this locally. The configuration values get loaded into the containers as they start. To see this work now, we can simply reapply our deployment using `kubectl apply -f k8s`. Once it is running, we can verify the results by querying against the database by trying a query in a different language:

```
curl <url>:80/translate/hello?language=arabic
```

Hopefully, you see the proper translation!

It's now Friday, two weeks since you started this whole project, and less than a day from the Kubernetes kickoff meeting. You sit down and draft a quick email to the team telling them your status and drafting your findings in a design document to help the team move forward. Smiling, you reflect on how far your company has come. You've helped create a culture of experimentation while maintaining standards and easing development. Everyone seems pleased, but you know it will not be perfect. Things will need to change, new applications will need to be developed, and hopefully you will be able to help.

Summary

- Kubernetes clusters abstract deployments across multiple servers managed by your team.
- Deployments create groups of containers called pods that can scale depending on demand or required availability.
- Services route calls to deployments.
- Secrets and configuration files can be used to populate environmental variables for application configuration.

11

The loop

This chapter covers

- Outlining the phases of startups and projects
- Working through extensions to core areas of improvement

"I honestly didn't think we would be able to pull this off. It is amazing what we've been able to change in just the past few weeks," the project manager says, beaming. "We are going to move all of our projects to this style of development. If we are lucky, we can start experimenting with smaller projects and faster release cycles. The cost of updating software is so much lighter now. We've also reduced our server costs by deploying small applications as functions and then migrating them to our Kubernetes cluster."

You can't help but smile too. The project manager still hasn't seen the future pay-out of this pattern. When automation came to textile creation, it changed a 100% manual job into a 2% manual job. The long-term effects were more jobs in textile manufacturing and more products for everyday consumers. By automating 98% of the workflow, your company will now be able to produce more products and tools to help your company grow.

The funny thing about this story is that it won't have an end. You may end up building a new product again. You may move up to managing a team of developers. You may end up leaving your company for another or go out on your own. What is important is that it starts over. This last chapter is called "The loop" because, if you remember from chapter 1, you will need to go back and design after you deliver. This happens for systems and processes as well. Each time a new project starts, you should consider what could have been better the last time or other ideas you want to explore. As this book comes to a close, we'll review each stage or part (startup, acceleration, cruising) that the book was broken down into as well as each element in that stage (process, test, deliver) and decide what to look for in the future.

11.1 Startup

It is obviously the goal for any project to be delivered early and under budget. This doesn't always happen, but when creating a new product or proof of concept, anything goes. We want to establish some processes and quality checks and not worry too much about scaling.

This is why we focused on development setup, unit tests, and serverless functions in the first section of this book. Getting developers on board will be the most important task. It's like organizing a worksite. If you have a clear outline of where things are and where they are going, you will spend less time giving direction and focus more on the development itself. In terms of where things were, we established a central repository and mechanism for moving code through our organization. This automated some of the work that our team needed to do and freed them up to focus on the code. Having this established early on is essential because it frees up developers to do other work. However, you should consider how often this task will need to be done before automating it. If you find yourself stopping your work more than once a week to do the same task, consider automating it.

Your software will change over time, but no more so than at the beginning of development. This is why simple tests that verify core functionality are a worthwhile investment rather than having end-to-end coverage right at the start. While some will scoff at accruing technical debt so early on in a project, I feel that if a project pivots or closes, it will be considered lost time. The trick is to recognize the turning point when a project is here to stay and tests should be improved. A good rule is to consider where you find bugs early on. If you find bugs or waste time with errors, maybe you should consider adding tests. Once you've crossed this horizon, a larger code cleanup plan should be considered. This can be a code cleanup blitz: everyone takes a section of code and adds tests and documentation.

Deployment should also be cheap and easy, which is why we selected FaaS and PaaS at the beginning. FaaS is more than capable of running your entire startup forever. You may find that you never need to switch from a FaaS because of how they scale and how your organization is structured. But at some point, you may find that it is cheaper to change to another deployment type. Or you may find that the functions aren't scaling

the way you want. In either case, you need to keep an eye on usage and metrics around these functions. All major cloud-hosting platforms provide this sort of insight and allow you to set alerts. Consider discussing what sort of alerts you want to have and coming up with a migration plan, if necessary. You will be happy you considered this and have a plan early on instead of doing a fire drill in the middle of the night on a Saturday.

The startup phase of application development is the equivalent of trailblazing. You may find you've walked in the wrong direction. You may find that you are heading in the right direction but haven't walked far enough. You may find that you shouldn't even be in this area at all. In all of these cases, it doesn't make sense to set down roots quite yet. Something temporary like a tent would suffice, so consider this phase the tent phase. You need to be mobile and temporary, not established. Once you feel the pain of the lack of durability, consider moving on to the next phase.

11.2   Acceleration

Once you are sure your product is here to stay, the next phase of development kicks in. This is the acceleration stage: you start to build rapidly. You're done blazing trails and have found a great place for a home base. You not only need to grow fast but grow in the right direction. That is why we focused on taking what we've built in the startup phase and expanding it. Now we put up walls and a roof on our tent and consider how the town will grow.

In this phase, we focused more on standardization and documentation. In building a home or an office, certain contractor standards are used. Boards are measured in feet or meters. Screws have a particular head type. Concrete needs certain proportions to set properly. We did the same with our linting and vetting procedures. We also wanted to establish better documentation to outline where our code is and how it is used. This is the equivalent of blueprints and schematics for our system.

We also focused on structuring our application to be modular. When you still need to be flexible within a constrained space, the last thing you need is a large and rigid item to maneuver. Having a modular system allows you to conform to the space in an easier way. Consider the difference between moving a couch and three chairs around a sitting room. Which is easier? In the same way, we structured our code to inject certain dependencies through the use of interfaces and tested them using mocked and stubbed tests. This way, each modular piece was tested independently, meaning we don't need to rewrite our tests unless the functionality changes in that one module.

We then took this new code and put it into a portable runtime using containers. First, Buildpacks were used to build optimized containers for Google's container runtime. Then we created our containers for developer use cases. Being able to ship our code around like this shows how teams may need to interact and share across different application boundaries. Having the ability to run and document dependencies in this way can alleviate integration problems in the future. Also consider the implications this can have on your ability to test your applications. QA departments or groups can create temporary deployments to run automated test scripts without affecting your production deployment.

Acceleration is used to describe this phase because it's important to not stop. You've figured out where to build, and now you need to expand. There is a certain speed that an object needs to reach to rid itself of the pull of gravity. This can only happen if you continue to accelerate. This is a compounding force, not just a static one. As you accelerate, you gain more and more speed, but it is harder and harder to get to that edge until, finally, you've escaped.

11.3 Cruising

Once you've escaped the pull of gravity, you no longer need to accelerate. Instead, you can cruise and explore. This does not mean that you're done. You've made it. You've gotten to a point where you can have the freedom to improve and explore. Course corrections will be needed, and mistakes will still happen.

When we got to this point, we were able to focus on making our applications flexible and stable. We can change the way our applications run based on the variables we put in. This functionality can be extended to move beyond adding default values or endpoints for database connections. Instead, you can use it to hide features that have not been completed. There are even ways to remotely manage these settings, meaning that you can simply flip a switch on a digital dashboard, and all of a sudden, your application will run differently.

Managing this flexibility is what makes your company succeed. After escaping the gravity of starting, you can now explore the vast reaches of your business. This becomes the key part of your success. In *The Lean Startup* (Currency, 2011), Eric Reise talks about the need to be flexible in a startup to find what the customer wants and do nothing more than that. This has been our guiding light throughout the book: keep it simple and keep changing. This helps us create the underlying tools necessary to deliver quickly and efficiently while continuing to improve. Once we are cruising, we can start building the process around how we develop features. We can use the behavior-driven development skills we learned in chapter 9 to help guide and focus our development. We can then start considering other forms of testing such as *exploratory testing*, wherein a team tries to break our system by generating tons of load or putting special characters into input fields. This can then be automated via user-simulated testing frameworks like Selenium or Cypress.

Hopefully, all of this leads you to find that you need to adjust your infrastructure. You'll know when you've reached this point when someone comes to you, says that your cloud bill is too high, and asks if there is something you can do about it. This will most likely come before anything else. This is because you are paying for the abstraction to have AWS or Google run your application for you. It's a convenience fee. Once at this point, you need to focus on infrastructure; only then does it make sense to look at cool tools like Kubernetes. This is not a hard-and-fast rule, but focus on simple rather than complex. If you don't have the team to support infrastructure like Kubernetes, you shouldn't worry about it. Focus on developing a product that you can show, and then worry about optimizing how and where it runs.

I say all of this from experience. I've been working in startups for around a decade and have seen how teams grow and where mistakes are made. All too often, developers and managers want to reach for a new and shiny technology or tool to get a job done when they don't need to. A former manager of mine once said, "People want to grab for a new tool all of the time but don't know how to use it. The old beat-up tools are old and beat up for a reason—it's because they work." This isn't to say that you shouldn't keep an eye on the new and shiny. In fact, you will need to incorporate them to keep growing and to keep up, as well as to keep your developers engaged. The skill lies in determining which tools to use and how to use them. As a team, you should discuss, plan, and research before starting down that path and think about supporting what you make for the future.

Here is an example of wasting time on something shiny from my recent past. I was working on an application that was very similar to applications I have built before. A message came in with some metric data, and I needed to normalize it to be displayed on various dashboards. I decided that I wanted to make this system totally event based and that all communication throughout the service would be asynchronous, so I built a complex system around a tool I've had my eyes on for a year or so. I was excited and happy with what I built—until I wasn't. I soon realized that I had built something more complex than what was needed, and while it would scale, it did not need to scale in the way I thought it would. Then I realized that the library I was using became deprecated within two weeks of development, and suddenly the timeline to refactor what I had just written was moved up.

The lesson is that I built something shiny and new for me, not for the customer. I over-designed and over-developed, and then I had to face the consequences of rebuilding what I had just built. This came from a lack of planning and discipline on my end. It's important to find a way to make sure that doesn't happen in the future. What was the mitigating tactic I came up with so this sort of problem doesn't happen again? I started writing design documents and placing them in a folder in my repo so that people can review designs before the work is done and referred to them to see how the system was built. These are known as RFCs, and they are very helpful in allowing teams to think about and discuss designs before they develop.

These are just some things you will experience as your project or product grows through the various stages. Let's now look at the various elements of each stage and discuss how you can go beyond what we covered in process, testing, and delivering.

11.4 Elements of development

When we started this book, I mentioned that what I present is not new—at least not new to the industry. The hope is that I provide a handbook to get you and your business started. Software development didn't click until I started reading comparisons between software development and manufacturing.

I can imagine my various coworkers at my startup all fulfilling different roles. Wearing hard hats and uniforms, I can see my manager directing a fellow developer on a forklift while my project manager moves folders with various orders from different

stations. Meanwhile, a QA team member is checking boxes on their clipboard, making note of the slightest imperfection. Finally, our Ops team comes by, loads it up on a truck, and ships it out of the building.

That was exactly how the teams were divided, and that's exactly how work flowed through our system. It took a lot of work for us to figure out how to work together, build good relationships, and establish trust. A few months before we were purchased, I came up with a plan to present how to streamline this work. The result was a pipeline similar to this book to help automate the process of taking an idea and making it real with a few clicks of a mouse.

When perusing the research for this idea, I found that some great books described CI/CD pipelines, testing methodologies, and code standardization practices but didn't put them together with examples. When I looked at the books, I organized them into process, testing, and delivery.

11.4.1 Process

Working on a team is hard, whether your team members are your best friends or complete strangers. Everyone does things differently, and it's up to you to figure out how to get along and make things together. Waste can cause problems in teams. When you waste someone's time with an incomplete feature, sloppy code, or an obvious bug, it can quickly escalate from annoying to disrespectful. Once disrespect for a coworker has set in, it becomes difficult for a team to mesh and collaborate.

Processes save time. By establishing standards and practices, you reduce the amount of waste produced by saving people's time and interactions. If a program can tell you that your code looks bad, that saves someone else the effort of telling you, and you will receive fast, concise feedback. Yet these simple but effective tools are often overlooked. The simple pipeline that we created at the beginning established our process, and we added to it throughout the book. Establishing a process of verifying, testing, and deploying automatically reduces the time wasted in handing off and getting to production. This pipeline is illustrated in figure 11.1.

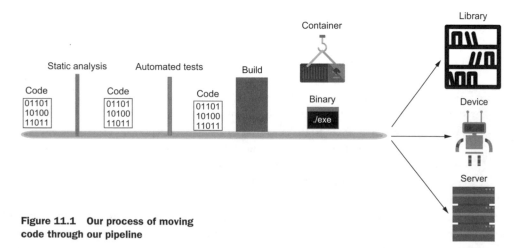

Figure 11.1   Our process of moving code through our pipeline

You should also have a process for your process. While this seems cyclical, it is helpful. Periodically evaluating how you are building and delivering your product will help you improve. This is known as *continuous improvement* (a different CI than the continuous integration we did earlier). Toyota realized that when they were able to increase their productivity, their employees were not at full capacity, meaning they could do additional work because their jobs had become simpler, so Toyota asked their employees to use this extra time to improve their process: to see where they were inefficient or falling short. This isn't done by picking some arbitrary area that you feel needs improvement. The employee and manager need metrics, evaluations, and designs before your improvement becomes part of a process.

What does this mean for your team? Ensure that you and your teammates are at full capacity and that you are allowing yourself some time to find areas of improvement. Setting up metrics around delivery time, build time, and response time can all be used to improve your application and your process. Think of how you want to use testing and how your pipeline is working. What are the ergonomics of your development environment? Is it hard to set up, or does it require someone else to get it working? Is your computer crashing if you don't run things a particular way? Does it make sense to develop another way?

Always be thinking of improving not only your software but also the way you develop software. One way of doing that is through targeted and appropriate testing.

11.4.2 *Testing*

Testing in startups is such a tricky thing to get right. Your code is changing so much and so often that your tests can sometimes get in the way of what you are developing. You spend all of your time writing tests for a given piece of code that changes within a week. Why should you spend time testing when it can go away in an instant?

Let me ask you this: How do you know if a particular piece of code will stay or go? You don't. While I've been on the end of deleting or rewriting my tests more often than I can remember, I can distinctly remember projects where we had zero test coverage and paid a penalty for it in the long run. We soon encountered so many bugs in production that the time would have been better spent writing the test code in the first place.

What should you do? Should you just not write tests until it's painful? Absolutely not! This will decrease your productivity and increase your overall lead time. To solve this problem, we need to think about testing throughout the process, not just at one particular stage. The overall trend of the book was to move from simple to complex. In the same way, your tests should evolve to become more complex and robust by checking various portions of the code in different ways. This saves you and the rest of your team time.

But how much should you test, and what should you test? The answer is to start simply with basic unit tests around deterministic sections of code. These are your typical algorithmic functions that calculate balances or error rates. You give it a set of data, and the same answer kicks out each time. This is done by using the basic unit tests and the mocking techniques we talked about in chapters 4 and 7. Chapter 10 explored integration-level testing against larger services. We didn't get to a full-system,

end-to-end, UI-to-API-level testing. All of this should reflect what we see in our testing pyramid (figure 11.2).

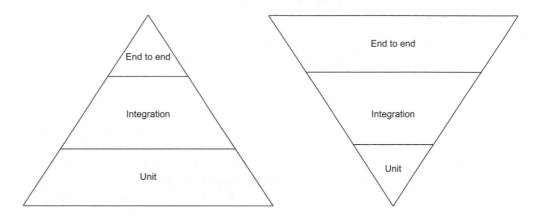

Figure 11.2 The testing pyramid focuses on building a foundation of unit tests.

By starting with the smaller chunks of work and building up, we build a solid foundation for testing. If you do anything, do automated unit tests. These are the foundation of your quality assessment of your product. Keep these quality checks as close to the code as possible in all cases, but specifically for the unit tests. If you find that your unit tests are breaking or getting in the way, you need to reconsider your testing process. Writing good unit tests is an art as much as it is a science. You find what to test and what not to test. Test-driven development, as mentioned in chapter 4, is extremely helpful in helping us whittle down tests to their core elements.

You may find that your approach to testing is fine but that you are constantly changing them. This is an indication of thrashing in other places. Do you have a grasp of the code you are writing? Are others writing quality tests? Are you getting the correct requirements? Is the project clearly defined? If any of these questions are answered "no," you should have a team meeting.

Testing brings to light more than just bugs in your code. It helps you find bugs in your process. As an example, I've worked for several companies that have had very complicated setups for writing tests. Entire test databases need to be loaded, certain software needs to be installed or running, and scripts need to run to set up your test environment. While these by themselves are not dangerous, they lead to frustration among team members because they struggle with the setup rather than writing the test. When you find that team members don't want to write tests or test locally due to local development environments, you have a bug in your process.

The eventual goal in all of this automated testing is the goal of any sort of automation: freeing others up to do more creative work. If you can build automated tests suites at all levels, your team will start to be able to explore areas of improvement such as these:

- Performance of different functions or systems
- Usability of the product
- Rare or extreme edge cases (before customers identify them)
- User workflow improvements

There are many other areas of improvement. The point is that testing is an essential part of creating a feedback loop that is only going to help your company grow. The only way to find out if it works as expected is to release it to the public.

11.4.3 *Delivering*

Options for delivering your products shift more quickly than sand dunes. Not too long ago, companies installed their own servers and hardware. Then it became the cloud with all of these virtualized servers. At the time, there were few options for cloud computing, but now there are many, and many more come out each month. Like electricity, computing is becoming a utility that is accessible to anyone with a computer and a credit card. Because of the vast expansion of cloud technologies, tools have been built to sit on top of this vast system of computational utilities. Platforms like Kubernetes and serverless frameworks are all operating within the context of abstracted computational resources (see figure 11.3).

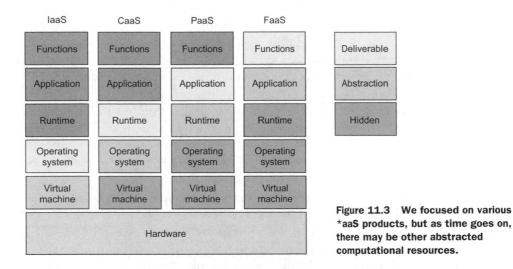

Figure 11.3 **We focused on various *aaS products, but as time goes on, there may be other abstracted computational resources.**

But we cannot expect the changes to stop there. While other concepts of process and testing will have small improvements and changes over time, the general principles will stay the same. How you deliver your product will change significantly in the future. We are already seeing trends in moving computational resources onto CDN networks, which were originally used for caching web pages. Now they can run lightweight APIs and computations on the "edge" of the network.

All of this is to say that in a few years, chapters 4, 7, and 10 may refer to outdated technology in the cloud world. In fact, I guarantee they will. But this doesn't mean that this book will become outdated. Like the other concepts, some core pieces are essential. First and foremost, your pipeline falls squarely in the realm of delivery. We started the book by talking about automated delivery and its importance. We also discussed the fact that delivery can mean multiple things depending on the technology. We focused on cloud technologies because they are a simple way to start. But delivery can happen in IoT devices by pushing software updates or just downloadable binaries or packages for people to install. Your pipeline should be able to take the code you write and deliver an artifact, pure and simple.

The delivery of cloud products will change, but those rules will also remain the same: start with the easiest and cheapest until you know more about how your product is used. In journalism, they tell you to follow the five Ws of investigation to get to the bottom of a story, and those apply here as well:

- *Who* will be using your product?
- *What* are they doing with your product?
- *Where* are people using the product?
- *When* are people using it the most?
- *Why* are people using your product?

All of these items are essential for delivering what a customer needs and wants. The questions almost seem repetitive in that sense, right? When you deliver your product, you need to find ways of investigating these areas. For example, if you find that most of your users are in Europe and not the United States, you should consider deploying in a cloud region in Europe until you can scale to multiple deployment zones. Only with metrics can you find these things out.

This was a core piece that I was not able to cover in the book, but it is essential. Metric gathering helps you determine where to take your product. It answers the investigation questions and helps you justify future work to your employer and team. Moving forward, it will be up to you to determine how to evolve your delivery and product over time.

11.5 The OODA loop

In the early 1960s, Colonel John Boyd developed a military strategy called the OODA loop:

- *Observe*—Collect data.
- *Orient*—Analyze the data.
- *Decide*—Determine the course of action based on your analysis of the data.
- *Act*—Act on what was decided.

The process repeats, which puts you back in the observation stage (figure 11.4).

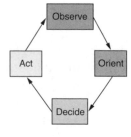

Figure 11.4
The OODA loop

I hope you can see the parallels with what we were able to accomplish in this book. The project manager observed the cost and maintenance of the old system. In orienting themselves with the data, they decided that a new service should be built at a lower cost. Then they acted by starting this project.

Then it looped!

You *observed* how the old system was built. Having been *oriented* in the current development process, you were able to decide that the lowest cost method is to write a simple API run through a FaaS for low cost and maintenance. You *acted* by creating a CI process that delivers this simple function.

It looped again!

You observed that your FaaS was a successful proof of concept. The analysis determined that the process would not scale to other teams. You decided to increase testing and create a portable application for other teams to use.

Then it looped again!

Driven by the success of your containerized product, management observed that others should do the same. To do this, we required increased levels of process and testing and needed to create a containerized deployment environment. We decided to add configuration management and integration testing to our process and create a Kubernetes cluster.

And the loop will continue!

When you think of your product development as a loop instead of a long line, you'll find that your development mindset changes. Just like a loop, products don't end. Instead, they evolve. Yes, just like all evolution, you will have products that go extinct, but evolution is full of victors and losers; that's just the way it is. It is those who cannot adapt that die. Instead, focus on how your product can adapt by observing, orienting, deciding, and acting.

11.6 Conclusion

I recently had lunch with a former manager of mine. We were discussing his role and how things had changed. "I don't get to do much development anymore, and I don't have any engineers report directly to me, so I don't see much code. But what I can't seem to get away from is our pipeline. I'm constantly checking and trying to improve it. I'm not sure why I can't leave it alone."

It made sense to me. He was now at a point where the details of the code were not important. What was important was the delivery and then shipping it to customers. He didn't need to know how a test was written or what language the product was written in. All he needed to see was that a certain standard was established and a process was being used. Beyond that, he needed to trust the rest of the team to do their jobs.

The journey up to this point has paralleled my career, along with that of many others. I started this book by saying that there wasn't anything new in these pages, and I hope you recognized some patterns or processes listed here. The success of a project lies outside the control of the developer or the company. The only thing you can do is make sure you deliver. Delivering a quality product that can quickly adapt to the

market and your customer needs is within your control. All you need is to build the tools to deliver, assemble a team around them, and explore.

11.7 Summary

- A product is a journey, not a destination.
- Pipelines help manage processes within a team without micromanaging.
- Change is inevitable, so you need to find a way to orient yourself within that change.

appendix A
Using Kotlin

Throughout the book, I have mentioned that software development and code maintenance patterns are not limited to a single language or technology, so the following sections will quickly demonstrate how to introduce these same processes using three popular languages, Kotlin, JavaScript, and Python, and present an alternate deployment option using tools from HashiCorp. To start, we'll look into Kotlin, a language built on the JVM and growing in popularity as it matures.

Kotlin has the benefit of being built on top of existing technologies in Java, which means that the tools and patterns are fairly mature. We will build a new CI pipeline using Kotlin-specific tools, but the steps will remain mostly the same in our Makefile. To start, we will build our hello-api again using Kotlin and Redis.

A.1 *Frameworks*

Frameworks both aid and hinder development teams. Sometimes a framework will help you launch your product quickly, but over time, you may find that you struggle against it, losing your momentum. Taking the time to research available frameworks and reassessing the ones you are using are very important. Look for these features:

- Ease of use
- Documentation quality
- Viability

All three are very important. You don't want to use a framework that is obscure and no longer supported because bugs and vulnerabilities may arise, and you will not be able to fix them. At the same time, you don't want to adopt a framework that doesn't support the technology you want to use. In the Java development world, an up-and-coming framework called Quarkus fits all these criteria. Luckily, this framework can be used with Kotlin and was built to run in container-based ecosystems.

Developed and supported by Red Hat, Quarkus provides many drivers and out-of-the-box tools to help rapidly build and test APIs. To set it up, follow these steps:

- Install Java (http://mng.bz/e1mz).
- Go to code.quarkus.io.
- Name the group com.manning and the artifact hello-api.
- Keep the Build Tool as Maven, Java Version 17.
- In the filters section, add Kotlin, RESTEasy Reactive Kotlin Serialization, and Redis Client.
- Click Generate your application, and open your project.

NOTE   Spring is a big player in Java/Kotlin frameworks and has excellent documentation in both Java and Kotlin.

Once these steps are complete, we can unzip our project and get started.

A.2   *Coding*

Quarkus gives us a lot without us needing to do anything. Like many modern JVM-based frameworks, Quarkus makes extensive use of annotations to take care of most of the wiring. This can be extremely helpful but also a mystery when it comes time for debugging. We first create four files in our com/manning/hello-api package. First is the main function, which we will call TranslationResource.kt. This will be our entry point for translations, as shown in the following listing.

Listing A.1   TranslationResource.kt

```
package com.manning.hello-api

import javax.inject.Inject
import javax.ws.rs.GET
import javax.ws.rs.Path
import javax.ws.rs.PathParam
import javax.ws.rs.Produces
import javax.ws.rs.QueryParam
import javax.ws.rs.core.MediaType

@Path("/translate")                                    ◁─┐ Base path for
class TranslationResource {                               │ the request

    @Inject                                            ◁─────── Dependency injection
    private lateinit var service: ITranslationService  │       of translation service

                                                       ┌── Subpath for
    @GET                                               │   request
    @Path("/{word}")                                ◁──┘
    @Produces(MediaType.APPLICATION_JSON)
    fun translate(
        @PathParam("word") word: String,
        @QueryParam("language") language: String?      │ Call service based on
    ) = service.translate(language, word)           ◁──┘ path and query params

}
```

REST GET method

When our application starts, Quarkus will look for all of our paths and add them to the main controller, just like we did manually in Go. There is nothing special about this code other than that we mount an interface as our service to handle the translation. This interface will act as a barrier behind the actual Redis implementation, just like we did in Go. That interface is defined in `ITranslationService.kt` as in the following listing.

Listing A.2 `ITranslationResource.kt`

```
package com.manning.hello-api

interface ITranslationService {
    fun translate(language: String?, word: String): Translation?
}
```

Defines interface method that returns optional translation object

Pretty simple, right? It's almost exactly the same as our Go interface. We optionally return a Translation type. This is defined in a separate `Translation.kt` file which will replicate our Translation struct from Go (see the following listing).

Listing A.3 `TranslationResource.kt`

```
package com.manning.hello-api

data class Translation(
    val language: String?,
    val translation: String?
)
```

Creates a data class or DTO for messages

Finally, we can get to the Redis connection. Here, we have a bit more code (see the next listing) and the actual retrieval from Redis itself.

Listing A.4 `RedisTranslationService.kt`

```
package com.manning.hello-api

import io.quarkus.redis.datasource.RedisDataSource
import org.eclipse.microprofile.config.inject.ConfigProperty
import javax.enterprise.context.ApplicationScoped
import javax.inject.Inject

@ApplicationScoped
class RedisTranslationService : ITranslationService {

    @Inject
    private lateinit var redisAPI: RedisDataSource

    @ConfigProperty(name = "default.language")
    var defaultLanguage: String? = "english"

    override fun translate(language: String?, word: String): Translation? {
        val commands = redisAPI?.string(String::class.java)
```

Injects Redis client

Sets default language from config

```
            val lang = language?.lowercase() ?: defaultLanguage
            val key = "$word:$lang"
            val translation = commands?.get(key)        ⟵⎯ Gets translation
            return if (translation == null) {               from Redis
                null
            } else {
                Translation(language = lang, translation = translation)
            }
        }
    }
}
```

In order for Redis to connect, we need to provide some properties that it can grab to connect. These values can be overridden, just like in Go, by passing in environmental variables. By default, we want to use localhost, so we will fill out our `resources/application.properties` file like this.

Listing A.5 `application.properties`

```
quarkus.redis.hosts=redis://localhost:6379    ⟵⎯ Default property of where
quarkus.redis.client-type=standalone             to connect to Redis
quarkus.datasource.jdbc=false

default.language=english
```

Now that we have the code, let's introduce how we build and run it. Then we will use this for testing. Finally, we'll wrap this all in a pipeline.

A.3 *Maven*

Maven is a build tool under the Apache project that allows Java developers to manage their project dependencies (like our `go.mod` file) as well as incorporate different build and testing scripts (like our Makefile). Other build tools such as Gradle can be used to fulfill similar tasks. In this section, we will focus on using Maven. Maven projects are managed by using a `pom.xml` file, which you will find at the root of the setup project you downloaded along with an `mvnw` script. This script is a wrapper around basic Maven tooling so that developers don't need to worry about environment-specific variables (e.g., their operating system and base Maven file).

We will use Maven to build, run, and test our code. First, let's run what we've written. Make sure you have your Redis database running, and then type in `./mvnw compile quarkus:dev` in a terminal window. You'll see a bunch of files being downloaded and then compiled, and finally you'll see a message that says the server is listening. At this point, try your trusty `curl` commands from previous chapters to test it.

Now that we have an understanding of how Maven looks, we will use it for running our unit tests.

A.4 *Testing*

For our testing example, we will jump right into integration tests because they give us a sense of how tests are written in Kotlin, and integration tests typically are more involved at setup and teardown. This will give us a great overview while providing a

jumping-off place to fill in the rest of the testing pyramid. For our test, we again use a container for the database and a library called RestAssured, which will give us a nice REST testing framework for verification. To get started, create a file called `TranslationTest.kt` in the test folder (see the following listing).

Listing A.6   `TranslationTest.kt`

```
package com.manning.hello-api

import io.quarkus.test.common.QuarkusTestResource
import io.quarkus.test.junit.QuarkusTest
import io.restassured.RestAssured.given
import org.hamcrest.CoreMatchers.equalTo
import org.junit.jupiter.api.Test

@QuarkusTestResource(RedisTestContainer::class)          ◁──┐ Depends on
@QuarkusTest           ◁──┐ Tells the build tool              a container
class TranslationTest {    │ that this is a test

    @Test
    fun testHelloEndpoint() {
        given()
            .`when`().get("/translate/hello")
            .then()
            .statusCode(200)
            .body("translation", equalTo("Hello"))
            .body("language", equalTo("english"))
    }

    @Test
    fun testHelloEndpointGerman() {         ┌─ Tests the request using
        given()                        ◁───┘   fluent assertion
            .`when`().get("/translate/hello?language=GERMAN")
            .then()
            .statusCode(200)
            .body("translation", equalTo("Hallo"))
            .body("language", equalTo("german"))
    }
}
```

The tests should seem familiar from earlier in the book. Now we need to create another file that tells our testing plugin that this particular test is an integration test. To do that, we simply create a file with the content in the following listing.

Listing A.7   `TranslationTest.kt`

```
package com.manning.hello-api

import io.quarkus.test.junit.QuarkusIntegrationTest

@QuarkusIntegrationTest           ◁──┐ Defines this test suite
class TranslationIT : TranslationTest()   │ as an integration test
```

That's it! Finally, we need our database container to run our tests against. To do this, we add a dependency to our pom.xml file. There, under dependencies, you will add the lines in the following listing.

Listing A.8   pom.xml

```xml
<dependency>
     <groupId>org.testcontainers</groupId>
     <artifactId>testcontainers</artifactId>
     <version>1.17.3</version>
     <scope>test</scope>
 </dependency>
```

Then we create a file called RedisTestContainer.kt and add the code in the following listing.

Listing A.9   RedisTestContainer.kt

```kotlin
package com.manning.hello-api

import io.quarkus.test.common.QuarkusTestResourceLifecycleManager
import org.testcontainers.containers.BindMode
import org.testcontainers.containers.GenericContainer
import org.testcontainers.utility.DockerImageName

class RedisTestContainer : QuarkusTestResourceLifecycleManager {

    private val redisContainer = GenericContainer(DockerImageName.parse(
    "redis:latest"))
        .withExposedPorts(6379)
        .withClasspathResourceMapping("data", "/data", BindMode.READ_ONLY)

    override fun start(): MutableMap<String, String> {
        println("STARTING redis ")
        redisContainer.start()
        println("redis://${redisContainer.getHost()}:${
    redisContainer.getMappedPort(6379)}")
        return mutableMapOf(Pair("quarkus.redis.hosts", "redis://${
    redisContainer.getHost()}:${
    redisContainer.getMappedPort(6379)}"))
    }

    override fun stop() {
        println("STOPPING redis")
        redisContainer.stop()
    }
}
```

Creates a redis container with the mounted data directory

Establishes a command map for retrieving messages

That's it! To test, run ./mvnw clean test, and you will see your test run successfully!

A.5 *Linting and the initial pipeline*

For linting, we use an open source tool called `ktlint`, which is written and maintained by Pinterest as an open source project. It supports both a downloadable, standalone app as well as a Maven plugin. Here, we will use the prebuilt binary to make installation a little more straightforward. We often make linting the first step of our pipeline because it is the simplest and often the fastest step to run. Let's create our pipeline up to build and deploy, which we will finalize in the next section.

Create a new workflow file in `.github/workflows/pipeline.yml` using the code in the following listing.

Listing A.10 `pipeline.kt`

```
name: Kotlin Checks

on:
  push:
    branches:
      - main
env:
  REGISTRY: ghcr.io
  IMAGE_NAME: ${{ github.repository }}

jobs:
  format-check:
    name: Check formatting
    runs-on: ubuntu-latest
    steps:
    - uses: actions/checkout@v3
    - uses: actions/setup-java@v3          Defines the
      with:                                Java version
        distribution: 'temurin'
        java-version: '17'
        cache: 'maven'                     Installs and
    - name: Download Ktlint                runs ktlint
      run: curl -sSLO https://github.com/pinterest/ktlint/releases/
      ↳download/0.47.1/ktlint && chmod a+x ktlint
    - name: Lint
      run: ./ktlint
  test:
    name: Test Application
    needs:
      - format-check
    runs-on: ubuntu-latest
    steps:
    - uses: actions/checkout@v3
    - uses: actions/setup-java@v3
      with:
        distribution: 'temurin'
        java-version: '17'
        cache: 'maven'
    - name: Run Test                       Deletes all old files
      run: ./mvnw clean test               and runs tests
```

If you commit your changes and push them, you should see the tests run and the lint pass!

A.6   *Containerizing*

The final step is putting this application into a container. To do this, we use another neat Quarkus trick. In recent years, specialized compilers have been developed to allow Java code to be compiled into native system code. This allows your containers and packages to be smaller in size and to run faster. Additionally, you no longer need to be as concerned about JVM security patches and updates; instead, you only need to worry about the OS's security problems. Quarkus has taken this technology and added it to the build system for Quarkus apps. Quarkus even provides you with the Maven steps and Docker container to use, so right away we can add the last job to our pipeline and verify that it works (see the following listing).

Listing A.11   `pipeline.kt`

```
name: Kotlin Checks

jobs:
...
  containerize:
    name: Build and Push Container
    runs-on: ubuntu-latest #
    needs: test
    steps:
    - uses: actions/checkout@v3
    - uses: actions/setup-java@v3
      with:
        distribution: 'temurin'
        java-version: '17'
        cache: 'maven'
    - name: Build
      run: ./mvnw package -Pnative -Dquarkus.native.container-build=true
    - name: Build Container
      run: docker build -f src/main/docker/Dockerfile.jvm -t
        gcr.io/${{ secrets.GCP_PROJECT_ID }}/hello-api:kotlin-latest
    - name: Set up Cloud SDK
      uses: google-github-actions/setup-gcloud@main
      with:
        project_id: ${{ secrets.GCP_PROJECT_ID }}
        service_account_key: ${{ secrets.gcp_credentials }}
        export_default_credentials: true
    - name: Configure Docker
      run: gcloud auth configure-docker --quiet
    - name: Push Docker image
      run: docker push gcr.io/${{ secrets.GCP_PROJECT_ID }}/hello-api:
        kotlin-latest
    - name: Log in to the GHCR
      uses: docker/login-action@master
      with:
        registry: ${{ env.REGISTRY }}
```

Builds a native Java binary — points to `run: ./mvnw package -Pnative -Dquarkus.native.container-build=true`

Uses an internal Dockerfile to build a container — points to `gcr.io/${{ secrets.GCP_PROJECT_ID }}/hello-api:kotlin-latest`

```
      username: ${{ github.actor }}
      password: ${{ secrets.GITHUB_TOKEN }}
  - name: Tag for Github
    run: docker image tag gcr.io/${{ secrets.GCP_PROJECT_ID }}/hello-api:
    ➥kotlin-latest ${{ env.REGISTRY }}/${{ env.IMAGE_NAME }}:
    ➥kotlin-latest
  - name: Push Docker image to GCP
    run: docker push ${{ env.REGISTRY }}/${{ env.IMAGE_NAME }}:
    ➥kotlin-latest
```

> Pushes the container to the registry

Once you've pushed this last change, download your container or deploy it to your Kubernetes cluster to see how it works!

Kotlin and Quarkus are both relatively new in the world of Java-based languages and frameworks. This makes them poised to meet the challenges of current software development. While this chapter just touches the surface, I encourage you to dig deeper and experiment more because JVM languages are not going away, and you may find a lot of work in helping migrate and improve Java applications in the future.

appendix B
Using Python

In this appendix, we will build an API and pipeline with Python-specific tools using Python 3.8 with `pip` installed. Please ensure that you have it installed (https://www.python.org/downloads/).

B.1 Poetry

Before we build our project, we need to create a repeatable environment to work in. Python follows a common practice of sharing libraries among several projects. Languages like C, Java, and even Go use a central repository of libraries that are downloaded and stored locally on your machine. The problem with this process is that if you are not keeping track of the versions, the next person who sets up their development environment may have different versions of libraries, which can introduce new issues or break current functionality. Most of these languages, therefore, store the version of the library so that the environment can be set up almost identically.

With Go, we have the `go.mod` file which will allow Go to redownload all dependencies for a given module. Python provides us with a very basic option called the virtual environment which allows developers to act like they are running on a fresh installation of Python with no additional libraries. Any subsequent libraries are installed using a tool called `pip`. After they are installed, you can create a requirements document. This is created by the `pip freeze` command which outputs all libraries installed. If we want something more explicit in our application dependency, it will require us to use a separate tool called Poetry to handle libraries, installation, and building.

First, we need to install Poetry by running this command:

```
curl -sSL https://install.python-poetry.org | python3 -
```

Then we create a new project by typing the command:

```
poetry new hello-api
```

Simple as that! Now let's write our API.

B.2 Coding

We will use a combination of tools to host our API. The framework that will create the handlers is called FastAPI, a relatively new routing library that is, well, fast. It will run on a uvicorn server. As before, our backend will require a Redis database, so we need those dependencies as well. To add those libraries to our project, we simply type this:

```
poetry add fastapi \
uvicorn redis
```

The libraries will be installed, and your pyproject.toml will be updated for these dependencies. Now we can create our application. Create a new file in the hello_api directory called app.py, and add the code in the following listing.

Listing B.1 app.py

```
from fastapi import FastAPI, Depends
import hello_api.deps as deps
from hello_api.repo import RepositoryInterface

app = FastAPI()          ←——| Creates a base handler

repo = deps.redis_client          ←——┐ Loads the
                                       | redis client
@app.get("/translate/{word}")
def translation(
    word: str, language: str = "english", repo: RepositoryInterface =
    ➥Depends(repo)
):                                 ←——| Injects the Redis client into the handler
    resp = repo.translate(language, word)
    return {"language": language.lower(), "translation": resp}
```

This handler should look familiar. Here, we create the app, a set of dependencies, and a route to translate the word. Our translation function requires an interface and a dependency to fulfill the interface, so let's create those. First, we create the interface in a file called repo.py with the code in the following listing.

Listing B.2 repo.py

```
class RepositoryInterface:          ←————————┐ Establishes an interface
    def translate(self, language: str, word: str) -> str:   | that can be duck typed
        """translates word into given language"""
        pass
```

While we name this an interface, it technically isn't because Python doesn't have explicit interface types. This is a simple way to leverage Python's duck-typing system, just like we did in Go. This interface is more like an abstract class in which the methods are not supposed to be implemented, only defined. All we need to do is implement the interface in our redis.py with the code in the following listing.

Listing B.3   `repo.py`

```python
import redis
import os
from hello_api.repo import RepositoryInterface

class RedisRepository(RepositoryInterface):            ◁─┐ Implements
                                                          │ the interface
    host: str = os.environ.get("DB_HOST", "localhost")
    port: str = os.environ.get("DB_PORT", "6379")
    default_language: str = os.environ.get("DEFAULT_LANGUAGE", "english")

    def __init__(self, client=None) -> None:                     ◁─────────────┐
        if client is None:                                                     │
            self.client = redis.Redis(host=self.host, port=self.port)          │
        else:                                          Instantiates the client or sets
            self.client = client                        an optional client variable │

    def translate(self, language: str, word: str) -> str:    ◁─┐ Satisfies
        """translates word into given language"""              │ the interface
        lang = language.lower() if language is not None else
        ➥self.default_language
        key = f"{word.lower()}:{lang}"
        return self.client.get(key)
```

Here, you can see that we extend the interface and implement its methods. We can create our connection and handle the requests. The last step is to leverage FastApi's dependency injection tool by creating a file called `deps.py`, which will house functions to fetch the required dependency to run the service with the code in the following listing.

Listing B.4   `deps.py`

```python
from hello_api.repo import RepositoryInterface
from hello_api.redis import RedisRepository

                                                    Required for FastAPI
                                                    dependency injection
def redis_client() -> RepositoryInterface:      ◁──┘
    return RedisRepository()
```

To run your application, type

```
uvicorn hello_api.app:app
```

and you should be in business! Now let's add our checks.

B.3   Testing

We will use a different approach to testing our Python application than what we did in the Go chapters. Instead of using a Redis container to simulate the database connection, we will instead use an in-memory Redis replacement called `redislite`. We will use dependency injection to replace the actual connection, and everything should be

the same. We need to add two testing libraries for our tests to work by running the following commands:

```
poetry add redislite \
requests
```

Create a directory called `tests`, and add the code in the following listing.

Listing B.5 `test_hello_api.py`

```python
from hello_api.app import app, repo
from fastapi.testclient import TestClient
from redislite import Redis

from hello_api.repo import RepositoryInterface
from hello_api.redis import RedisRepository
import unittest


class AppIntegrationTest(unittest.TestCase):
    def redis_client(self) -> RepositoryInterface:          # Internal function to create
        self.fake_redis = Redis()                           # a mock redis client
        self.fake_redis.set("hello:german", "Hallo")
        self.fake_redis.set("hello:english", "Hello")

        return RedisRepository(client=self.fake_redis)

    def setUp(self):                                        # Sets up
        self.repo = self.redis_client()                     # the test
        self.client = TestClient(app)
        app.dependency_overrides[repo] = self.redis_client  # Overrides the
                                                            # dependency function
                                                            # with an internal function
    def test_english_translation(self):
        response = self.client.get("/translate/hello")
        assert response.status_code == 200
        assert response.json() == {"language": "english", "translation":
        "Hello"}

    def test_german_translation(self):
        response = self.client.get("/translate/hello?language=GERMAN")
        assert response.status_code == 200
        assert response.json() == {"language": "german", "translation":
        "Hallo"}
```

Now we should be able to verify that our tests work. To do this, we will use a tool to help us keep our tests and formatting standardized.

B.4 Nox

Nox is an open source tool that allows you to organize and standardize your testing and linting scripts. To use this tool, you must install Nox globally, so open a new terminal window, and type the following commands:

```
pip install --user --upgrade nox
```

Next, we create a `noxfile.py` file at the root of the project. We then add the options in the next listing to the file.

Listing B.6 `noxfile.py`

```
import nox

nox.options.sessions = "lint", "tests"        ◁──┐  Jobs that can
locations = "hello_api", "tests", "noxfile.py"    │  be completed
                                               ◁──┐  Files the jobs can
@nox.session                                      │  be completed on
def tests(session):
    session.run("poetry", "install", external=True)   ◁──┐  Runs the
    session.run("pytest")                                 │  command

@nox.session
def lint(session):
    args = session.posargs or locations
    session.install("flake8", "flake8-black")
    session.run("flake8", *args)
```

That's it! Notice that Nox uses `flake8` as our linter. We want to configure it a bit, and to do this, we need to create a `.flake8` file and add the code in the following listing.

Listing B.7 `\.flake8`

```
[flake8]
select = E123,W456        ◁──┐  Defines rules
max-line-length = 88         │  for linting
                          ◁──┐  Sets the max
                             │  line width
```

Nox will take care of the rest for us. To lint and test, we need to run the following commands:

```
nox -rs lint
nox -rs tests
```

You will see the script run through each of these stages with the proper output. We have the linting and testing incorporated, which are the last steps before the pipeline defines the container it should run in.

B.5 *Defining the container*

Packaging scripting languages are a bit different than packaging compiled languages. In our Go and Kotlin examples, we built the application and were left with a file that we could distribute and copy around. In languages such as Python and JavaScript, it becomes more important to set up the environment correctly for the scripts to run; otherwise, they will fail on startup or in the middle of a request. This is why we chose a package and dependency manager like Poetry. It will manage all of this for us. Let's define our container, as in the next listing.

Listing B.8   Dockerfile

```
FROM python:3.10.7-slim-bullseye as base

ENV PYTHONFAULTHANDLER=1 \
    PYTHONHASHSEED=random \
    PYTHONUNBUFFERED=1

WORKDIR /app

FROM base as builder

ENV PIP_DEFAULT_TIMEOUT=100 \
    PIP_DISABLE_PIP_VERSION_CHECK=1 \
    PIP_NO_CACHE_DIR=1 \
    POETRY_VERSION=1.1.15

RUN pip install "poetry==$POETRY_VERSION"
COPY pyproject.toml poetry.lock ./
RUN poetry config virtualenvs.create false \
  && poetry install
COPY hello_api hello_api
ENV PORT 8080
EXPOSE 8080
CMD ["uvicorn","hello_api.app:app","--port","8080","--host","0.0.0.0"]
```

Annotations in listing:
- **Production-level environmental variables for container** (pointing to ENV PYTHONFAULTHANDLER block)
- **Installs poetry** (pointing to RUN pip install line)
- **Runs server** (pointing to CMD line)

We have our Dockerfile and can move on to our pipeline.

B.6   Creating the pipeline

This pipeline will lint, test, and build the container. To get started, create a new workflow file in `.github/workflows/pipeline.yml` and add the following code. First we will set up Nox to run our linter (see the following listing).

Listing B.9   `pipeline.yml`

```
name: Python Checks

on:
  push:
    branches:
      - main

env:
  REGISTRY: ghcr.io
  IMAGE_NAME: ${{ github.repository }}

jobs:
  format-check:
    name: Check formatting
    runs-on: ubuntu-latest
    steps:
    - uses: actions/checkout@v3
    - uses: actions/setup-python@v4
```

```
  with:
    python-version: '3.10'
- run: pip install --user --upgrade nox    ◁── Installs Nox
- name: Run Check Lint
  run: nox -rs lint    ◁── Runs Nox lint
```

Then, in the next listing, we will use Nox to run our tests.

Listing B.10 pipeline.yml

```
name: Python Checks
...
jobs:
...
  test:
    name: Test
    runs-on: ubuntu-latest
    needs: format-check
    steps:
        - uses: actions/checkout@v3
    - uses: actions/setup-python@v4
      with:
        python-version: '3.10'
    - run: pip install --user --upgrade nox
    - name: Run Tests
      run: nox -rs tests    ◁── Uses Nox to run tests
```

Finally, we will build and ship our container in the following listing.

Listing B.11 pipeline.yml

```
name: Python Checks
...
jobs:
...
  containerize:
    name: Build and Push Container
    runs-on: ubuntu-latest #
    needs: test
    steps:
    - uses: actions/checkout@v3
    - name: Build Container
      run: docker build -t gcr.io/${{ secrets.GCP_PROJECT_ID }}/hello-
      ➥api:python-latest .    ◁── Builds a Docker image
    - name: Set up Cloud SDK
      uses: google-github-actions/setup-gcloud@main
      with:
        project_id: ${{ secrets.GCP_PROJECT_ID }}
        service_account_key: ${{ secrets.gcp_credentials }}
        export_default_credentials: true
    - name: Configure Docker
      run: gcloud auth configure-docker --quiet
    - name: Push Docker image
```

```
    run: docker push gcr.io/${{ secrets.GCP_PROJECT_ID }}/hello-
    ➥api:python-latest
  - name: Log in to the GHCR
    uses: docker/login-action@master
    with:
      registry: ${{ env.REGISTRY }}
      username: ${{ github.actor }}
      password: ${{ secrets.GITHUB_TOKEN }}
  - name: Tag for Github
    run: docker image tag gcr.io/${{ secrets.GCP_PROJECT_ID }}/hello-
    ➥api:python-latest ${{ env.REGISTRY }}/${{ env.IMAGE_NAME }}:
    ➥python-latest
  - name: Push Docker image to GCP
    run: docker push ${{ env.REGISTRY }}/${{ env.IMAGE_NAME }}:python-
    ➥latest
```

Due to how large the Python ecosystem is, at this point there may be a bunch of other ways to create and deploy your Python application. The point is that tools and processes can be put in place to protect your code and reduce bugs. This is especially important for languages like Python because they trade type safety and compile time errors for flexibility, allowing for rapid development.

appendix C
Using JavaScript

Node.js is a JavaScript runtime that allows developers to write applications to run outside of the web browser. This has led to the growth of JavaScript libraries, helping developers write backend services. We can use tools to connect to databases and create APIs. Let's get started.

C.1 *Node Package Manager*

NPM, or the Node Package Manager, is the central build and dependency management tool we'll use for our API. We will use the Express library. First, make sure you have Node installed from https://nodejs.org/en/download/; then install the Express Generator application:

```
npm install express-generator -g
express hello-api
```

Once the code has been generated, edit the package.json file using the code in the following listing.

Listing C.1 package.json

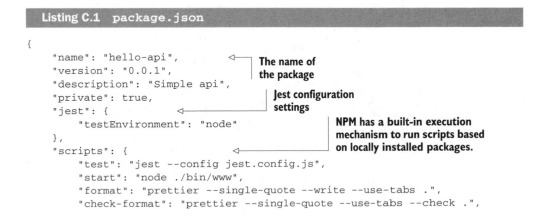

```json
{
    "name": "hello-api",                    ◁── The name of
    "version": "0.0.1",                          the package
    "description": "Simple api",
    "private": true,                        Jest configuration
    "jest": {                    ◁──        settings
        "testEnvironment": "node"           NPM has a built-in execution
    },                                      mechanism to run scripts based
    "scripts": {                 ◁──        on locally installed packages.
        "test": "jest --config jest.config.js",
        "start": "node ./bin/www",
        "format": "prettier --single-quote --write --use-tabs .",
        "check-format": "prettier --single-quote --use-tabs --check .",
```

```
          "lint": "eslint \"**/*.js\" --max-warnings 0 --ignore-pattern
      ➥node_modules/"
  },
  "author": "Joel Holmes",
  "license": "MIT",                    ┌── Libraries required to
  "dependencies": {          ◁─────┘    run the application
      "debug": "^4.3.4",
      "express": "^4.18.1",
      "morgan": "^1.10.0",
      "redis": "^4.3.0"
  },                                   ┌── Libraries to test or
  "devDependencies": {       ◁─────┘    develop the application
      "eslint": "^8.23.0",
      "eslint-plugin-jest": "^27.0.1",
      "jest": "^29.0.0",
      "prettier": "^2.7.1",
      "supertest": "^6.2.4",
      "testcontainers": "^8.13.1"
  }
}
```

The `package.json` file houses all of the dependencies and scripts needed to test, build, and run our application. After making these changes, type `npm install` to add all of these dependencies to our project. We have set up the basic structure and can now start coding.

C.2 Coding

You'll notice that Express generated a lot of files for you. The main one is `app.js`. This is your entry route to your API. Open it, and replace it with the code in the following listing.

Listing C.2 app.js

```
let express = require('express');       ◁──┐  Imports express
let logger = require('morgan');            │  framework
                                                          ┌── Imports translation
let translateRouter = require('./routes/translation');   │   handler
                                              ◁─────────┘
const { Repository } = require('./repository/translation');  ◁──┐ Imports
                                                                 │ repository
class App {
    app = express();
    repo = undefined;
    constructor(host, port) {        ◁──┐  Constructs
        this.app.use(logger('dev'));    │  application class
        this.app.use(express.json());
        this.app.use(express.urlencoded({ extended: false }));
        this.repo = new Repository(host, port);
        this.app.get('/translate/:word', translateRouter(this.repo));
    }

    async close() {
        return this.repo.close();
    }
```

```
}
module.exports = { App };
```

Exports the app to be used
by the running application

Hopefully, you notice the difference between the generated code and what you wrote. We use the object-oriented paradigm of JavaScript to help us with future unit testing.

We have a router and repository to define. Let's define the router first. Create a directory called `routes`. This will house our `translation.js` file and will be the location of any other routes or groups of routes that you want to define. Create the file, and add the code in the following listing.

Listing C.3 translation.js

```
const translation = (translationService) => {
    return async (req, res) => {
        let language = req.query.language || 'english';
        const resp = await translationService.translate(language,
        ➥ req.params.word);
        resp
            ? res.json({ language: language.toLowerCase(), translation:
            ➥ resp })
            : res.status(404).send('Missing translation');
    };
};

module.exports = translation;
```

Functional definition
for handler

If a response
is given, return
it; otherwise,
it returns 404.

If a query parameter
is not passed,
default to English.

As you can see, this function requires the translation service to be passed to the function. This is different from what we do in other languages with dependency injection and stronger type checks. Instead, we pass the function in to handle the business logic. Alternatively, we could have created a class, as we did with the main app.

> **NOTE** We are organizing our files by function and not by domain, meaning we place all routes in a directory and all repository methods in each directory. An alternate way is to have a `translation` directory with a `repo.js` and a `route.js` file.

Now we need to define the translation repository. Create a directory called `repository` and a file called `translation.js`, and add the code in the following listing.

Listing C.4 translation.js

```
const redis = require('redis');

class Repository {
    constructor(host, port) {
        this.host = host ? host : process.env.DB_HOST || 'localhost';
        this.port = port ? port : process.env.DB_PORT || '6379';
        this.defaultLanguage = process.env.DEFAULT_LANGUAGE || 'english';
        const connectionURL = `redis://${this.host}:${this.port}`;
        console.log(`connecting to ${connectionURL}`);
```

```
        this.client = redis.createClient({ url: connectionURL });
        this.client.on('connect', () => {
            console.log('connected to redis');      Adds logging when the
        });                                          database is connected
        this.client.on('error', (err) => console.log('client error',
            err));
        this.client.connect();
    }

    async translate(language, word) {
        const lang = language
            ? language.toLowerCase()                 Checks for language; if not
            : this.defaultLanguage.toLowerCase();    specified, uses the default
        const key = `${word.toLowerCase()}:${lang}`;
        const val = await this.client.get(key);
        return val;
    }
    async close() {
        this.client.quit();
    }
}

module.exports = { Repository };
```

Adds logging for errors

Here, we build a connection to the Redis database and a function to retrieve the translation. To test this, open a terminal window and type `npm start`. We have a functioning API; let's test it.

C.3 Testing

We will jump right into an integration test using the testing framework Jest and a container library called `testcontainers`, which will provide us with a Redis database. Before we write our tests, we want to create a configuration file for our test framework Jest. Create a `jest.config.js` file, and add the following code:

```
module.exports = {
    testTimeout: 30000,
};
```

This will give our container time to start before our tests. Now we can write our integration test using the code in the following listing.

Listing C.5 app.test.js

```
const { GenericContainer } = require('testcontainers');
const { App } = require('./app');
const request = require('supertest');

let container;
let app;
let api;
                                          Sets up tests by
beforeAll(async () => {                    starting a container
    container = await new GenericContainer('redis')
```

```
            .withExposedPorts(6379)
            .withCopyFileToContainer('./data/dump.rdb', '/data/dump.rdb')
            .start();
        const port = container.getMappedPort(6379);
        const host = container.getHost();
        api = new App(host, port);          ◁─┐ Passes values to
        app = api.app;                          │ construct the app
    });

    afterAll(async () => {
        await api.close();
        await container.stop();
    });                                                     Writes a test to
                                                            call the endpoint
    describe('Translate', () => {
        test('hello translation in english to be hello', async () => {   ◁──────┘
            const response = await request(app).get('/translate/hello');
            expect(response.body).toEqual({
                translation: 'Hello',
                language: 'english',
            });
            expect(response.statusCode).toBe(200);
            return response;
        });
        test('hello translation in german to be hallo', async () => {
            const response = await request(app).get(
            ➥'/translate/hello?language=GERMAN');
            expect(response.body).toEqual({ translation: 'Hallo', language:
            ➥'german' });
            expect(response.statusCode).toBe(200);
            return response;
        });
    });
});
```

Now run npm test to see your tests pass.

C.4   Linting

Our next step is to check formatting and static code analysis. We will use Prettier and ESLint to help us with these steps. In the package .json code, we added scripts for running these libraries for formatting, checking format, and linting. To run these, simply type the following commands:

```
npm run format
npm run check-format
```

For linting, we need to create a configuration file for our linter (see the next listing).

Listing C.6   \.eslintrc.json

```
{
    "env": {                    ◁─┐ Defines the
        "node": true,              │ environment
        "commonjs": true,
```

```
        "es2021": true
    },
    "extends": "eslint:recommended",          ⟵┐  Passes in Jest
    "overrides": [                                 formatting rules
        {
            "files": ["**/*.test.js"],
            "env": {
                "jest": true
            },
            "plugins": ["jest"],
            "rules": {
                "jest/no-disabled-tests": "warn",
                "jest/no-focused-tests": "error",
                "jest/no-identical-title": "error",
                "jest/prefer-to-have-length": "warn",
                "jest/valid-expect": "error"
            }
        }
    ],
    "parserOptions": {
        "ecmaVersion": "latest"              Defines additional
    },                                   ⟵┐  formatting rules
    "rules": {
        "indent": ["error", "tab"],
        "linebreak-style": ["error", "unix"],
        "quotes": ["error", "single"],
        "semi": ["error", "always"]
    }
}
```

Now you can run the lint step by typing

```
npm run lint
```

It was pretty simple to incorporate these steps right into our script. This shows the power of having a single tool that can fulfill multiple areas of our pipeline. The final step before we assemble our pipeline is to define the container.

C.5 *Defining the container*

Much like the Python container we made in appendix B, JavaScript requires an environment to be set up for the scripts to run. NPM is installed as part of the base image so that we can run the install process for our dependencies and run the main app. The following listing shows our container definition.

Listing C.7 Dockerfile

```
FROM node:17          ⟵┐  Base
                          image
# Create app directory
WORKDIR /usr/src/app

# Install app dependencies
COPY package*.json ./
```

```
RUN npm ci --only=production        ◁─┐  Cleans and installs dependent
                                       └  packages required for production
# Bundle app source
COPY . ./
ENV PORT 8080
ENV NODE_ENV production
EXPOSE 8080                            ┌  Runs using a wrapper script
CMD [ "node", "./bin/www" ]         ◁─┘  provided by Express
```

Finally, we can build our pipeline.

C.6   *Building the pipeline*

This pipeline is similar to those in the other chapters in that it will have linting, testing, and container steps, as shown in the following listing.

Listing C.8 `pipeline.yml`

```
name: JavaScript Checks

on:
  push:
    branches:
      - main
env:
  REGISTRY: ghcr.io
  IMAGE_NAME: ${{ github.repository }}

jobs:
  format-check:
    name: Check formatting
    runs-on: ubuntu-latest
    steps:
    - uses: actions/checkout@v3
    - uses: actions/setup-node@v3
      with:
        node-version: 17        ┌  Cleans and installs
    - run: npm ci            ◁──┘  dependencies
    - name: Run Check Format               ┌  Runs format
      run: npm run check-format         ◁──┘  check
    - name: Run Check Lint
      run: npm run lint        ◁──┤ Runs lint
```

First we will do a simple clean, install, and format checking before we move on to our integration tests (see the following listing).

Listing C.9 `pipeline.yml`

```
name: JavaScript Checks
...
jobs:
...
  test:
```

```
    name: Test
    runs-on: ubuntu-latest
    needs: format-check
    steps:
    - uses: actions/checkout@v3
    - uses: actions/setup-node@v3
      with:
       node-version: 17
    - run: npm ci
    - name: Test
      run: npm run test
```

Runs tests using
npm script

When the integration tests have completed, we can finally build our container to ship
(see the next listing).

Listing C.10   pipeline.yml

```
name: JavaScript Checks
...
jobs:
...
  containerize:
    name: Build and Push Container
    runs-on: ubuntu-latest #
    needs: test
    steps:
    - uses: actions/checkout@v3
    - name: Build Container
      run: docker build -t gcr.io/${{ secrets.GCP_PROJECT_ID }}/hello-api:
          ➥javascript-latest .
    - name: Set up Cloud SDK
      uses: google-github-actions/setup-gcloud@main
      with:
        project_id: ${{ secrets.GCP_PROJECT_ID }}
        service_account_key: ${{ secrets.gcp_credentials }}
        export_default_credentials: true
    - name: Configure Docker
      run: gcloud auth configure-docker --quiet
    - name: Push Docker image
      run: docker push gcr.io/${{ secrets.GCP_PROJECT_ID }}/hello-api:
          ➥javascript-latest
    - name: Log in to the GHCR
      uses: docker/login-action@master
      with:
        registry: ${{ env.REGISTRY }}
        username: ${{ github.actor }}
        password: ${{ secrets.GITHUB_TOKEN }}
    - name: Tag for Github
      run: docker image tag gcr.io/${{ secrets.GCP_PROJECT_ID }}/hello-api:
          ➥javascript-latest ${{ env.REGISTRY }}/${{ env.IMAGE_NAME }}:
          ➥javascript-latest
    - name: Push Docker image to GCP
      run: docker push ${{ env.REGISTRY }}/${{ env.IMAGE_NAME }}:
          ➥javascript-latest
```

Builds a
container

appendix D
Using Terraform

Infrastructure as code is not a new concept, but over the years, the tools have changed from scripts and images that are on physical hardware your company owns to tools built to work in the cloud. Kubernetes and serverless platforms have taken the spotlight off of other tools that help build infrastructure within these various cloud environments. There are trade-offs and benefits to all different types of deployments. In this appendix, examples are provided for one last tool to give you a broad overview of the deployment landscape.

D.1 Building the image

My first job was with the IT department in high school. While working there, I was able to assist in unboxing and wiring the computer labs. After all the computers were unboxed and plugged in, I would turn them all on, rapidly tapping on keys to enable network mode. Within a few minutes, I would see an installer start to run, and within the hour, we had 20 identical machines. Every week I would repeat this magic with amazement.

The amazement hasn't worn off. Today we need to do the same task in the cloud with our applications. Instead of unboxing physical servers, we push our images to ephemeral ones. When you create a server in the cloud, it is a virtual machine on a larger server cluster. It can go down and start right back up on a completely different box in a completely different part of the building it's in.

To build the image, we will use Packer (https://www.packer.io/), a tool by HashiCorp that builds server images based on the specifications provided. Then we will create a Packer image definition with the code in the following listing.

Listing D.1 `hello-api.pkr.hcl`

```
variable "project_id" {          Input variables
  type    = string               needed for the build
}
```

216

```
variable "git_sha" {
  type    = string
  default = "UNKNOWN"
}

source "googlecompute" "hello-api" {
  project_id = ${var.project_id}
  source_image_family = "ubuntu-2204-lts"
  image_name = "hello-api-${var.git_sha}"
  ssh_username = "packer"
  zone = "us-central1-a"
}

build {
  sources = [sources.googlecompute.hello]

  provisioner "file" {
    destination = "/home/ubuntu/hello-api"
    source      = "api"
  }

  post-processor "manifest" {
    output = "manifest.json"
    strip_path = true
    custom_data = {
      sha = "${var.git_sha}"
    }
  }
}
```

The base image we will be building from

The name of the image we are going to create

Special builder that copies our binary over to the image

This will build an image with the name of the commit that was merged. Next, we need to adjust our account to be able to deploy images. Run the commands in the following listing.

Listing D.2   `hello-api.pkr.hcl`

```
gcloud projects add-iam-policy-binding YOUR_GCP_PROJECT \
    --member=serviceAccount:GITHUB_SERVICE_ACCOUNT_NAME@YOUR_GCP_PROJECT.
    ➥iam.gserviceaccount.com \
    --role=roles/compute.instanceAdmin.v1

gcloud projects add-iam-policy-binding YOUR_GCP_PROJECT \
    --member=serviceAccount:GITHUB_SERVICE_ACCOUNT_NAME@YOUR_GCP_PROJECT.
    ➥iam.gserviceaccount.com \
    --role=roles/iam.serviceAccountUser

gcloud projects add-iam-policy-binding YOUR_GCP_PROJECT \
    --member=serviceAccount:GITHUB_SERVICE_ACCOUNT_NAME@YOUR_GCP_PROJECT.
    ➥iam.gserviceaccount.com \
    --role=roles/iap.tunnelResourceAccessor
```

This will allow our GitHub pipeline to use Packer to build the image. Next, we will write the server to run the image.

D.2   *Deploying the image*

To define our infrastructure, we use Terraform (https://www.terraform.io/), another HashiCorp tool. Terraform provides a language to define servers, load balancers, databases, and more. It also keeps track of the state of your infrastructure, which will be important when you need to change or delete a service. We need to install Terraform locally so that we can set up a few necessary pieces. To begin, create a directory called `infra` and then a sub-directory called `global`. In these, we will add the code in the following listing to a `main.tf` file.

Listing D.3   main.tf

```
resource "google_storage_bucket" "default" {          ◁─┐   Defines a state bucket to store
  name          = "hello-api-bucket-tfstate"              │   our current infrastructure values
  force_destroy = false
  location      = "US"
  storage_class = "STANDARD"
  versioning {
    enabled = true
  }
}
```

Then run `terraform apply` and confirm. This bucket will hold the state of our entire system so that we can make changes. If this file were to be stored on a laptop, no one else could make changes. If the file were lost, you would lose the state of your infrastructure and would need to modify it by hand.

Next, we will define the server and variables needed to deploy. Create a directory called `infra/server`, and add the code in the following listing.

Listing D.4   main.tf

```
terraform {                           ◁─┐   Defines the backend we
 backend "gcs" {                         │   will use and the state file
   bucket = "hello-api-bucket-tfstate
   prefix = "terraform/state"
 }
}

resource "google_compute_instance" "hello_api" {     ◁─┐  Creates the
  name          = "hello-api"                            │  server instance
  machine_type = "f1-micro"
  zone          = "us-east1-a"

  boot_disk {
    initialize_params {
      image = ${var.image_name}      ◁─┐   Inputs the
    }                                    │   image name
  }
  lifecycle {
    create_before_destroy = true
  }
```

```
metadata_startup_script = "sudo chmod +x /home/ubuntu/hello-api && sudo
➥ /home/ubuntu/hello-api"                          ◁─┐  The script that runs
}                                                      │  when the server starts

resource "google_compute_firewall" "hello_api" {   ◁──  Creates a hole in the firewall
  name    = "hello-api-firewall"                         to access the service
  network = "default"

  allow {
    protocol = "tcp"
    ports    = ["8080"]
  }
  source_ranges = ["0.0.0.0/0"]
}
                                         ┌─  Output endpoint
output "public_dns" {       ◁───┘            to call the API
  value = google_compute_instance.hello_api.public_dns
}
```

Now we can create our pipeline.

D.3 Creating the pipeline

Our pipeline will compile our binary, package it with Packer, and then create a server. Upon any commit, the server will redeploy (see the next listing).

Listing D.5 `pipeline.yml`

```yaml
name: Terraform Depoyment

on:
  push:
    branches:
      - main

jobs:
  build-image:
    name: Build image
    runs-on: ubuntu-latest
    steps:
    - name: Set up Go 1.x #
      uses: actions/setup-go@v2
      with:
        go-version: ^1.18
    - name: Check out code into the Go module directory #
      uses: actions/checkout@v2
    - name: Build
      run: make build #
    - name: Build Artifact
      uses: hashicorp/packer-github-actions@master
      with:
          command: build
          arguments: "-color=false -on-error=abort"
```

```
            target: packer.pkr.hcl
            working_directory: infrastructure/packer
        env:
            PACKER_LOG: 1
            PKR_VAR_git_sha: $(git rev-parse --short "$GITHUB_SHA")
            PKR_VAR_project_id: ${{ secrets.GCP_PROJECT_ID }}
    deploy-server:
      name: Deploy Server
      runs-on: ubuntu-latest
      steps:
      - uses: hashicorp/setup-terraform@v2
      - name: Init
        run: terraform init
      - run: export TF_VAR_image_name=hello-api-$(git rev-parse --short
        ➥"$GITHUB_SHA")
      - name: install
        run: terraform apply -auto-approve
```

Infrastructure can get complicated, and this pipeline only shows a simple way of creating a continuous deployment. It differs from chapter 10 because this infrastructure code is automatically deployed instead of being integrated manually. In the output of the pipeline, you find the endpoint you need to call the service.

index

MANNING

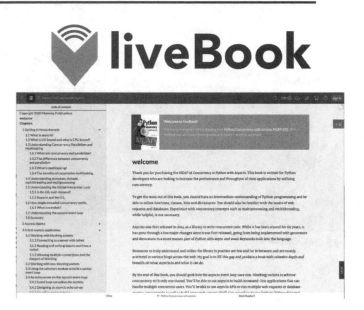

A new online reading experience

liveBook, our online reading platform, adds a new dimension to your Manning books, with features that make reading, learning, and sharing easier than ever. A liveBook version of your book is included FREE with every Manning book.

This next generation book platform is more than an online reader. It's packed with unique features to upgrade and enhance your learning experience.

- Add your own notes and bookmarks
- One-click code copy
- Learn from other readers in the discussion forum
- Audio recordings and interactive exercises
- Read all your purchased Manning content in any browser, anytime, anywhere

As an added bonus, you can search every Manning book and video in liveBook—even ones you don't yet own. Open any liveBook, and you'll be able to browse the content and read anything you like.*

Find out more at www.manning.com/livebook-program.

*Open reading is limited to 10 minutes per book daily

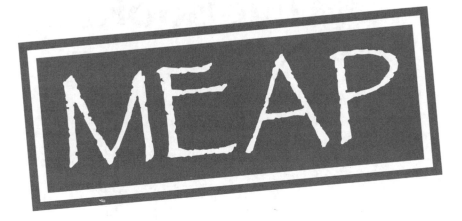

The Manning Early Access Program

Don't wait to start learning! In MEAP, the Manning Early Access Program, you can read books as they're being created and long before they're available in stores.

Here's how MEAP works.

- **Start now.** Buy a MEAP and you'll get all available chapters in PDF, ePub, Kindle, and liveBook formats.

- **Regular updates.** New chapters are released as soon as they're written. We'll let you know when fresh content is available.

- **Finish faster.** MEAP customers are the first to get final versions of all books! Pre-order the print book, and it'll ship as soon as it's off the press.

- **Contribute to the process.** The feedback you share with authors makes the end product better.

- **No risk.** You get a full refund or exchange if we ever have to cancel a MEAP.

Explore dozens of titles in MEAP at www.manning.com.